Spectral Multi-Detector Computed Tomography (sMDCT)

X-ray computed tomography (CT) has been one of the most popular diagnostic imaging modalities for decades in the clinic for saving patients' lives or improving their quality of life. This book is an introductory one-stop shop for technological and clinical topics in multi-detector computed tomography (MDCT).

Starting with MDCT's fundamentals in physics and mathematics, the book provides an in-depth introduction to its system architecture and imaging chain, signal detection via energy-integration and photon-counting mechanisms, clinical application-driven scan modes and protocols, analytic and iterative image reconstruction solutions, and spectral imaging – the latest technological advancement in MDCT. The book extends its coverage on image quality assessment under the theory of signal detection and statistical decision. In recognition of its clinical relevance for conspicuity enhancement in angiographic and parenchymal imaging applications, the book features a chapter dedicated to the fundamental (chemical, physical and physicochemical) properties and clinical administration of iodinated contrast agent. The book ends with an outlook of the contrast agents that are novel in material and delivery, and their synergy with spectral MDCT to elevate CT's contrast resolution in cardiovascular, neurovascular and oncologic applications.

This book will be an invaluable reference for researchers, engineers, radiological physicians and technologists, and graduate and senior undergraduate students.

Features

- Provides an accessible introduction to the subject
- Up to date with the latest advances in emerging technologies and procedures
- Provides a historical overview of CT technology

Xiangyang Tang, PhD, is an imaging scientist with extensive research and development experience in industry (GE Healthcare), academia (Emory University School of Medicine) and the clinic (Emory Healthcare).

With a focus on computed tomography, Tang has been working in the field of medical imaging for more than 20 years. He is a professor of radiology and imaging sciences at Emory University School of Medicine, Fellow of SPIE (International Society for Optics and Photonics) and Fellow of AAPM (American Association of Physicists in Medicine). Along with the publication of more than 200 papers in leading scientific journals and conferences, his contributions to the scientific community include serving as associate editor for a number of prestigious journals, in addition to working on the scientific committees of leading conferences and panels for numerous federal and foundational study sections.

Series in Medical Physics and Biomedical Engineering

Series Editors: Kwan-Hoong Ng, E. Russell Ritenour, and Slavik Tabakov

Recent books in the series:

Modelling Radiotherapy Side Effects Practical Applications for Planning Optimisation
Tiziana Rancati, Claudio Fiorino

Proton Therapy Physics, Second Edition
Harald Paganetti (Ed)

e-Learning in Medical Physics and Engineering: Building Educational Modules with Moodle
Vassilka Tabakova

Diagnostic Radiology Physics with MATLAB®: A Problem-Solving Approach
Johan Helmenkamp, Robert Bujila, Gavin Poludniowski (Eds)

Auto-Segmentation for Radiation Oncology: State of the Art
Jinzhong Yang, Gregory C. Sharp, Mark Gooding

Clinical Nuclear Medicine Physics with MATLAB: A Problem Solving Approach
Maria Lyra Georgosopoulou (Ed)

Handbook of Nuclear Medicine and Molecular Imaging for Physicists – Three Volume Set Volume I: Instrumentation and Imaging Procedures
Michael Ljungberg (Ed)

Practical Biomedical Signal Analysis Using MATLAB®
Katarzyna J. Blinowska, Jaroslaw Zygierewicz

Handbook of Nuclear Medicine and Molecular Imaging for Physicists – Three Volume Set Volume II: Modelling, Dosimetry and Radiation Protection
Michael Ljungberg (Ed)

Handbook of Nuclear Medicine and Molecular Imaging for Physicists – Three Volume Set Volume III: Radiopharmaceuticals and Clinical Applications
Michael Ljungberg (Ed)

Electrical Impedance Tomography: Methods, History and Applications, Second Edition
David Holder and Andy Adler (Eds)

Introduction to Medical Physics
Cornelius Lewis, Stephen Keevil, Anthony Greener, Slavik Tabakov, Renato Padovani

Calculating X-ray Tube Spectra: Analytical and Monte Carlo Approaches
Gavin Poludniowski, Artur Omar, Pedro Andreo

Problems and Solutions in Medical Physics: Radiotherapy Physics
Kwan-Hoong Ng, Ngie Min Ung, Robin Hill

Biomedical Photonics for Diabetes Research
Andrey Dunaev and Valery Tuchin (Eds)

Spectral Multi-Detector Computed Tomography (sMDCT): Data Acquisition, Image Formation, Quality Assessment and Contrast Enhancement
Xiangyang Tang

For more information about this series, please visit: https://www.routledge.com/Series-in-Medical-Physics-and-Biomedical-Engineering/book-series/CHMEPHBIOENG

Spectral Multi-Detector Computed Tomography (sMDCT)

Data Acquisition, Image Formation, Quality Assessment and Contrast Enhancement

Xiangyang Tang

CRC Press
Taylor & Francis Group
Boca Raton London New York

CRC Press is an imprint of the
Taylor & Francis Group, an **informa** business

First edition published 2023
by CRC Press
2385 NW Executive Center Drive, Suite 320, Boca Raton, FL 33431

and by CRC Press
4 Park Square, Milton Park, Abingdon, Oxon, OX14 4RN

CRC Press is an imprint of Taylor & Francis Group, LLC

© 2024 Taylor & Francis Group, LLC

Library of Congress Cataloging-in-Publication Data

Names: Tang, Xiangyang (Imaging scientist), author.
Title: Spectral multi-detector computed tomography (sMDCT) : data acquisition, image formation, quality assessment and contrast enhancement / Xiangyang Tang.
Other titles: Series in medical physics and biomedical engineering.
Description: First edition. | Boca Raton : CRC Press, 2023. | Series: Series in medical physics and biomedical engineering | Includes bibliographical references and index Identifiers: LCCN 2022060171 | ISBN 9780367137533 (hardback) | ISBN 9781032518220 (paperback) | ISBN 9780429028465 (ebook)
Subjects: MESH: Multidetector Computed Tomography | Image Enhancement
Classification: LCC RC78.7.T6 | NLM WN 206 | DDC 616.07/5722--dc23/eng/20230429
LC record available at https://lccn.loc.gov/2022060171

ISBN: 9780367137533 (hbk)
ISBN: 9781032518220 (pbk)
ISBN: 9780429028465 (ebk)

DOI: 10.1201/9780429028465

Typeset in Times
by Deanta Global Publishing Services, Chennai, India

To

Yujun, my father, who lost his life when I was 6 years old, for the intelligence that enables me to make a life and career in the US;

Jieli, my wife, for all the years since we knew each other on the first day of middle school and the kids we have;

Leonardo and Sylvia, two fresh college graduates, for the joy since you were born;

Junwen, my brother, for the love and taking care of Mom since I left home at age 16;

Suwen, my Mom, for the motherhood and kindness that accompany me along the way.

Contents

Contents

Preface

As a scientist in both industry (Applied Science Lab of GE Healthcare) and academia (Emory University School of Medicine), and an American Board of Radiology–certified medical physicist in clinics (Emory Healthcare), I've been engaged in medical imaging research focused on computed tomography (CT) for more than 20 years. With hands-on experience in development of CT imaging systems and methods, and the clinical practice of medical physics, I was encouraged to write a book on CT with coverage on the major topics that I've worked on. The writing of this book has been partially concurrent with the worldwide COVID pandemic and finally comes out with ten chapters emphasizing the sciences and technologies relevant to spectral multi-detector CT (sMDCT), especially those that may elevate MDCT's contrast resolution – the capability of detecting pathologies at subtle contrast against their normal surroundings.

This book is aimed at providing a coverage on the sciences and technologies underlying MDCT in a manner that differs from others in the literature. Hopefully, by reading through the chapters, readers, including scientists, researchers, clinicians and medical physicists who are currently working in the field, and graduates or senior college students who major in biomedical engineering and/or medical physics, may find an entrance to the topics that are more specific and relevant to their work or study. Following is a brief delineation of each chapter.

Starting with a chronicle review of the technological milestones, such as system geometry, architecture and data acquisition scheme (scan), in CT's development over half a century, a survey of CT's clinical utilities for saving patients' lives or improving the quality of their lives in diagnosis of cardiovascular, neurovascular and oncological diseases and assessment of the therapeutic response and/or efficacy is given in Chapter 1.

Chapter 2 presents the mathematical fundamentals related to the two-dimensional/three-dimensional (2D/3D) X-ray transform, Radon transform, Radon space and their relationship with the Fourier transform and Fourier space via the Fourier slice theorem. As such, the data sufficiency condition associated with MDCT's data acquisition (scan) scheme, such as the axial and spiral/helical scan in clinical practice, can be readily understood.

By going through each loop of MDCT's imaging chain, Chapter 3 concerns the nonideal physical properties, such as scattering and beam hardening, of X-ray as the medium of generating and carrying the signals in MDCT and the resultant artifacts. To help readers understand the limitation and potential of MDCT over clinical applications, the detection of signals carried by X-ray via energy integration and photon counting and their pros and cons are also elucidated in this chapter.

In Chapter 4, readers are exposed to the filtered back-projection (FBP)–based analytic image reconstruction solutions that are being employed in MDCT over various data acquisition (scan) schemes demanded by diversified clinical applications, ranging from single-detector row to 4, 16, 64, 128, 192, 256 or even more detector rows, under both axial and spiral/helical scans and data range of 360° (full), 180° + fan-angle (half) or between (partial).

Chapter 5 provides readers with a concise introduction to the iterative reconstruction algorithms that can be utilized in MDCT for image formation, from the earliest ART (algebraic reconstruction technique) to statistical iterative image reconstruction with regularization and the latest optimization-based approaches. Hopefully, readers may find access in this chapter to a realm that has recently been evolving at an expedited pace.

CT is one of the major imaging modalities for the community of medical imaging to reach consensus that the assessment of image quality should be carried out in the theory of signal detection and decision-making. Nevertheless, with CT as one of the most established modalities, it has become increasingly common that only pixel-wise metrics, such as signal-to-noise and contrast-to-noise ratios, are used as the figures of merit (FOMs) for image quality assessment. This practice may lead to inaccurate or biased conclusions, especially in scenarios wherein contrast resolution is the major concern, e.g., in assessing the advantages of iterative reconstruction over FBP, or sMDCT over the conventional MDCT. To address these issues, the methods and associated FOMs for image quality assessment via observer studies, including ideal observer, human observer and model observer, and the relationship among them, are visited in depth in Chapter 6.

Chapter 7 and Chapter 8 are dedicated to sMDCT – the latest advancement in CT technologies – implemented via either energy integration or photon counting. Starting from the conventional two-material decomposition-based sMDCT, these two chapters extend their coverage on multi-material decomposition-based sMDCT, ranging from the physical fundamentals, data acquisition schemes and image formation solutions to image presentation approaches. With an emphasis on photon-counting implementation, Chapter 8 digs into the approaches for optimizing the image quality of sMDCT, by taking multiple factors into account, such as the material space dimensionality, the condition of the basis materials, the condition of spectral channelization, the noise correlation in material-specific images, and the task-dependent spectral channelization and spectral weighting. Chapter 8 ends with surveying the clinical utility of energy-integration sMDCT in current clinical practice and foreseeing the potential clinical utility of photon-counting sMDCT in future clinical applications.

From the very beginning, iodinated contrast agents have played an indispensable role to conventional MDCT's success in diagnostic imaging of both angiographic and parenchymal lesions. Looking forward, the clinical role played by iodinated contrast agents will continue in sMDCT. Hence, not only radiologists but also others who are motivated to make contributions to the technological and/or clinical advancement of MDCT should have good understanding of the properties of iodinated contrast agents in physics, chemistry, physicochemistry and chemotoxicity, as well as their administration in clinical settings, such as protocoling of agent injection, concerting with the MDCT scan and dealing with incidental adverse reactions. Also, professionals in the field should be updated with the latest progression in exploration of more MDCT contrast agents that are novel in material, structure and delivery approach. Hopefully, Chapter 9 may serve those purposes.

The book concludes in Chapter 10 with a viewing of the technological challenges, clinical potentials and research opportunities associated with photon-counting sMDCT, especially in light of exploration of biomarker targeted contrast agents and the fast evolution of deep-learning (machine-learning) technologies.

Finally, I'd like to extend my appreciation to Carolyn C. Meltzer, MD, for the opportunity for career development at the Department of Radiology and Imaging Sciences, Emory University School of Medicine. Also, I'd like to express my appreciation to my mentors, colleagues and professional peers for their advice, support and help, giving me opportunities and sharing over the years. In particular, my thanks go to Huiqiao Xie, PhD, Yan Ren, PhD, and Shaojie Tang, PhD, for their work presented in this book; and other lab members, Yi Yang, PhD, and Wenting Long, PhD, for their work over the years.

About the Series

The *Series in Medical Physics and Biomedical Engineering* describes the applications of physical sciences, engineering, and mathematics in medicine and clinical research.

The series seeks (but is not restricted to) publications in the following topics:

- Artificial organs
- Assistive technology
- Bioinformatics
- Bioinstrumentation
- Biomaterials
- Biomechanics
- Biomedical engineering
- Clinical engineering
- Imaging
- Implants
- Medical computing and mathematics
- Medical/surgical devices
- Patient monitoring
- Physiological measurement
- Prosthetics
- Radiation protection, health physics, and dosimetry
- Regulatory issues
- Rehabilitation engineering
- Sports medicine
- Systems physiology
- Telemedicine
- Tissue engineering
- Treatment

The *Series in Medical Physics and Biomedical Engineering* is an international series that meets the need for up-to-date texts in this rapidly developing field. Books in the series range in level from introductory graduate textbooks and practical handbooks to more advanced expositions of current research.

The *Series in Medical Physics and Biomedical Engineering* is the official book series of the International Organization for Medical Physics.

The International Organization for Medical Physics

The International Organization for Medical Physics (IOMP) represents over 18,000 medical physicists worldwide and has a membership of 80 national and six regional organizations, together with a number of corporate members. Individual medical physicists of all national member organisations are also automatically members.

The mission of IOMP is to advance medical physics practice worldwide by disseminating scientific and technical information, fostering the educational and professional development of medical physics and promoting the highest quality medical physics services for patients.

A World Congress on Medical Physics and Biomedical Engineering is held every three years in cooperation with International Federation for Medical and Biological Engineering (IFMBE) and International Union for Physics and Engineering Sciences in Medicine (IUPESM). A regionally based international conference, the International Congress of Medical Physics (ICMP) is held between world congresses. IOMP also sponsors international conferences, workshops and courses.

The IOMP has several programmes to assist medical physicists in developing countries. The joint IOMP Library Programme supports 75 active libraries in 43 developing countries, and the Used Equipment Programme coordinates equipment donations. The Travel Assistance Programme provides a limited number of grants to enable physicists to attend the world congresses.

IOMP co-sponsors the *Journal of Applied Clinical Medical Physics.* The IOMP publishes, twice a year, an electronic bulletin, *Medical Physics World.* IOMP also publishes e-Zine, an electronic news letter about six times a year. IOMP has an agreement with Taylor & Francis for the publication of the *Medical Physics and Biomedical Engineering* series of textbooks. IOMP members receive a discount.

IOMP collaborates with international organizations, such as the World Health Organisation (WHO), the International Atomic Energy Agency (IAEA) and other international professional bodies such as the International Radiation Protection Association (IRPA) and the International Commission on Radiological Protection (ICRP), to promote the development of medical physics and the safe use of radiation and medical devices.

Guidance on education, training and professional development of medical physicists is issued by IOMP, which is collaborating with other professional organizations in development of a professional certification system for medical physicists that can be implemented on a global basis.

The IOMP website (www.iomp.org) contains information on all the activities of the IOMP, policy statements 1 and 2 and the 'IOMP: Review and Way Forward' which outlines all the activities of IOMP and plans for the future.

1 Introduction

For more than half a century, enormous effort has been devoted by scientists and researchers in the field to make X-ray computed tomography (CT) increasingly capable of assisting in diagnoses and interventions, and assessing the therapeutic efficacy of diseases in cardiovascular, neurovascular and oncological applications. Objectively speaking, each aspect of CT's imaging performance may not be the best compared to other imaging modalities in clinics (Tang 2014; Tang and Xie 2018). For example, as we know, the contrast resolution of CT in differentiation of soft tissues may not be as high as that of PET/SPECT or MRI. The root cause underlying the limitation of CT's contrast resolution is that the subject contrast between pathophysiologic lesions and surrounding tissues in CT is generated by energetic X-ray flux at an atomic level. The vast majority of the atomic constituents of soft tissues are hydrogen, oxygen, carbon and nitrogen that are of relatively small atomic number and thus differ only moderately in their photoelectric absorption and Compton scattering – the two major generators of contrast in X-ray–related, including CT, imaging modalities. Meanwhile, the temporal resolution of CT may be inferior to that of MRI when special pulse sequences, e.g., echo planner imaging (EPI), are employed. Furthermore, the spatial resolution of CT may not be as good as that of sonography when only a small and shallow region of interest (ROI) is being imaged, e.g., imaging the carotid via intravascular ultrasound. However, putting all the aspects of image quality together, it is quite fair to claim that CT is the best and most robust imaging modality to fulfill the requirements imposed by the vast majority of clinical applications for saving lives or improving quality of life.

1.1 CHRONICLE REVIEW OF X-RAY COMPUTED TOMOGRAPHY

Since its advent in the early 1970s (Hounsfield 1973), CT has advanced substantially in every aspect of its capability for clinical applications, with the most remarkable being its speed of data acquisition and image formation. In the very beginning, it took about 5 minutes for first-generation CT to acquire a full set of data for one single CT image (Figure 1.1a). Nowadays, on average, roughly 1 millisecond is needed in state-of-the-art multi-detector row CT (MDCT) to acquire the data for generating one image, which, notably, is a 300,000-fold $((5 \times 60)/(1/1000) = 300,000)$ increase in the speed.

Thus far, at least four major milestones have been passed in the advancement of CT technologies. The first one was the evolution from first-/second-generation geometry (Figure 1.1a and Figure 1.1b) to third-/fourth-generation geometry (Figure 1.1c and Figure 1.1d) under circular source trajectory (termed *axial scan* henceforth). The narrow pencil (Figure 1.1a) or small fan beam (Figure 1.1b) has expanded into a large fan beam that can accommodate the entire body of a patient, enabling substantially

DOI: 10.1201/9780429028465-1

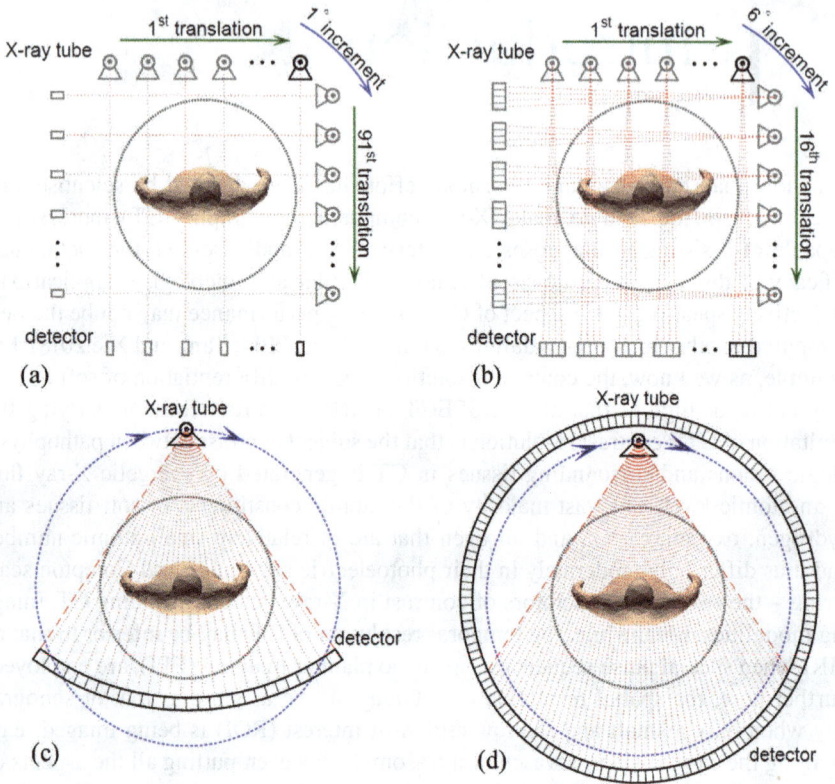

FIGURE 1.1   Schematic diagrams showing the architecture of CT in the (a) first, (b) second, (c) third and (d) fourth generations.

faster CT gantry rotation, thus speeding data acquisition. Under third-generation geometry, a one-dimensional (1D) curved array (arc) of detector elements (termed *channels* henceforth) was used to implement the fan beam, while that spanning the entire circle was used under fourth-generation geometry. Both of them were then called single-detector row CT (SDCT), and, apparently, they had to work at the step-and-shoot mode to longitudinally scan the large organs or extremities of the human body, which commonly resulted in an inter-scan delay, involuntary patient visceral motion and patient discomfort under clinical settings.

The second milestone was the advent of spiral/helical CT empowered by slip-ring technology in 1990 (Figure 1.2), in which the 180°-interpolation or 360°-interpolation approach was used for projection data synthesis and then image reconstruction (Kalender et al. 1989, 1990; Crawford and King 1990). The elimination of the step-and-shoot scan mode and the resultant inter-scan delay marked the entrance of CT technologies and applications into a new era of unprecedented clinical excellence in patient throughput and comfort, saving of contrast agent, and reduction of motion artifact or spatial mis-registration. The clinical community hailed the overwhelming

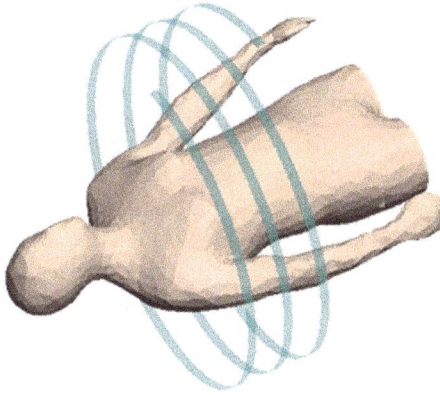

FIGURE 1.2 Schematic diagram showing the spiral/helical source trajectory of a single-detector row CT.

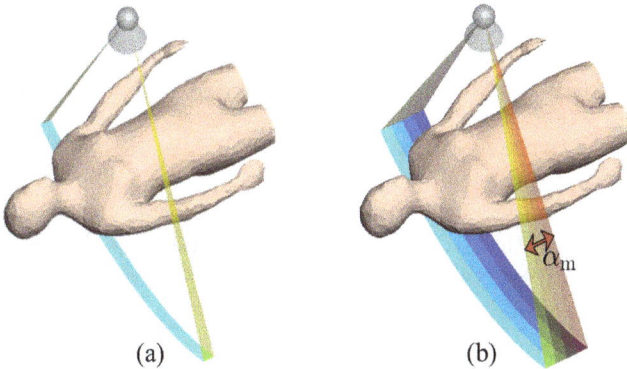

(a) (b)

FIGURE 1.3 Schematic diagrams showing the geometries of a (a) fan beam in SDCT and (b) cone beam in MDCT for either data acquisition or image reconstruction.

success of spiral/helical CT over extensive applications, which drove all major CT manufacturers to deliver their spiral/helical CT products within a short period of time at the beginning of the 1990s.

The third major milestone was MDCT based on multi-detector row technology (Figure 1.3b). The initial attempt to transition from SDCT to MDCT was the twin-detector row CT offered by Elscint (Elscint Twin) in 1992 (Liang and Kruger 1996; Kalayoglu 2011). Six years later, all major vendors were unveiling MDCT technologies that supported simultaneous formation of four transectional images from the data acquired along the circular source trajectory (termed *axial scan* henceforth) (Hu 1998; Taguchi and Aradate 1998) at the Radiological Society of North America's (RSNA's) 84th Scientific Assembly and Annual Meeting held in 1998 at the Exhibition Hall of the McCormick Place in Chicago. With the launching of four-detector CT in the marketplace, CT technology based on fourth-generation geometry was forced out, as the hardware costs associated with the two-dimensional (2D) detector array along the entire CT gantry made MDCT based on such a geometry competitively disadvantaged against those based on third-generation geometry. By 2002, all major CT vendors were marketing their 16-detector row flagship MDCT scanners (Flohr et al. 2003), which turned the submillimeter craniocaudal spatial resolution and three-dimensional (3D) isotropic spatial resolution into reality, enabling numerous advanced clinical applications, e.g., the imaging of temporal bone and coronary artery angiographies. Note that the leap from the simultaneous generation of four transactional image slices to sixteen slices took only about four years, while about eight years elapsed from one to four slices. Just three years later, all major CT manufacturers had launched their flagship 64-detector row MDCT scanners (Flohr et al. 2005) – an even larger leap in the number of detector rows in 2005 – and made the scan of large organs or extremities readily feasible within one breath hold. Since then, the major CT manufacturers have competed fiercely by launching their flagship products at a variety of detector rows, e.g., the 128-detector row MDCT in 2007, 256-detetor row MDCT in 2007 and 320-detector row MDCT in 2008 (Rybicki et al. 2008). The field has observed a race in the number of detector rows among rival CT vendors (also called the "slice war") since the mid-1990s, driven by the desire to scan a patient's entire heart and other large organs without table movement (Figure 1.4). As such, the radiation dose, contrast agent dose and inter-slab artifact can be substantially reduced, in addition to the efficiency of utilizing the output power of the X-ray source (usually an X-ray tube).

It is interesting to speculate on how large an X-ray beam's longitudinal aperture will eventually be in MDCT. Clearly, the longitudinal beam aperture is dependent on the desire to cover large organs/tissues in the human body with one gantry rotation

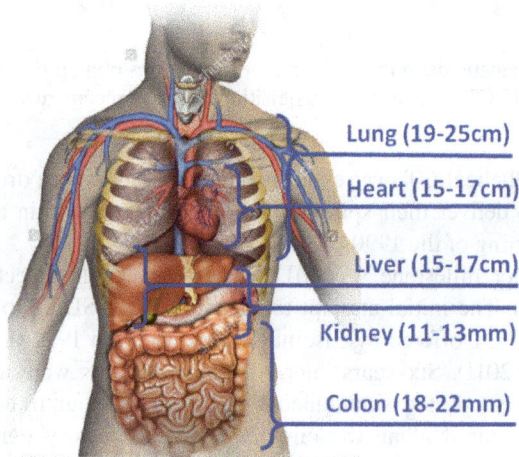

Lung (19-25cm)

Heart (15-17cm)

Liver (15-17cm)

Kidney (11-13mm)

Colon (18-22mm)

FIGURE 1.4 Diagram showing the longitudinal range of the major organs in the human body. (Drawing adopted with permission from Shutterstock.)

and the cost of CT detector fabrication. Presented in Figure 1.4 are the typical longitudinal ranges corresponding to major organs/tissues in the human body. For cardiac imaging, the goal of MDCT is to cover the entire heart in one gantry rotation so the inter-slab discontinuity caused by inconsistencies in cardiac motion or contrast agent circulation can be avoided. The longitudinal size of the heart in the vast majority of the population is approximately 160 mm. Hence, the number of detector rows is 320 or 256, when the detector row width projected to the axis of rotation is 0.5 mm or 0.625 mm, respectively, as we have already witnessed in the marketplace. Organs larger than the heart can be readily scanned by the spiral/helical modes of MDCT, as routinely practiced in clinics on a daily basis (Tang 2014; Tang and Xie 2018).

The fourth milestone was the advent of dual-source–dual-detector (DSDD) MDCT (Figure 1.5) launched by Siemens Healthineers (then Siemens Healthcare) in 2008 (Flohr et al. 2008; Petersilka et al. 2008), which not only enabled cardiovascular imaging at almost doubled the temporal resolution but also material-specific imaging (Alvarez and Macovski 1976) and virtual monochromatic imaging (Alvarez and Seppi 1979) (termed *spectral imaging* henceforth) via material decomposition with each of its X-ray sources simultaneously working at high and low peak voltages. In principle, the material decomposition should be carried out in the projection domain (Alvarez and Macovski 1976) (pre-reconstruction), but its conversion into an implementation in the image domain (post-reconstruction) was very successful with DSDD MDCT (see more detail in Section 1.2.3). Recognizing its clinical relevance and potential, this spectral CT technology was also implemented in the

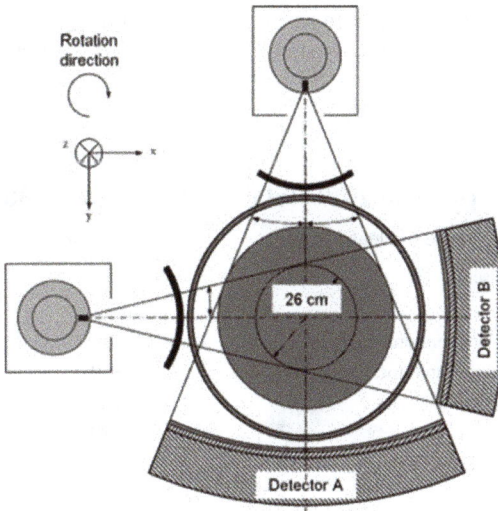

FIGURE 1.5 Schematic diagram showing the architecture of dual-source–dual-detector MDCT. (Adopted with permission from Petersilka et al. 2008.)

conventional single-source–single-detector (SSSD) MDCT by other major vendors through the techniques of fast kVp-switching (Chandra and Langan 2011), dual-layer X-ray detection (Vlassenbroek 2011) or slow kVp-switching (Hounsfield 1973). Since then, regardless of the implementation approach, spectral imaging has been adding significant value to the clinical practice of MDCT, especially in advanced clinical applications, such as the differentiation between malignant and benign lesions in oncologic cases or between hemorrhage and calcification in neurovascular cases.

1.2 CLINICAL APPLICATIONS OF STATE-OF-THE-ART MDCT FOR DIAGNOSTIC IMAGING

Worldwide, the number of CT installations per 100,000 population in a country has become one of the indicators of its level of healthcare and welfare. Notably, in recent years, the increment in CT installments in developing countries has been outpacing the growth of their economy, while that in developed countries remains at the plateau. Each year, more than 80 million CT scans and/or procedures are carried out in the US. As one of the most popular imaging modalities, CT has played an indispensable role for excellence in clinical practice, especially in supporting diagnostic and therapeutic intervention decision-making of those diseases or traumatic injuries that are ranked as the five leading causes of death in the nation (Table 1.1).

1.2.1 TYPICAL CLINICAL APPLICATIONS OF MDCT

Through clinical trials, numerous studies have been conducted to evaluate and verify MDCT's clinical utility in detection and characterization of vascular and parenchymal anomalies and/or lesions. With sensitivity and specificity and/or other clinically relevant metrics as the figures of merit, a large body of introductory, review and

---

TABLE 1.1
Leading Causes of Death in 2019 (Total Mortality: 2,854,838)

Rank	Cause of Death	Number of Deaths	% of All Deaths
1	Heart diseases	659,041	23.1
2	Cancer	599,601	21.0
3	Accidents (unintentional injuries)	173,040	6.1
4	Chronic lower respiratory diseases	156,979	5.5
5	Cerebrovascular diseases	150,005	5.3
6	Alzheimer diseases	121,499	4.3
7	Diabetes mellitus	87,674	3.1
8	Nephropathy	51,565	1.8
9	Influenza and pneumonia	49,783	1.7
10	Intentional self-harm	47,511	1.7

Source: Adopted from National Vital Statistics reports (Heron 2021).

---

research papers on MDCT's clinical utility and/or relevance in cardiovascular, neu-rovascular, thoracic, abdominal/pelvic and extremity imaging has been published in the literature (Rydberg et al. 2000). For readers to have a broader impression about the significant role being played by MDCT in the clinic, a number of typical, routine and important applications of MDCT for diagnostic imaging are presented in Figure 1.6, as exemplification of its versatile utility and relevance on a daily basis in clinical practice.

1.2.2 Dual-Source–Dual-Detector MDCT for Cardiovascular Imaging

With the increasing number of detector rows, MDCT is becoming one of the most popular modalities for cardiac imaging, e.g., the diagnosis of stenosis in coro-nary arteries, in addition to the gold standard of practice via fluoroscopy-guided

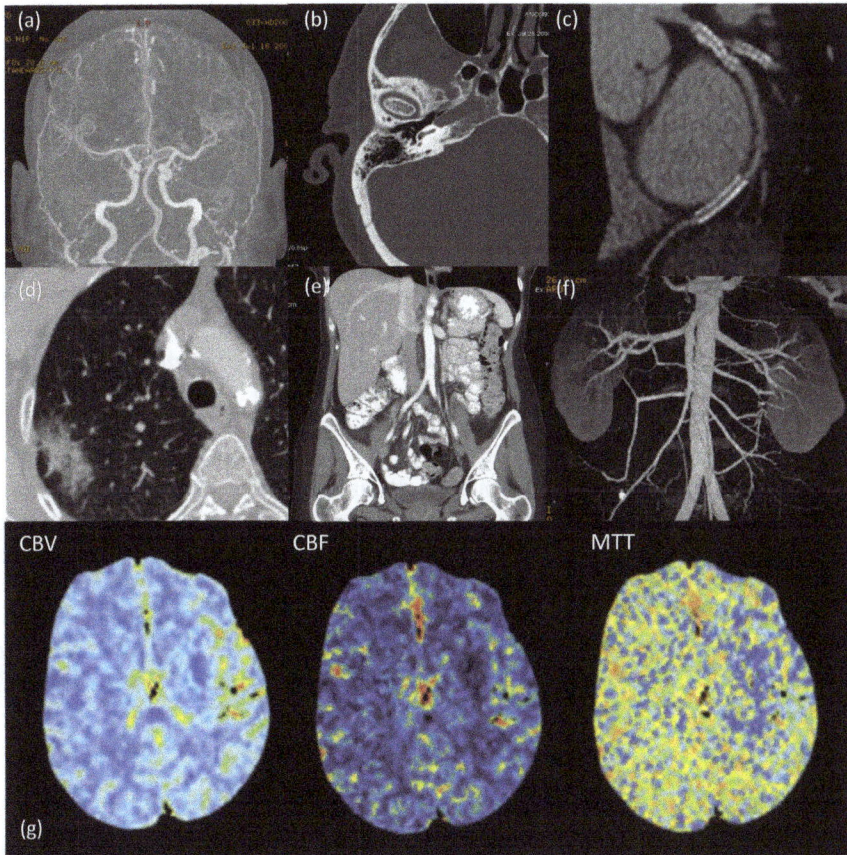

FIGURE 1.6 Typical clinical applications of MDCT: (a) head CT angiography, (b) temporal bone, (c) coronal artery stent, (d) lung cancer, (e) abdominal/pelvic, (f) renal angiography and (g) CT perfusion for acute ischemic stroke.

catheterization. To take a snapshot of the heart in a cyclic motion, the temporal resolution becomes the most critical imaging performance (Ohnesorge et al. 2000b; Flohr et al. 2000; Vembar 2003; Tang and Pan 2004; Taguchi et al. 2006; Hsieh et al. 2006; Flohr and Ohnesorge 2008; Tang et al. 2008a). The temporal resolution of an MDCT scanner is dependent on the duration of time during which the projection data are acquired. Accordingly, the short scan mode is usually employed for cardiovascular imaging. If, for instance, the time for an MDCT gantry to rotate one circle is 0.3 sec, the temporal resolution is $0.3 \times (55° + 180°)/360°$ sec ≈ 0.2 sec, which is sufficient for imaging a heart that beats fewer than 65 times in a minute, i.e., 65 beats/minute (b/m). For patients with a higher heartbeat rate, which occurs frequently in the clinic, beta-blocker is usually administered to decrease the heartbeat rate until it is stably lower than 65 b/m. However, the avoidance of beta-blocker is of clinical relevance, especially for patients with suspected myocardial infarction. Therefore, in addition to a short scan, more methods to improve the temporal resolution for clinical excellence are needed. A straightforward way to do so is to increase the gantry rotation speed of MDCT. For instance, if the gantry rotation speed can increase to 0.2 sec per rotation (s/r), the temporal resolution would be $0.2 \times (55° + 180°)/360°$ sec ≈ 130 ms. However, to reach a 0.2 s/r gantry speed, the G-force in a typical MDCT would be larger than 70 g, leading to extreme challenges and high cost in MDCT gantry fabrication.

An alternative way is to acquire the projection data in an inter-cycle multi-sector fashion (Taguchi et al. 2006; Flohr and Ohnesorge 2008; Tang et al. 2008a). Since the heart physiologically repeats itself, the projection data can be acquired over multiple cycles at an appropriate phase gated by the ECG signal. For example, an ideal case may occur in the two-cycle data acquisition, in which half of the data come from cardiac cycle I and the rest from cycle II. It is not hard to imagine, however, that the ideal case rarely occurs in reality, because the temporal relationship between the two cycles is jointly determined by the MDCT's gantry rotation speed and patient's heartbeat rate and initial phase, which seldom guarantees a perfect lineup in timing, not to mention the fact that the patient's heartbeat rate variation may further complicate the situation. In principle, the effective temporal resolution (T_{eff}) of a two-cycle data acquisition and image reconstruction can be defined as $T_{eff} = max(T_I, T_{II})$, where T_I and T_{II} are the duration of time to acquire the data in cycles I and II, respectively, and $max(\cdot,\cdot)$ denotes an operation to select the larger of the two variables. Hence, only the ideal case can ensure a doubled temporal resolution, and all other cases are between the best (doubled temporal resolution) and worst (no gain in temporal resolution) scenarios (Tang et al. 2008a).

In general, the larger the difference in the temporal span during which the projection data are acquired from each individual cycle, the less the gain in temporal resolution. It should also be realized that, although ECG may repeat itself, the mechanical state of the heart never repeats itself exactly, particularly for MDCT imaging at spatial resolution that is significantly better than that in SPECT or PET, wherein the assumption on the heart's repetition in the mechanical state may be reasonable. Fortunately, however, if the data corresponding to each sector come from an identical cardiac cycle with an equal period of time for data acquisition, then a doubled temporal resolution is guaranteed (see the schematic on the right of Figure 1.7). It should be emphasized that there is no chance for the heart rate arrhythmia to degrade the temporal resolution, because all the data come from the same single cardiac cycle. Using a DSDD MDCT, the heartbeat rate of a patient can readily exceed 65 b/m, as demonstrated by the images of the coronary arteries presented in Figure 1.8.

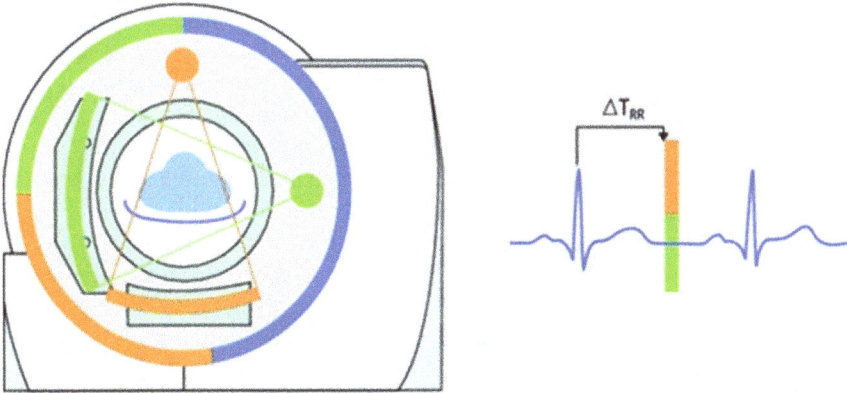

FIGURE 1.7   Diagrams showing the schematic of data acquisition in a dual-source–dual-detector CT to ensure the ideal case always occurs, with the data corresponding to both sectors came from the identical cycle. (Adopted with permission from Flohr and Ohnesorge 2008.)

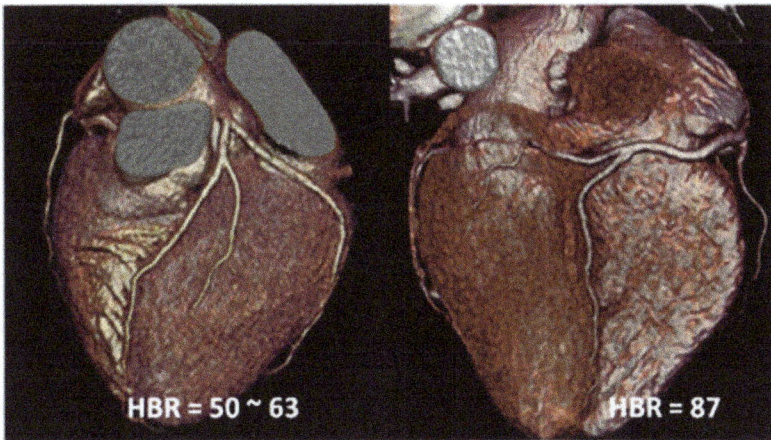

FIGURE 1.8   The 3D surface rendering of the heart generated by (a) a single-source–single-detector MDCT and (b) a dual-source–dual-detector MDCT.

1.2.3 Dual-Energy Imaging in MDCT: A Form of Spectral Imaging

Given a single peak voltage (kVp; also called the maximum energy) of an X-ray source, usually an X-ray tube, CT images can be formed by reconstruction from the projection data that have been adequately corrected for the non-linearity due to the so-called beam-hardening effect. The CT images are presented in the Hounsfield unit (HU) that is converted from the material's linear attenuation coefficient, in which the intensities of water and air are calibrated to 0 HU and −1000 HU, respectively. As to be elucidated in Chapter 3, a material's attenuation of X-ray is determined by its linear attenuation coefficient that is jointly dependent on the material's mass attenuation coefficient and electron density, respectively. It is often the case that the linear attenuation coefficient of different materials, e.g., an iodinated contrast agent and calcification existing in atherosclerotic plaques, may possess almost identical linear attenuation coefficients and thus lead to difficulties in making diagnostic decisions under clinical settings (see Chapter 7, Figure 7.5 for more information).

In DSDD MDCT, corresponding to the projection data acquired at low and high kVps, respectively, a pair of CT images can be obtained to facilitate the differentiation of tissues, organs and contrast agents. As illustrated in the renal case displayed in Figure 1.9, the calcification (Ca^{++}) is hardly differentiable from the uric acid in the CT image corresponding to the high kVp (vertical projection onto the abscissa), while the iodine is hardly differentiable from the calcification in the image acquired at low kVp (horizontal projection onto the coordinate). In fact, by carrying out a pixel-wise analysis in the 2D space spanned by the HUs acquired at low and high kVps, respectively, the difficulties in differentiation between calcification and iodine or between uric acid and calcification become much smaller (Sodickson et al. 2021).

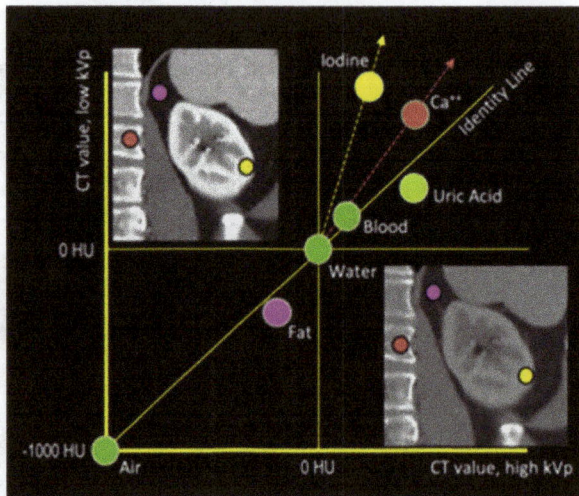

FIGURE 1.9 A diagram shows the schematic of material analysis carried out in a DSDD MDCT using its DECT functionality. (Adopted with permission from Sodickson et al. 2021.)

This imaging approach offered in DSDD MDCT is called dual-energy CT (DECT) and is the most straightforward implementation of material-specific imaging, which, along with virtual monochromatic imaging and analysis, are the two primary forms of spectral CT – the major subject to be covered in this book.

1.3 PHOTON-COUNTING SPECTRAL MDCT: THE LATEST LEAP IN CT TECHNOLOGY

Until recently, the signal generated by the attenuating object in the X-ray beam in CT is detected through the mechanism of energy integration, regardless of whether it is in the form of a gas-chamber or solid-state detector. Presently, CT technology is approaching or passing by its fifth milestone by adopting the mechanism of photon-counting detection of X-rays in MDCT. Mainly due to its advantages in spectral channelization (Roessl and Proksa 2007b; Ren et al. 2020) and spectral weighting (Tapiovaara and Wagner 1985; Cahn 1999; Giersch 2004; Niederlöhner 2005; Wang and Pelc 2011), X-ray photon-counting detection technology offers unprecedented opportunities for MDCT to fulfill its clinical potentials, as exemplified by the case of temporal bone examination presented in Figure 1.10. Clearly, photon-counting MDCT outperforms energy-integration MDCT substantially in anatomic delineation of the fine bony structure, especially the incudostapedial joint, and integrity assessment of the neurological functionality, even at a lowered radiation dose (Benson et al. 2022).

As witnessed in the past one and a half decades, by making a paradigm shift in the clinical practice of MDCT, the energy-integration spectral MDCT has added significant value to MDCT's clinical utility for oncologic, cardiovascular and neurovascular applications. Now, it is exciting to see another leap in CT technology that makes the photon-counting spectral CT ready for clinical missions. It is anticipated

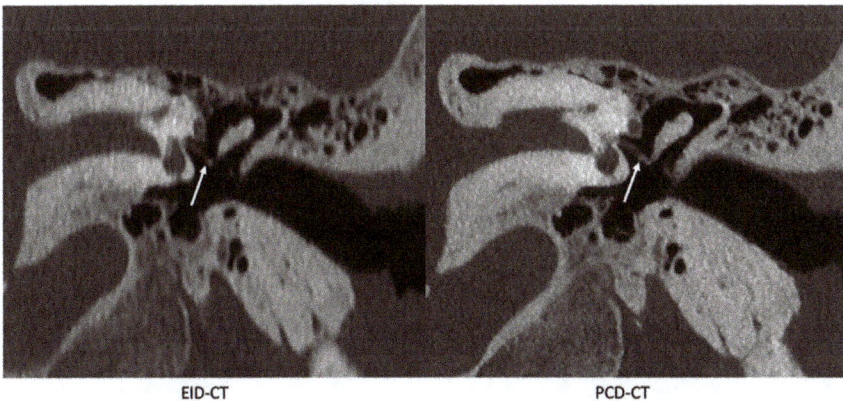

EID-CT   PCD-CT

FIGURE 1.10 Delineation of the incudostapedial joint (arrows) in the temporal bony structures: (left) energy-integration MDCT versus (right) photon-counting MDCT. (Images adopted from Benson et al. 2022 with permission.)

that photon-counting spectral MDCT will have higher potential to boost the contrast resolution and spatial resolution in comparison to its energy-integration counterpart. To translate this leap in MDCT technology into a leap in MDCT's clinical utility, tremendous efforts are needed from the community that comprises clinicians, researchers, specialists and engineers. To be successful in making such a translation, engaged professionals should have knowledge of the fundamentals in mathematics and physics related to MDCT and an in-depth understanding of MDCT system architecture, imaging chain, data acquisition, image formation, contrast agents for conspicuity enhancement and the approaches to assess image quality. This book serves all these purposes.

Prior to ending this introductory chapter, I want to make some editorial comments. Historically, spectral MDCT implemented via energy-integration X-ray detection has been named dual-energy CT. However, in recognition of their common ground in physics, making such a distinction between them is arbitrary from my point of view, especially in light of the fact that the realistic spectral response of the photon-counting detector in MDCT (see Chapter 7 and Chapter 8) is far from ideal. Hence, from now on throughout the book, I will make no distinction of spectral MDCT in its implementation between photon-counting and energy-integration X-ray detection, unless such a distinction is necessary. Also, as a quantitative tomographic imaging modality, MDCT has also been called multi-slice or multi-section CT (MSCT). Unless otherwise specified, I refer to multi-slice, multi-section and multi-detector row CT as multi-detector CT (MDCT) from now on throughout the book for clarification and consistence in expression. Moreover, in general, I refer to CT as either MDCT or SDCT (single-detector CT) if no distinction between them is necessary in the context.

2 Fundamentals in Mathematics for MDCT

X-ray photons interact with materials while they propagate in a medium and get attenuated on their way passing through it. Statistically, if N_0 monochromatic X-ray photons transverse one single attenuating material of thickness l, the number of X-ray photons that survive the attenuation is

$$N = N_0 e^{-\mu l} \tag{2.1}$$

where μ is the material's linear attenuation coefficient (LAC). As we know, the LAC of material varies as a function of the energy of X-ray photons. Then, taking the polychromatic nature of the X-ray source under clinical settings into account, Equation 2.1 should be modified to

$$N = N_0(E) e^{-\mu(E)l} \tag{2.2}$$

where $\mu(E)$ is the LAC of the material at energy E.

In computed tomography (CT), we are interested in reconstruction of the LAC distribution $\mu(E, \rho, \vec{n})$ of an object from its projections, where $\vec{n}$ denotes the unit directional vector of a point within the object and ρ the distance of the point from the coordinate origin O along $\vec{n}$. Without losing generality, from now on we denote the LAC distribution as a function $f(E; \rho, \vec{n})$. In the case of monochromatic energy, $f(E; \rho, \vec{n})$ can be denoted as $f(\rho, \vec{n})$ and thus the attenuation of X-ray photons passing through the object can be determined as

$$N = N_0 e^{-\int_L f(\rho, \vec{n}) dl} \tag{2.3}$$

where L represents the route of the X-ray beam. If the X-ray's polychromatism is taken into account, Equation 2.3 should be modified to

$$N = N_0(E) e^{-\int_E \int_L f(E; \rho, \vec{n}) dl dE} \tag{2.4}$$

where E denotes the spectrum of the X-ray source.

DOI: 10.1201/9780429028465-2

2.1 2D X-RAY TRANSFORM, RADON TRANSFORM AND RADON SPACE

Let's assume monochromatism at this moment. Originating from Equation 2.3, the X-ray transform of a two-dimensional (2D) object function $f(\rho,\vec{n})$ along route L at any direction is defined as

$$Xf(\rho,\vec{n}) = \int_L f(\rho,\vec{n})d\rho = -\log\left(\frac{N}{N_0}\right) \qquad (2.5)$$

That is, the X-ray transform of the object function $f(\rho,\vec{n})$ is an integral and can be measured as $-\log\left(\frac{N}{N_0}\right)$ in practice. On the other hand, as illustrated in Figure 2.1, the Radon transform of the 2D object function $f(\rho,\vec{n})$ along $\vec{n}$ is defined as

$$Rf(\rho,\vec{n}) = \int_{\vec{r}\cdot\vec{n}} f(\vec{r})d\vec{r} \qquad (2.6)$$

which is an integral along the line orthogonal to $\vec{n}$ at distance ρ from the origin (see the Radon line defined in Figure 2.1) and corresponds to a vector $(\vec{n},\rho)$ in the 2D Radon domain.

Specifically, Equation 2.6 can be rewritten as

$$Rf(\rho,\vec{n}) = \int_{-\pi}^{\pi}\int_0^{\infty} f(\vec{r})\delta(\vec{r}\cdot\vec{n}-\rho)\rho\,d\rho\,d\theta \qquad (2.7)$$

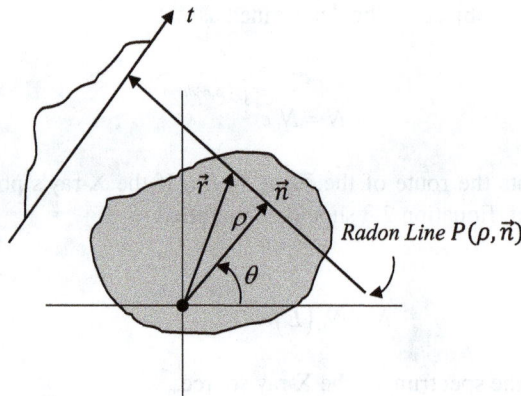

FIGURE 2.1 A schematic diagram illustrating a 2D object function $f(\vec{r})$ in 2D real space $\mathcal{R}^2$ and a Radon line intersecting it.

If all the Radon domain information $Rf(\rho,\bar{n})$ of a 2D object function is available from its X-ray transforms defined in Equation 2.5 (also called projection data), the 2D object function $f(\bar{r})$ can be obtained by reconstruction from $Rf(\rho,\bar{n})$ via the 2D inverse Radon transform

$$f(\bar{r}) = \frac{1}{4\pi^2} \int_{-\pi}^{\pi} \int_{0}^{\infty} Rf(\rho,\bar{n}) \frac{1}{\bar{r}\cdot\bar{n}-\rho} d\rho d\theta \qquad (2.8)$$

Notably, the 2D Radon transform pair (Equations 2.7 and 2.8) provides the mathematical foundation for us to understand the concepts of tomography, data insufficiency and redundancy in single-detector CT (SDCT). In practice, however, the inverse Radon transform (Equation 2.8) has not been commonly employed for image reconstruction, mainly because of the existence of other efficient and computationally tractable algorithms, such as the filtered back-projection (FBP) algorithm or Fourier transform-based (or convolution-based) algorithms. As the focus of this book is on MDCT, we stop the coverage on SDCT right here, but readers who are interested in learning more details of SDCT, especially the adequate handling of data insufficiency and redundancy over various application-driven scan modes, e.g., half-scan, partial-scan, full-scan or over-scan and their associated image reconstruction algorithms, are referred to the classical textbooks (Kak and Slaney 1988) and papers published in the literature (Parker 1982; Crawford and King 1990; Silver 2000).

2.2 3D X-RAY TRANSFORM, RADON TRANSFORM AND RADON SPACE

With an increasing number of detector rows in MDCT under circular source trajectory (*axial MDCT* henceforth), the cone angle of X-ray beams in data acquisition becomes formidably large, which may lead to severe cone-beam (CB) artifacts in reconstructed images (Tuy 1983; Smith 1985, 1990; Natterer 1986; Rizo et al. 1991; Chen 1992; Clack and Defrise 1994). The root cause of CB artifacts in axial MDCT is the fact that the data acquisition by the cone-shaped X-ray beam cannot meet the data sufficiency condition (DSC). As stated by Tuy and Smith in their most widely cited papers (Tuy 1983; Smith 1985, 1990), "For every plane that intersects the object to be imaged it intersects the source trajectory at least once". However, it may be hard for one to fully understand the Tuy–Smith DSC stated in the spatial domain with respect to why a cone-shaped X-ray beam in axial MDCT cannot provide sufficient data for theoretically exact image reconstruction (i.e., data insufficiency). In a more straightforward manner, the Tuy–Smith DSC can be geometrically perceived as the fact that a pair of conjugate rays in a cone-shaped X-ray beam in axial MDCT are not collinear (i.e., data inconsistency) (Feldkamp 1984; Tang et al. 2005), except for those located within the central plane determined by the circular trajectory. Note that the distinction made between data insufficiency and inconsistency is arbitrary and only serves the purpose of providing two different perspectives to look at the same problem.

2.2.1 3D X-Ray Transform, Radon Transform, Radon Shell and Radon Space

In fact, a better view of data insufficiency or inconsistency in axial MDCT can be made in the Radon domain, in which a null space (or missed zone) cannot be filled by the projection data acquired by a cone-shaped X-ray beam along the circular trajectory. Letting $f(\vec{r})\left(\vec{r}=(\varphi,\theta,r)\right)$ denote an object function in three-dimensional (3D) real space $\mathcal{R}^3$ under the spherical coordinate system, the 3D X-ray transform of object function $f(\vec{r})$ is defined as the integral along line L

$$Xf(\vec{r}) = \int_L df(\vec{r}) = \int_{-\infty}^{\infty} f\left(\vec{r}_0 + \vec{k}\cdot\vec{l}\right)d\vec{l} \tag{2.9}$$

where $\vec{r}_0$ denotes the vector connecting a point in line L and the origin of the coordinate system, and $\vec{k}$ is the unit vector with its direction parallel to line L. Furthermore, the 3D Radon transform of the object function $f(\vec{r})$ is defined as (Buzug 2008)

$$Rf(\vec{r}) = \int_{0}^{2\pi} \int_{-\frac{\pi}{2}}^{\frac{\pi}{2}} \int_{0}^{\infty} f(\vec{r})\delta(\vec{r}\cdot\vec{n}-\rho)\rho d\rho d\theta \tag{2.10}$$

As illustrated in Figure 2.2, the Radon transform of a 3D object function is an integral on the plane that is jointly determined by the norm $\vec{n}$ and distance ρ from the origin O, and such a plane is called the Radon plane, with its norm defined as

$$\vec{n} = \left(\sin\theta\cos\varphi, \sin\theta\sin\varphi, \cos\theta\right) \tag{2.11}$$

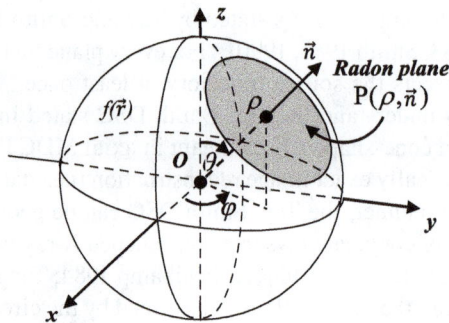

FIGURE 2.2 Schematic of an object function $f(\vec{r})$ in 3D real space $\mathcal{R}^3$ and a Radon plane $P(\rho,\vec{n})$ intersecting the point denoted by $p(\rho,\vec{n})$.

Theoretically, if all the information in the Radon domain is known, the 3D object function $f(\vec{r})$ can be reconstructed from $Rf(\vec{r})$ using the 3D inverse Radon transform (Buzug 2008)

$$f(\vec{r}) = \frac{-1}{8\pi} \int\limits_{-\pi/2}^{\pi/2} \int\limits_{0}^{2\pi} \int\limits_{0}^{\infty} \frac{\partial^2}{\partial\rho^2} Rf(\vec{r}) r\, dr\, d\beta\, d\alpha \tag{2.12}$$

where $(r\sin\alpha\,\cos\beta, r\sin\alpha\,\cos\beta, r\cos\beta)$ is defined in the Radon space, and vector $\vec{r}$ is defined in the 3D real space as

$$\vec{r} = \rho\left(\sin\theta\cos\varphi, \sin\theta\sin\varphi, \cos\theta\right) \tag{2.13}$$

It should be straightforward to imagine that, given a point $p(\vec{r})$ in $\mathcal{R}^3$, the locus of norms of all the Radon planes passing through point $p(\vec{r})$ forms a shell with vector $\overline{OP}$ as its diameter (see more in Section 2.2.3 and Figure 2.4). Hence, a point in a 3D object to be reconstructed can contribute to all the data on a shell in the Radon domain, and thus the shell is called a Radon shell (Tuy 1983; Rizo 1991). Moreover, it is very important to understand that the support of the Radon transform of a spherical object function in the 3D spatial domain is still a sphere with the same diameter in the 3D Radon domain.

2.2.2 3D FOURIER TRANSFORM AND FOURIER SLICE THEOREM

There exists a correspondence between the 3D Radon transform and 3D Fourier transform of an object function $f(\vec{r})$ that is known as the Fourier slice theorem (Buzug 2008). It states that the 1D Fourier transform of data along a radial line in the 3D Radon domain of $f(\vec{r})$ is equal to the data along the same radial line in the 3D Fourier transform of $f(\vec{r})$. The 3D Fourier slice theorem offers an analytic perspective of the Tuy–Smith DSC. Under the polar coordinate system in the 3D Radon domain and Cartesian coordinate system in the 3D Fourier domain (Figure 2.3), the Fourier slice theorem can be analytically expressed as

$$F_\rho\left(Rf(\rho,\vec{n})\right) = F\left(u,v,w\right)\big|_{(\rho,\vec{n})} \tag{2.14}$$

where $F(\cdot)$ denotes a 1D Fourier transform along the radial line defined by $(\rho,\vec{n})$ (Figure 2.3a), and $F(u,v,w)\big|_{(\rho,\vec{n})}$ is the Fourier transform of the 3D object function $f(\vec{r})$ along the identical radial line $(\rho,\vec{n})$. Note that, specifically, we have

$$\begin{aligned} u &= \rho'\sin\theta'\cos\varphi' \\ v &= \rho'\sin\theta'\sin\varphi' \\ w &= \rho'\cos\theta' \end{aligned} \tag{2.15}$$

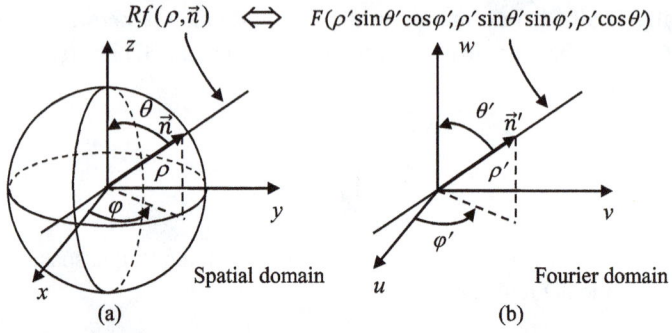

$$Rf(\rho,\vec{n}) \quad \Longleftrightarrow \quad F(\rho'\sin\theta'\cos\varphi', \rho'\sin\theta'\sin\varphi', \rho'\cos\theta')$$

Spatial domain

Fourier domain

(a)   (b)

FIGURE 2.3 Correspondence between the 3D Radon domain and 3D Fourier domain established by the 3D Fourier slice theorem.

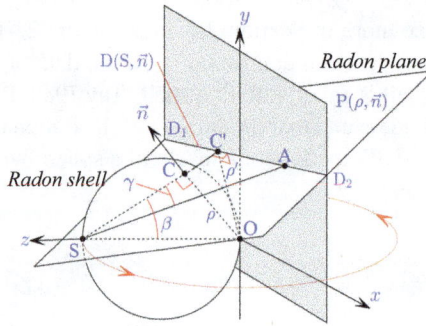

FIGURE 2.4 Schematic showing the geometry of axial CBCT data acquisition by a cone-shaped X-ray beam and a flat-panel detector, and the relationship among detector, X-ray transform (e.g., the line integral along *SA*), Radon plane and Radon shell.

2.2.3 DATA INSUFFICIENCY VIEWED IN 3D RADON AND FOURIER SPACES

For a simple geometric illustration, suppose we have a 2D flat-panel detector for data acquisition as the example to illustrate the data insufficiency in axial MDCT (Figure 2.4), wherein S denotes the X-ray beam's focal spot. The Radon plane that intersects S and the detector along line D_1D_2 corresponds to a point in the 3D Radon domain. Given an ideal 2D detector (i.e., its dimension and sampling rate are infinite), it should not be hard to understand that all the Radon planes intersecting the source S and the detector determine the data in the Radon domain on the Radon shell with SO as its diameter. The Radon shell sweeps circularly in the Radon domain twice and forms a torus with a data redundancy of two (Figure 2.5a), while the cone-shaped X-ray beam and detector assembly proceed in the spatial domain along a circular trajectory. Apparently, no matter how many turns the assembly rotates, there exists

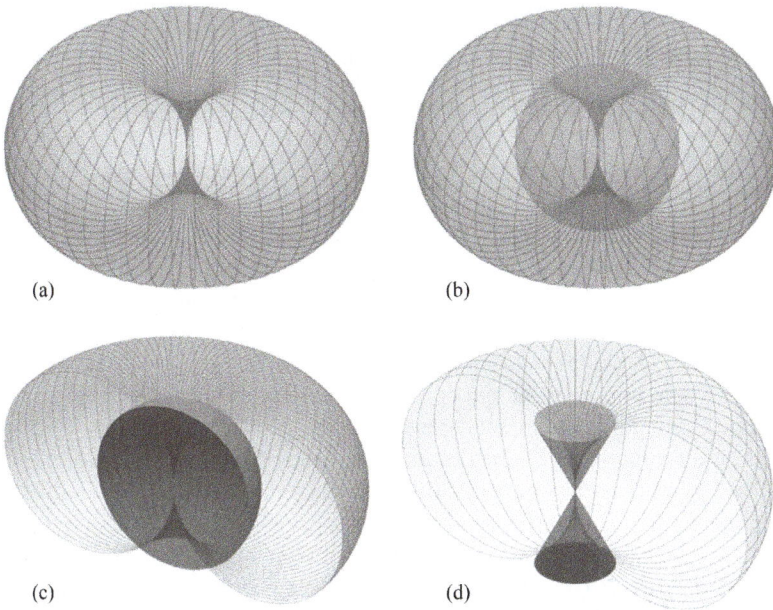

(a)   (b)

(c)   (d)

FIGURE 2.5   The data distributed over a torus in the 3D Radon domain correspond to the projection data acquired along a circular source trajectory (a); the shadowed sphere in (b) denotes the Radon data corresponding to a spherical object of identical diameter in the spatial domain, (c) shows a sectional view of (b), and (d) illustrates the cone-shaped null space in the 3D Fourier domain.

a missed zone, or more rigorously speaking in mathematics, a null space, in the Radon domain, as illustrated in Figure 2.5a–c. Such a null space is the root cause of data insufficiency in axial MDCT and the resultant CB artifacts. It should be noted that, for geometric clarification, the aforementioned reasoning is presented under the setting of a flat-panel detector that is usually utilized in cone-beam CT (CBCT), but it holds for the setting of a cylindrical multi-row detector used in MDCT, after a straightforward geometric transformation.

According to the 3D Fourier slice theorem, the data insufficiency in axial MDCT can also be viewed in the Fourier domain, as illustrated in Figure 2.5d (Zeng and Gullberg 1992; Buzug 2008). The null space in the Fourier domain becomes a cone with the half angle determined by $\sin^{-1}(R/D)$, where R denotes the radius of the object to be imaged, and D is the distance from the X-ray source to the axis of rotation. Note that the null space in the Fourier domain morphologically differs from that in the Radon domain (Tuy 1983; Rizo 1991). The larger the object to be imaged (i.e., the larger R), the larger the null space in the Fourier domain, leading to more severe CB artifacts.

2.3 SOURCE TRAJECTORIES IN MDCT THAT MEET DATA SUFFICIENCY CONDITION

With all the points presented earlier, it is time to ask: What would be the source trajectory or trajectories in MDCT to meet the Tuy–Smith DSC? It turns out that the most feasible and efficient approach is the spiral/helical scan, since, as illustrated in Figure 2.6a, it sweeps the 3D Radon domain seamlessly at adequately designed pitch and thus meets the DSC (Rizo 1991; Kudo and Saito 1991; Yan and Leahy 1992; Wang et al. 1993; Tang et al 2006). This is probably the most fortunate coincidence and thus beneficial to the entire community of CT. Being indispensably supported by the CT industry, the spiral/helical CT scan has indeed been the most meritorious and thus most widely utilized scan mode over clinical applications for more than 30 years, and, more important, it can continue to remain as the most meritorious and thus most widely utilized scan mode in the future.

In addition to the spiral/helical scan, a number of supplemental source trajectories have been proposed to fulfill the DSC, including the circle-plus-line (Zeng and Gullberg 1992; Hu 1995, 1997), circle-plus-arc (Wang and Ning 1999), circle-plus-two-arcs (Tang 2001; Tang and Ning 2001; Ning et al. 2003), dual orthogonal circles (Nett et al. 2007; Zhuang et al. 2008), dual orthogonal circles plus line (Kudo and Saito 1994a), and dual elliptical (Noo et al. 1998). As an example, the schematic of a circle-plus-two-arc source trajectory is presented in Figure 2.7, and filling the null space in the Radon domain is illustrated in Figure 2.6b. Apparently, these circle-plus scan modes demand extra source trajectories that may incur resistance to their wide acceptance, even though they may be meritorious in certain special and dedicated clinical applications. This may be the fundamental reason underlying the fact that so far no circle-plus scan mode has been viable in the clinical environment.

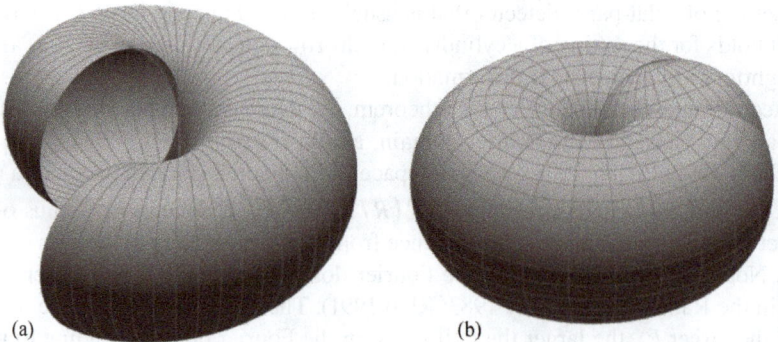

(a) (b)

FIGURE 2.6 The data in the Radon domain provided by the projection data acquired by a cone-shaped X-ray beam along the (a) spiral/helical trajectory and the (b) circle-plus-arc trajectory.

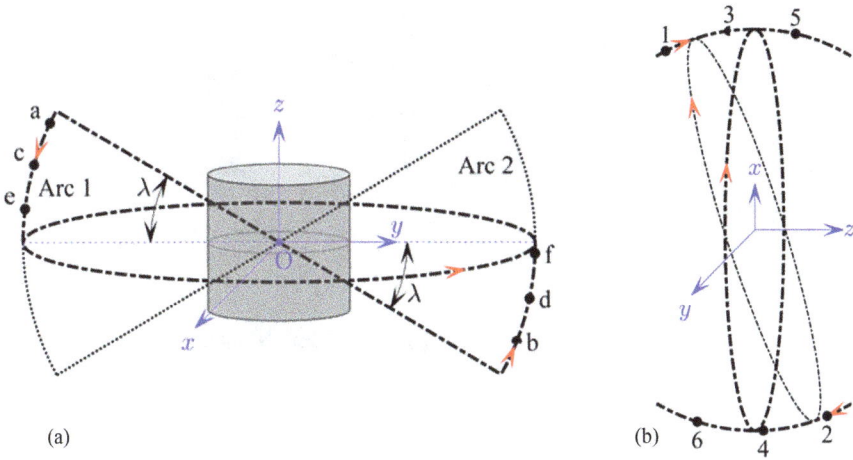

(a)   (b)

FIGURE 2.7   (a) The circle-plus-two-arc source trajectory, where vertexes a, b, c, d, e and f indicate the sequence of projection data acquisition along the arc sub-orbits. (b) The "quasi" spiral mode to implement the circle-plus-two-arc trajectory, in which CB projection is sequentially acquired.

2.4 CONE-BEAM ARTIFACTS IN AXIAL MDCT DUE TO DATA INSUFFICIENCY

Having had an in-depth understanding of the Tuy–Smith DSC associated with axial MDCT/CBCT in the spatial domain and the existence of a null space in the Radon and Fourier domains, we are ready to analyze the mechanisms at which each type of CB artifact is rendered and their morphology. As illustrated in Figure 2.8, the CB artifacts rendered by data insufficiency can be exemplified in the spatial domain using the computer-simulated Defrise phantom, which consists of seven identical ellipsoids deployed along the CT's axis of rotation (AOR) (Figure 2.8a). The semi-axes of the ellipsoids are 100 mm, 100 mm and 7.5 mm, respectively. A central coronal view (intersecting the AOR) of the reconstructed Defrise phantom is shown in Figure 2.8b. Visually, with increasing distance from the central plane determined by the source trajectory, the CB artifacts (i.e., reconstruction inaccuracy) manifest themselves as (i) geometric distortion in the discs' shapes and (ii) dropping of the discs' intensities. As quantitatively confirmed by the profiles plotted in Figure 2.8b, the distortion in shape and drop in intensity become increasingly prominent, while approaching the last disc at the top and bottom (approximately corresponding to 10° in cone angle), respectively. Notably, as no anatomic structure in the human body mimics it, the Defrise phantom may exaggerate the severity of CB artifacts, but it does serve as a reminder of the existence of CB artifacts in reality.

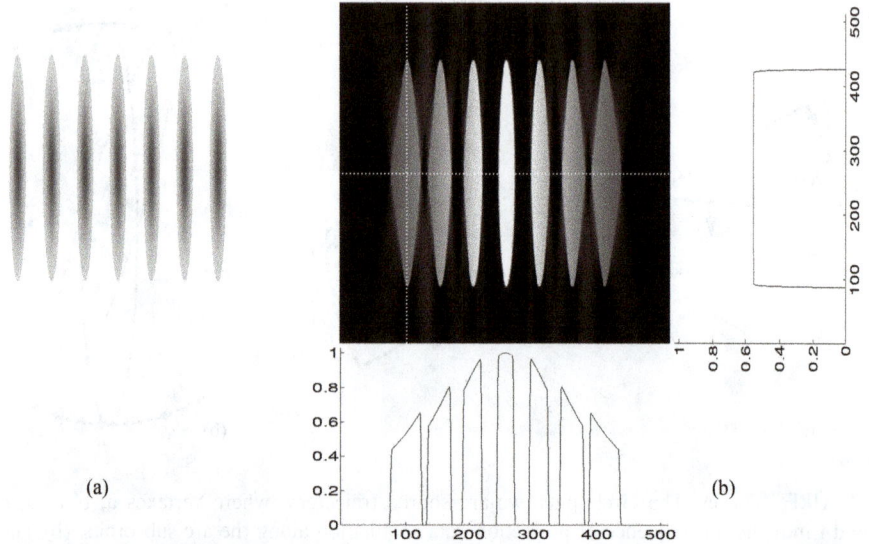

FIGURE 2.8 (a) Schematic of the Defrise phantom at linear attenuation coefficient equivalent to water and (b) its central coronal view reconstructed by the Feldkamp–Davis–Kress (FDK) algorithm and the cross-center profiles.

2.5 IMAGE FORMATION IN MDCT THAT MEETS DATA SUFFICIENCY CONDITION

We have observed the morphology of CB artifacts and the mechanism through which the artifacts are rendered, along with the understanding that the root cause of the CB artifacts is the X-ray beam's cone angle in data acquisition. As indicated earlier, the data insufficiency and inconsistency are intrinsic in axial MDCT data acquisition, i.e., the CB artifacts still appear if the detector used in data acquisition is ideal. In reality, however, no ideal detector is available for data acquisition in axial MDCT. For example, the detector used in axial MDCT is inevitably truncated along the longitudinal direction and leads to data truncation-induced artifacts, while the longitudinal spatial sampling rate may be insufficient and lead to aliasing artifacts. In fact, both the longitudinal data truncation and insufficient spatial sampling rate are indirectly associated with the X-ray beam's cone angle in data acquisition. Due to space limitations, however, we will only discuss the artifacts that are an immediate consequence of the cone angle in this chapter.

As indicated in Section 2.2.3 and especially illustrated in Figure 2.5, the Radon information corresponding to a spherical object in the 3D spatial domain occupies a sphere of identical radius in the 3D Radon domain (Tuy 1983; Rizo 1991; Tang 2001). Moreover, the 2D radon transform is a planar integral that may transform an abrupt variation in the 3D spatial domain into a moderate variation in the 3D Radon domain, providing an opportunity for filling the null space via interpolation if the dimension of the object to be imaged is relatively small. Early efforts attempted to fill the null space via interpolation (Hu 1996; Yang et al. 2005) with limited success. More important, it should be noted that the object to be imaged in the clinic, e.g., the head, trunk or extremities, is of large longitudinal dimension, which may generate information occupying a large sphere in the Radon domain.

2.5.1 MDCT Scanned in Circle-Plus Source Trajectories

Recognizing the limitations associated with the interpolation approach, a straight-forward step to overcome the difficulty in satisfying the Tuy–Smith DSC is to fill the null space in the Radon space with data acquired from the trajectory supplemental to the circular one. As indicated in Section 2.3, a number of circle-plus source trajectories have been proposed to enable CT to meet the DSC, but none of them have been implemented by the CT industry or are viable in the clinic, due to their potential impact on clinical workflow, challenges in electromechanics or simply the inconvenience they may cause. In principle, circle-plus source trajectories can do a good job of suppressing CB artifacts by filling the null space in the 3D Radon domain (Defrise and Clack 1994; Kudo and Saito 1991, 1994b; Yan and Leahy 1992; Wang and Ning 1999; Tang and Ning 2001). Figure 2.9 presents the case of circle-plus-two-arc (see Figure 2.7) as an example to demonstrate how a circle-plus source trajectory can suppress the cone-angle-induced artifacts in the spatial domain, while it fills the null space in the Radon domain as illustrated in Figure 2.6b.

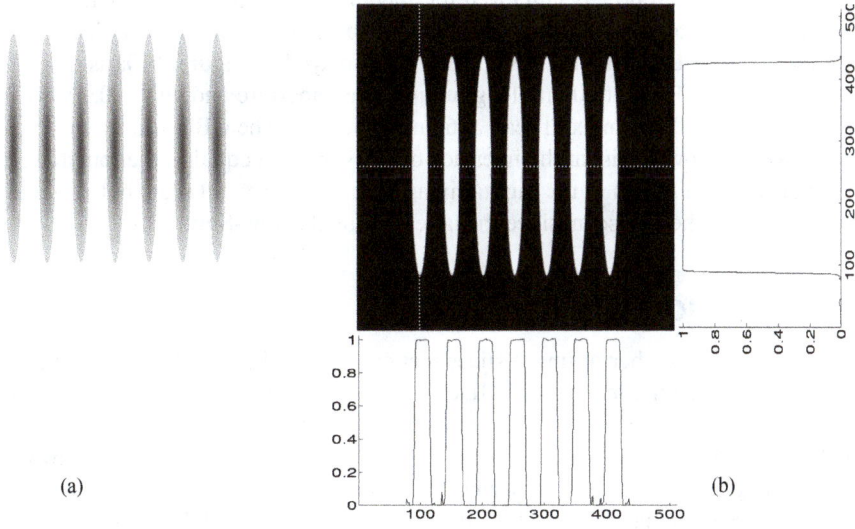

(a)   (b)

FIGURE 2.9   (a) Schematic of the Defrise phantom at linear attenuation coefficient equivalent to water and (b) the central coronal view of the image reconstructed by the CB-FBP algorithm from projection data acquired along a circle-plus-two-arc trajectory and the cross-center profile.

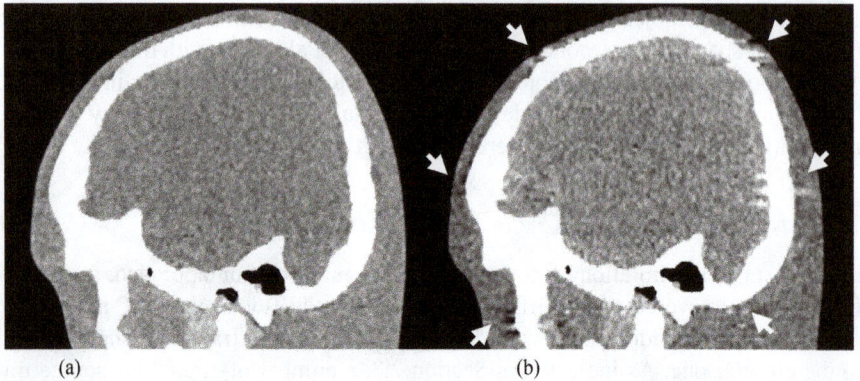

FIGURE 2.10 Sagittal images of an anthropomorphic pediatric head phantom generated by (a) helical scan at 2 cm longitudinal beam aperture and (b) axial scan at 6 cm longitudinal beam aperture.

2.5.2 MDCT SCANNED IN SPIRAL/HELICAL SOURCE TRAJECTORY

As stated in Section 2.3 and illustrated in Figure 2.6a, the spiral/helical scan of MDCT actually meets the Tuy–Smith DSC, as long as the effective spiral/helical pitch is within a reasonable range. The allowable spiral/helical pitch in an MDCT scan is dependent on gantry geometry and detector deployment, and a spiral/helical pitch up to 1.5:1 is routinely employed for diagnostic imaging over clinical applications (Taguchi et al. 2004; Tang et al. 2006, 2008b; Heuscher et al. 2004; Stierstorfer et al. 2004). For example, the sagittal image displayed in Figure 2.10a is a spiral/helical scan in MDCT at 20 mm longitudinal beam aperture and pitch ~0.9:1, while that in Figure 2.10b is an axial scan at 60 mm aperture. The CB artifacts, indicated by the white arrows, exist at the interface of slabs that are equal to the longitudinal beam aperture in length in the sagittal image generated in axial scan, but not in the image by spiral/helical scan, since the latter fulfills the Tuy–Smith DSC.

2.6 DISCUSSION

The race for the number of image slices that can be simultaneously formed in axial MDCT has driven the majority of MDCT vendors to increase the number of detector rows in their flagship MDCT products, which has enormously benefited the healthcare industry and patients in the past two and a half decades. Meanwhile, the image quality of MDCT, in terms of contrast, spatial, temporal and, recently, spectral resolution, has advanced at almost the same pace. Both hardware and software are the keys to enable the translation of MDCT's advancement in technologies into clinical applications. In particular, the hardware-based methods, such as the dual-source–dual-detector MDCT and/or faster MDCT gantry rotation speed for improving the temporal resolution of cardiovascular imaging, and photon-counting

X-ray detection, which is on the horizon, for suppressing electronic noise, spectral weighting (see Chapter 8) and thus improving the contrast resolution, are the pillars for MDCT technologies to advance.

Though the number of detector rows in MDCT continues to increase, the number of detector rows used for spiral/helical scanning in the clinic is usually 64 or 128. This means that the increment in the number of detector rows in MDCT is mainly to benefit the axial scan for coverage of large organs/tissues in one gantry rotation. One underlying reason is that, given the spiral/helical pitch, detector row width and gantry rotation speed (e.g., 1:1, 0.625 mm and 0.5 s/r, respectively), and an X-ray beam aperture larger than 128×0.625 mm (80 mm) may lead to patient table movement at a speed of 160 mm/sec, which may cause unacceptable patient discomfort, especially for those with illness, due to acceleration at the start and deceleration at the end of the scan. Moreover, a patient table proceeding at such a high speed may run ahead of the contrast agent, making chasing the bolus no longer feasible. Still one more consequence of the spiral/helical scan at super high speed in the clinic would be unexpected involuntary visceral motion.

In addition to the aforementioned disadvantages, the spiral/helical scan is intrinsically not apt to deal with the intercycle and/or involuntary motion and resultant inconsistencies in projection data, hindering the diagnoses and/or characterization of pathophysiology that demand multi-cycle, multi-phasic and/or cine scans. Hence, axial MDCT, especially axial MDCT at large cone angles, has become the method of choice for functional imaging under clinical settings, which drives the community to explore solutions to overcome the difficulties associated with cone-angle-induced data insufficiency. Focusing on the CB artifacts in axial MDCT, this chapter reviewed its root cause, rendering mechanism, morphology and possible solutions to suppress CB artifacts. Under the theoretical framework of control systems, the CB artifacts rendered via data insufficiency or data inconsistency in axial MDCT are due to the axial source trajectory's inability of making observation. Fortunately, as we will see in Chapter 4, the CB artifacts due to data insufficiency or data inconsistency can be substantially suppressed by cone-angle-dependent 3D weighting schemes if the cone angle is moderate, or by artifact correction using two-pass CB reconstruction or iterative CB image reconstruction with adequate regularizations if the cone angle is relatively large.

Other artifacts, such as X-ray polychromatism and Compton scattering, may occur in axial MDCT too, and in-depth coverage of them can be found in Chapter 3. The CB artifacts rendered via longitudinal data truncation and insufficient sampling rate are due to the CT detector's measurement incapabilities. In other words, the CB artifacts rendered via longitudinal data truncation and insufficient sampling rate can be removed or substantially reduced if improvements are made in CT detector properties (e.g., using a detector that is wide enough to avoid longitudinal truncation at very fine [i.e., 0.1 mm or better] detector pitch, depending on targeted applications).

It should be noted that the Tuy–Smith DSC is specified under the condition where the 2D detector used for data acquisition is ideal (i.e., its dimension is sufficient to accommodate the entire object to be imaged at a spatial sampling rate that is at least twice the highest spatial frequency possessed by the object, thus fulfilling the requirement imposed by the Nyquist–Shannon theorem). If, however, either the dimension, spatial sampling rate or both is insufficient in practice, additional artifacts arise via data truncation and/or aliasing, respectively. In practice, the truncation can be either latitudinal, longitudinal or both. The artifacts caused by latitudinal truncation and its suppression have been extensively studied and reported in the literature (Ohnesorge et al. 2000a; Hsieh 2004), and thus we constrain our focus to longitudinal truncation in this chapter. Since they would disappear if the X-ray beam in data acquisition is fan-shaped, the additional artifacts caused by longitudinal truncation and insufficient sampling are also counted as CB artifacts. To fully understand CB artifacts' root causes, rendering mechanisms and their correlations, interested readers are referred to publications in the literature (Tang et al. 2018).

Prior to ending this chapter, let's talk a little bit more about the data sufficiency condition. In addition to the Tuy–Smith DSC, a few other versions have been proposed over the years. The earliest credit the work by Kirillov in 1961 (Krillov 1961), which was mathematically oriented and can only be met by an infinitely extended source trajectory. Another important early work was published by Orlov in 1975 (Orlov 1975), in which a parallel beam, rather than a cone beam, is assumed in data acquisition. Smith's version is a modification of Kirillov's and no longer needs to be fulfilled by an infinitely extended source trajectory (Smith 1985). Tuy and Smith pay more attention to the reconstruction of a region of interest (ROI) within an object (Tuy 1983; Smith 1990; Rizo 1991). Grangeat proposed a data sufficiency condition, based on his breakthrough equation between the first-order derivative of X-ray transform and the first-order derivative of 3D Radon transform (Grangeat 1991), which was later refined by Defrise and Clack (1994) and Kudo and Saito (Kudo and Saito 1994b). Thus far, almost all of them are closely associated with a specific CB reconstruction algorithm.

3 Fundamentals in Physics for MDCT

In theory, if the projection data acquired in multi-detector computed tomography (MDCT) meet the data sufficiency condition and the data redundancy is appropriately handled, the formed tomographic images should be accurate or "perfect", since the analytic image reconstruction algorithms are in theory exact (see Chapter 4 for details). However, if the projection data (also called raw data) would be directly used for image reconstruction, the formed images would be far from perfect and useless for any clinical applications. As to be illustrated in this chapter, intrinsic nonlinearity exists in the physical properties of detectors in MDCT, and the inconsistency over millions of detector channels (elements) and their variation over environmental factors may contaminate the projection data, and thus create intensive inaccuracy in formed tomographic images that manifest themselves as severe artifacts. Notably, those environmental factors can be thermal due to variation in the status of ventilation in MDCT's gantry and/or mechanics due to gravity's modulation on the centrifugal force experienced by the source-detector assembly while the gantry is rotating.

The most primary contamination on the raw projection data of MDCT is attributed to the Compton scatter that plays a dual role in both signal generation and interference, leading to severe inaccuracy in the Hounsfield unit (also called CT number) or non-uniformity (cupping or capping artifacts; see Section 3.5.2) in reconstructed tomographic images. Another primary contamination is attributed to the beam-hardening effect that is a consequence of the polychromatism of the X-ray source, leading to streaking and/or shading artifacts. Still another primary contamination is caused by the inter-channel gain inconsistency, especially along the latitudinal direction, leading to strong ring artifacts that may bury all the clinically relevant information. All these artifacts may undermine MDCT's clinical utility as a quantitative modality for diagnostic imaging. Hence, the importance of cleaning the contamination sufficiently from the raw projection data can never be overstated.

Notably, removal of the contamination from the projection data is technically challenging, since the X-ray is far from perfect as a source of signal generation and signal detection, which may be the underlying reason that there so few MDCT vendors in the world. Some of the artifacts may be very strong and stable and thus are relatively easy to address, while others may be really subtle, unstable and accordingly hard to deal with. A full understanding of the root causes and appreciation of the rationales behind the approaches to address these issues need to be grounded on an in-depth understanding of the essential physics of MDCT, its system architecture, imaging chain, and in particular, the mechanisms of signal generation and signal detection, which is the primary purpose of this chapter.

DOI: 10.1201/9780429028465-3

3.1 FUNDAMENTALS OF PHYSICS IN CONVENTIONAL CT

To fully understand and appreciate CT technologies and their latest advances in spectral CT, it is necessary for us to have a concise but deep review of the physics underlying conventional CT.

3.1.1 INTERACTIONS BETWEEN X-RAY PHOTONS AND MATERIALS

In the energy range for diagnostic imaging (15–150 kVp) and above the K-edge, the mass attenuation coefficient of a material can be decomposed as (Alvarez and Macovski 1976; Alvarez and Seppi 1979)

$$\mu(x,y;E) = \alpha(x,y) f_p(E) + \beta(x,y) f_c(E) \tag{3.1}$$

where $\alpha(x,y)$ and $\beta(x,y)$ are characteristic coefficients of the material at location (x, y) (supposed in the 2D coordinate system herein) within an object to be imaged. In fact (Johns and Cunningham 1983),

$$f_p(E) \cong \frac{1}{E^{3.2}} \tag{3.2}$$

characterizes the energy dependency of photoelectric absorption and

$$f_c(E) \cong C_0 \left\{ \frac{1+\gamma}{\gamma^2} \left[\frac{2(1+\gamma)}{1+2\gamma} - \frac{1}{\gamma} \ln(1+2\lambda) \right] + \frac{1}{2\lambda} \ln(1+2\gamma) - \frac{1+3\gamma}{(1+2\gamma)^2} \right\} \tag{3.3}$$

is the Compton scattering's (Klein–Nishina formula) dependency on energy, where $\gamma = E/510.975$ and

$$C_0 = 2\pi \left[\frac{\mu_0 e^2}{4\pi n} \right]^2 = 2\pi r_0 \tag{3.4}$$

Furthermore, $\alpha(x,y)$ and $\beta(x,y)$ have been empirically determined as (Johns and Cunningham 1983)

$$\alpha(x,y) \cong K_1 \frac{\rho}{A} Z^{3.8} \tag{3.5}$$

$$\beta(x,y) \cong K_2 \frac{\rho}{A} Z \tag{3.6}$$

where Z denotes the material's atomic number and A the mass number. Parameter ρ denotes the mass density, and K_1 and K_2 are constants. Note that, given a material, Z/A is virtually a constant and thus $\alpha(x,y)$ is determined by the atomic number, while $\beta(x,y)$ is dominated by its mass density. The profiles plotted in Figure 3.1 illustrates the variation of typical materials in the mass attenuation coefficient over

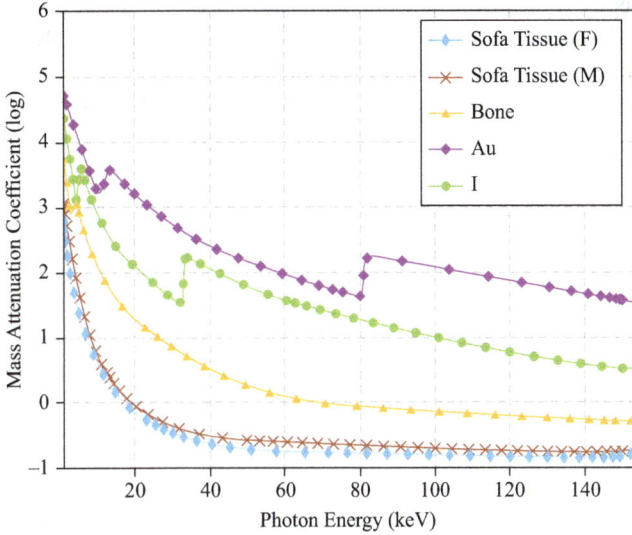

FIGURE 3.1 The mass attenuation coefficients of soft tissue, bone, iodine and gold over the energy range 20–140 keV for diagnostic imaging.

energy up to 150 keV. The X-ray mass attenuation coefficient for all elements and their mixtures can be consulted at NIST's online publication (Hubbell JH and Seltzer SM 2004) or other authoritative data (Woodard and White 1986; Cullen 1997). At a specific energy, the contrast between those materials is determined by the difference in their linear attenuation coefficients that is the product of the mass attenuation coefficient and mass density.

3.1.2 IDEAL CT WITH MONOCHROMATIC X-RAY SOURCE

Suppose $N_0(E)$ and $N(E)$ denote the number of X-ray photons possessing energy E incident on and transmitted through an object with its attenuation characterized by the linear attenuation coefficient $\mu(x, y; E)$, the Beer–Lambert law states that

$$N(E) = N_0(E)e^{-\int_L \mu(x,y;E)dl} \tag{3.7}$$

where (x, y) again denotes the location within the object to be imaged. Tomographic images of an object can be obtained by reconstruction of the attenuation distribution from its projection data acquired via either energy integration or photon counting (see Sections 3.4.1–3.4.3). In the energy-integration mode, an electric current proportional to the total energy carried by the X-ray photons impinging upon a detector element is recorded, while in the photon-counting mode, the electric pulse corresponding to an interaction between X-ray photon and detector material at each element is counted, whereby the height of each pulse is proportional to the energy of each absorbed X-ray photon. A threshold in the pulse height can be set to suppress electronic noise, and a range in the pulse height can endow each detector element with spectral resolution (or termed the *energy bin*).

Regardless of the detection mode, after taking the –log operation

$$I(E) = -\ln\left(N(E)\Big/N_0(E)\right) \tag{3.8}$$

the CT with monochromatic X-ray source, which is the ideal case and thus termed the *ideal CT*, can be conceived as reconstructing the 2D distribution μ $(x, y; E)$ from its projection

$$\int_L \mu(x,y;E)dl = \int_L \left[\alpha(x,y)f_c(E) + \beta(x,y)f_p(E)\right]dl \tag{3.9}$$

where $\int_L \cdot \, dl$ denotes the line integrals along L, a family of lines passing through

(x, y) along all orientations. As long as the data sufficiency condition (Tuy 1983; Smith 1985, 1990) (see Chapter 2, Section 2.2) is met, numerous algorithms can be employed to reconstruct μ $(x, y; E)$, although the filtered back-projection (FBP) algorithms have been preferably adopted in the CT industry because of their efficient data flow in image generation and reservation of spatial resolution that is mainly determined by the pitch of the detector element.

3.1.3 Energy-Integration CT with Polychromatic X-Ray Source

Though the pursuit of the monochromatic X-ray source never stops, no viable technology that can provide sufficient power for diagnostic imaging has been available thus far. Consequently, a polychromatic X-ray source is always used in practice, in which the energy of X-ray photons spreads over a spectrum up to the peak voltage E_{kVp} applied on the anode of the X-ray tube anode. Thus, we have

$$I(E) = \int_0^{E_{kVp}} S_{kVp}(E)e^{-\int_L \mu(x,y;E)dl} D(E)dE \tag{3.10}$$

Fundamentals in Physics for MDCT31

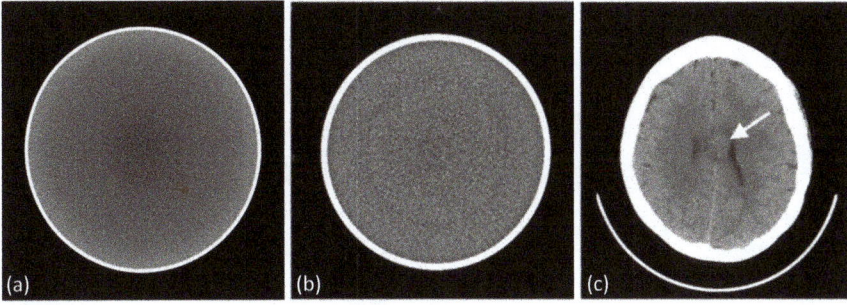

FIGURE 3.2 The artifacts caused by the polychromatism of the X-ray source in MDCT: (a) cupping artifacts in a cylindrical water phantom, (b) spectral artifacts in a cylindrical water phantom, and (c) bone (skull)-induced spectral artifacts in a head scan.

where $\int_0^{E_{kVp}} S_{kVp}(E)[\cdot]dl$ denotes the integration over the energy range $[0\ E_{kVp}]$.

Note that, the non-linearity of $f_c(E)$ and $f_p(E)$ manifests itself as the beam-hardening effect, which may result in streaking and shading artifacts that may interfere with diagnosis in clinics, because all existing image reconstruction algorithms assume Equation 3.9, rather than Equation 3.11. The cupping artifacts in Figure 3.2a and the subtle ring artifacts in Figure 3.2b and Figure 3.2c are examples of the typical spectral artifacts caused by the X-ray beam-hardening effect, which are usually removed in state-of-the-art MDCT via empirical correction algorithms that are proprietary to the vendors.

3.2 MDCT SYSTEM ARCHITECTURE AND IMAGING CHAIN

The 3D effect display of an X-ray CT scan is illustrated in Figure 3.3a, and a schematic of its imaging chain is shown in Figure 3.3b. The MDCT imaging chain comprises seven major components or subsystems: (i) the X-ray source generating the X-ray fluency to penetrate a patient, (ii) an X-ray filtration removing the low-energy X-ray photons that do not contribute to image formation and shaping the beam's intensity to conform to the patient's body contour for radiation dose reduction and noise uniformity, (iii) the post-patient collimator removing the Compton scattering that degrades image contrast and CT number (Hounsfield unit) accuracy, (iv) a scintillator detector array that converts the X-ray photons into light photons, (v) a data acquisition system (DAS) collecting the current generated by diodes and converting it into digital data and transferring it for data storage, (vi) an image reconstruction engine for data pre-processing and generating transverse image slices, and (vii) a computation engine for image presentation, such as coronal and sagittal multi-planar reformatting, maximum intensity projection (MIP), and volume and surface rendering.

(a)

(b)

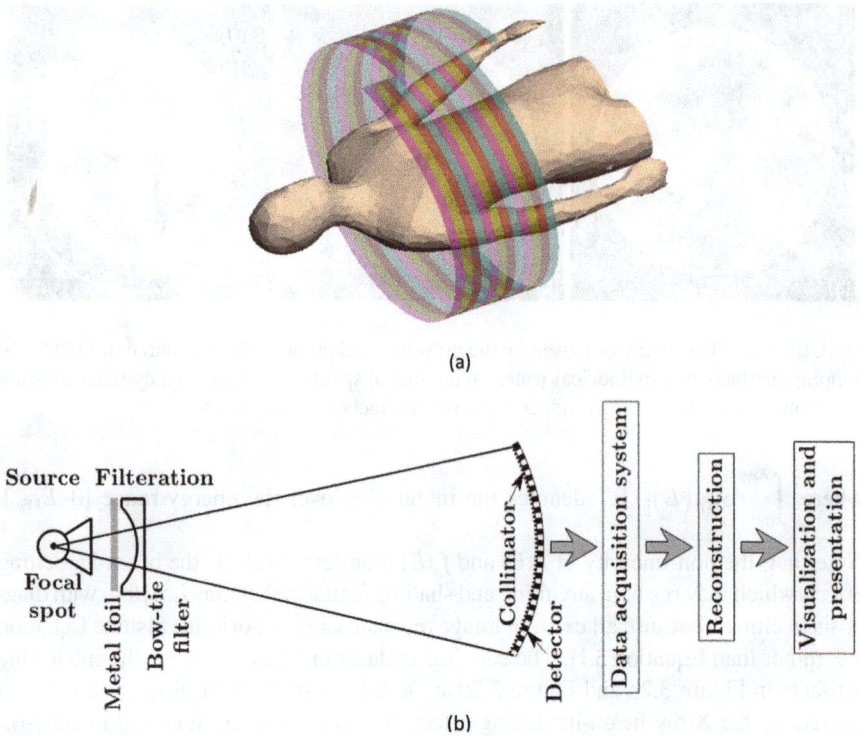

FIGURE 3.3　Diagrams showing (a) the schematic of an MDCT for diagnostic imaging and (b) its imaging chain.

3.3　PRIMARY LOOPS IN MDCT IMAGING CHAIN

Every component in the MDCT imaging chain plays an indispensable role, no matter if it is costly or virtually costless. For example, the X-ray filtration is just a thin layer of aluminum, copper or molybdenum on top of the bowtie filter's graphite substrate, but it is critical to determine the low contrast detectability and dose efficiency of MDCT in diagnostic imaging. Similar to the fact that the strength of a chain is determined by its weakest loop, the overall quality of an MDCT image is subject to the component in the imaging chain with the poorest performance. Thus, an adequate balance and trade-off over the spatial, contrast, temporal and spectral resolutions is the key to reach the best possible image quality that can be achieved in MDCT. What follows is a concise introduction to each of the key components of the MDCT imaging chain.

3.3.1　X-Ray Tube and Spectrum Shaping

Though the pursuit of a monochromatic X-ray source continues, no such viable technology that can provide sufficient intensity for diagnostic imaging in the clinical environment has thus far been available. Displayed in Figure 3.4a is the schematic of the latest X-ray tube technology employed in state-of-the-art MDCT. Differing from the conventional X-ray tube technology in which the tube's envelope is fixed, this novel tube's envelope rotates, which improves the tube's heat capacity substantially and thus avoids bulky metal mass for heat dissipation (Schardt 2004). However, it should be noted that both the conventional and latest X-ray tube work at the bremsstrahlung mechanism behave similarly, as illustrated in Figure 3.4b. In general, the X-ray photons at the low-energy end have no chance to penetrate the human body and thus generate no signal at the X-ray detector but deliver a radiation dose to the patient, especially if the patient's habitus is large. Therefore, thin metal foil made of aluminum, copper or molybdenum, or their combinations, is commonly utilized for spectrum shaping, i.e., removing the photons at the low-energy end from the beam as illustrated in Figure 3.4b, which may benefit a patient in the scanner by avoiding a significant amount of unnecessary radiation dose. Moreover, the removal of low-energy X-ray photons by the metal filtration may mitigate the likelihood of artifacts induced by Compton scattering and/or beam-hardening effect, as they are prone to occur while the X-ray photons are of relatively low energy. Notably, the adequacy in the metal foil's thickness is critical to the trade-off between dose-saving and imaging performance, since an over-hardened X-ray beam may reduce the subject contrast substantially (Huda 2016; Bushberg 2012).

3.3.2 BEAM SHAPING FOR RADIATION EQUALIZATION OVER SCAN FIELD OF VIEW

The beam-forming device in MDCT is utilized to shape the natural intensity distribution of an X-ray tube into one that fits the habitus of a patient to be scanned, in addition to the fact that such a device can also shape the spectrum of the X-ray beam, though to a less significant extent. The two major rationales underlying the adoption of the beam-shaping device are (i) making efficient use of the MDCT detector's

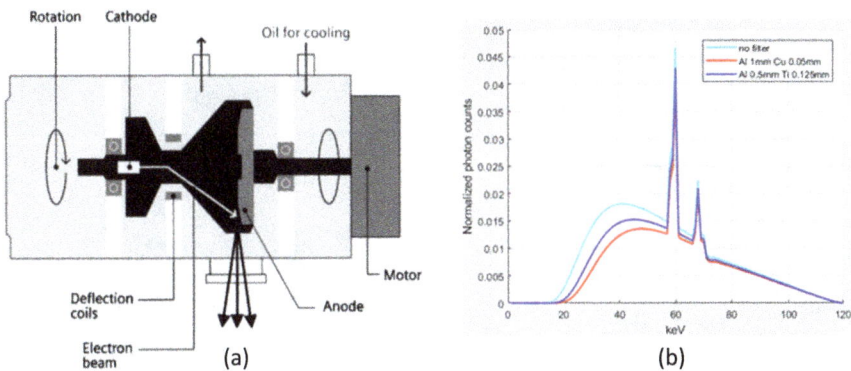

FIGURE 3.4 Schematics showing (a) the structure of an X-ray tube in MDCT and (b) the process of shaping the spectrum via metal foils. (Drawing in panel a is adopted with permission from Schardt 2004).

dynamic range and (ii) balancing the noise distribution across the scan field of view (sFOV). Displayed in Figure 3.5a is a diagram showing the schematic of the beam-forming device (usually called a bowtie in the community) and its geometric relationship with other major components (a detector array and a 20 cm circular water phantom to be scanned), while that in Figure 3.5b is the intensity distribution of the water phantom with and without the bowtie in place. It is unambiguously observed that the dynamic range needed to accommodate the projection data of the phantom has indeed been substantially reduced, as indicated by the solid arrows. Shown in Figure 3.5c is a profile of the water phantom after the –log operation, i.e., the projection in the sonogram. Again, it is clearly seen that the product of the line length and linear attenuation coefficient becomes substantially more uniform while the bowtie is in place than when without the bowtie, and thus the noise distribution in the reconstructed image is anticipated to become uniform (Toth 2007). Note that all the bowtie filters used in currently available MDCT in clinical settings are fixed in shape and hence cannot accommodate the human body habitus optimally over the entire 360° range. Research and development on the dynamic bowtie with its shape altering in data acquisition to fit the human habitus at any angle are being carried out in the field and readers interested in the details are referred to recent reports in the literature (Hsieh and Pelc 2013; Szczykutowicz and Mistretta 2013a, 2013b).

3.3.3 ANTI-SCATTER GRID

The radiation beam gets attenuated and thus generate a signal while the X-ray photons undergo the Compton scattering that alters their original emanating direction.

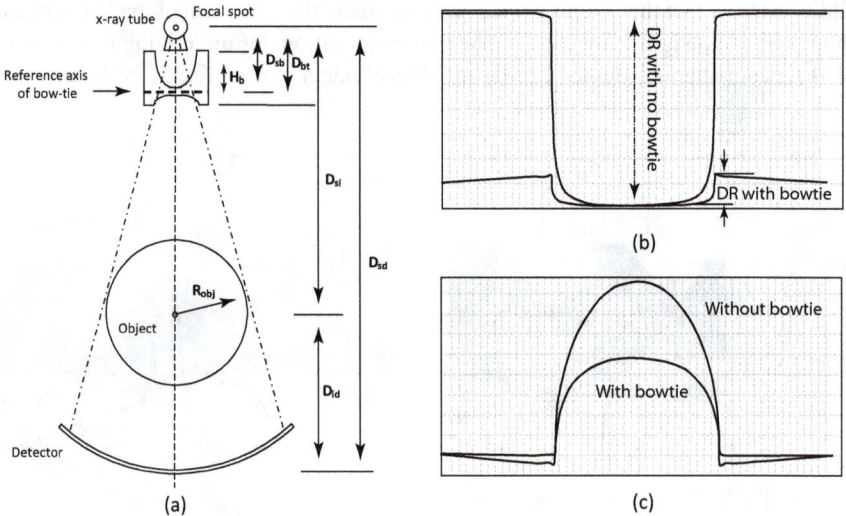

FIGURE 3.5 Schematic diagrams showing (a) the installation of a bowtie in a CT, and the projection of a 20 cm diameter water phantom (b) prior to and (c) post the –log operation (Equation 3.8; DR: dynamic range).

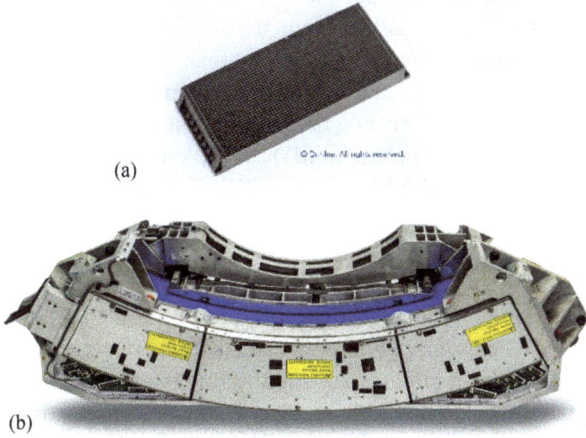

(a)

(b)

FIGURE 3.6   The zoomed view of (a) a 2D anti-scatter grid module that may be installed into (b) the detector assembly of an MDCT. (Pictures are adopted from Dunlee with Permissions).

Simultaneously, on the other hand, the deviated X-ray photons interfere with the detection of signals at neighboring detector channels, which generates shading artifacts that are morphologically similar to that caused by the beam-hardening effect as presented in Section 3.5.2. Usually, the beam-hardening-induced shading artifacts can be mitigated via algorithmic approaches to the extent that meets the requirements imposed by quantitative imaging in the clinic (e.g., Kyriakou et al. 2010). However, if the beam hardening is entangled with the Compton scattering, the task to such a software-based solution becomes much more challenging. Fortunately, using a post-patient anti-scatter grid installed in front of the detector array, the hardware-based approach can readily decouple the problems related to Compton scattering from that caused by beam hardening. In practice, a one-dimensional (1D) anti-scatter grid (ASG) works very well in an MDCT with beam aperture up to 20 mm. If a supplementary algorithmic solution is adopted, the 1D ASG can also work satisfactorily in MDCT with its beam aperture up to 40 mm. Nevertheless, for MDCT with a beam aperture exceeding 40 mm, a 2D ASG (Figure 3.6a) may have to be adopted to make MDCT meet the CT number uniformity specification over the large, e.g., 50 cm, sFOV. In general, a 2D ASG may impose much tougher challenges in terms of patient radiation dose since it attenuates more primary X-ray photons than a 1D ASG while it removes more scattered X-ray photons from the beam. Notably, also, the requirement on the accuracy of the mechanical alignment between the X-ray source and detector assembly (see an example in Figure 3.6b) that encloses a 2D ASG is significantly more stringent than the case in which a 1D ASG is installed.

3.4 DETECTION OF SIGNAL IN MDCT

The X-ray detector used in MDCT for data acquisition works either via energy integration or photon counting. Photon counting has been the most fundamental approach for radiation detection since the discovery of radiation and is the method of choice for data acquisition in nuclear medicine (PET/SPECT). However, the counting rate in CT is much higher (10^2- to 10^3-folds) than that in PET/SPECT, leading to the fact that detection of X-rays in CT has been implemented via energy integration for almost 50 years, until the recent emergence of photon-counting technology that is capable of counting X-ray photons in MDCT while managing the pulse pile-up to an acceptable extent (Ehn 2017; Flohr et al. 2020; Danielsson et al. 2021).

3.4.1 Detection of X-Rays in MDCT: Energy Integration

In the energy-integration mode, light photons proportional to the total energy carried by the X-ray fluency impinging upon a detector element are generated in the scintillator. Then, the light photons are captured by the photodiode and an electric current is generated. Apparently, this mode of X-ray detection is indirect, since the X-ray photons impinging on each detector element are converted into light photons and then electric current (signals). The diagram in Figure 3.7a is the schematic of an indirect detection of X-ray photons in a state-of-the-art energy-integration MDCT, in which the ceramic type GOS (gadolinium oxysulfide: Gd_2O_2S) is the scintillating material. Usually, the scintillating material is of high atomic number and can stop almost all X-ray photons incident on the detector, i.e., ~100% absorption efficiency, though a small fraction of the converted light photons may get lost on their way to the photodiode. The electrons induced by X-ray photons, as well as the dark current and the electronic noise caused by thermal shots, are collected and integrated (indicated by the single output) during signal detection.

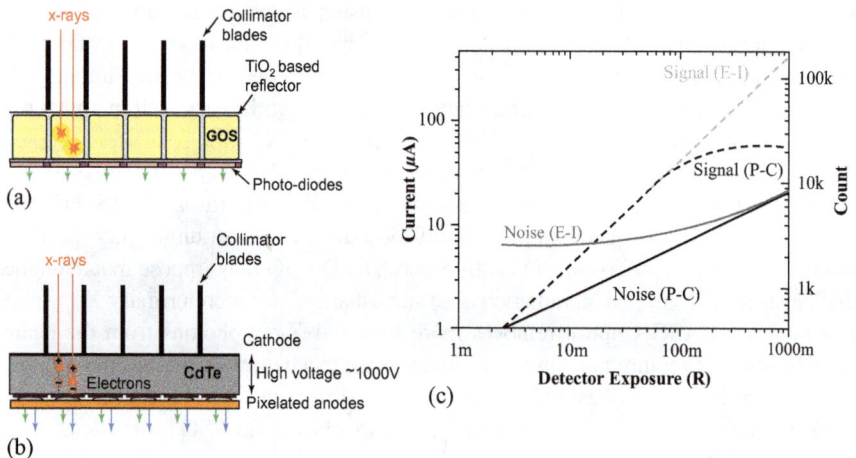

FIGURE 3.7 Schematic illustration of X-ray detection in CT by (a) indirect energy integration with a GOS scintillator and (b) direct photon counting implemented via CdTe, and comparison of their performance in signal and noise detection. (Drawings in (a) and (b) are adopted with permission from Flohr et al. 2020; E-I: energy-integration; P-C: photon-counting).

3.4.2 Detection of X-Rays in MDCT: Photon Counting

In the photon-counting mode, the electric pulse generated by an interaction between an X-ray photon and the detector material at each cell is counted, whereby the pulse height is proportional to the energy deposited by the X-ray photon. Consequently, a threshold and range in the pulse height can be set to not only suppress the electronic noise, but also to endow each detector cell with energy resolution. Figure 3.7b shows the schematic of photon-counting-based X-ray detection, in which the X-ray photons generate hole–electron pairs in the material called CdTe (cadmium telluride), and the electrons are collected by electrodes on which high voltage is applied. Since the X-ray photons are converted to electrons directly, such a signal detection mode is direct, in contrast to the indirect mode discussed earlier. The quantum efficiency of direct detection is intrinsically higher than that of indirect detection since almost no energy carried by the X-ray photons get lost in the former. Moreover, thresholding in pulse height can remove the electronic noise and a series of thresholdings can implement energy binning that offers the opportunity for spectral weighting to improve spectral CT performance, as to be elaborated later in this book (see Chapter 7 and Chapter 8).

3.4.3 Pros and Cons: Photon Counting vs. Energy Integration

A schematic view and comparison of the signal detection property between energy-integration and photon-counting modes is presented in Figure 3.7c, in which the coordinate to the right is "count" (corresponding to photon counting) and that to the left is "current" (corresponding to energy integration). Notably, the noise in photon-counting detection is quantum-dependent and goes down to zero, whereas there is a noise floor in energy-integration detection. In theory, there are four major advantages of the photon-counting detector over the energy-integration detector: (i) intrinsic separation of X-ray source spectra implemented via energy binning, which can substantially improve the performance of spectral CT; (ii) avoidance of electronic noise and Swank sink (Swank 1973), leading to substantially improved imaging performance in situations in which X-ray exposure is extremely low; (iii) matching between the detector's spectral response with the signal's spectral property (mainly determined by photoelectric absorption) via spectral weighting, leading to significantly improved efficiency in X-ray detection; (iv) facilitation of multiple material decomposition, e.g., multi-material decomposition, as elaborated in Section 8.3. Only a brief introduction to the photon-counting detector is given here; in-depth coverage is deferred to Chapters 7 and 8.

As illustrated in Figure 3.7c, the signal in photon counting starts to deviate from the linear mode and becomes damped with increasing X-ray exposure (termed *pulse pile-up* in the nomenclature), whereas virtually no saturation occurs in the energy-integration mode. This used to be the most challenging problem in spectral CT with photon counting for data acquisition, and the underlying reason is the fact that the X-ray photon flux rate in CT ($10^9/mm^2$ s) is roughly three orders higher than that in PET/SPECT ($10^6/mm^2$ s). Recently, due to finer pitch of detector elements and other techniques (Taguchi and Iwanczyk 2013), the risks in image quality associated with pulse pile-up has been mitigated to an extent that is acceptable for clinical imaging (Flohr et al 2020; Danielsson et al 2021).

3.5 COMMON ARTIFACTS DUE TO IMPERFECTIONS IN IMAGING CHAIN

Being the key components of the MDCT imaging chain, neither the X-ray source nor detector is perfect in its properties, leading to numerous artifacts in CT images if the root causes are not found and adequately addressed. Each major MDCT vendor has its own solutions, which are business proprietary, to reduce, if not eliminate, those artifacts. An exhaustion of all possible artifacts and their corresponding solutions are beyond the scope of this chapter. Only the most common artifacts, including their root causes and the principles in addressing them, are concisely covered here.

3.5.1 ARTIFACTS CAUSED BY INTER-CHANNEL GAIN INCONSISTENCE

The most common artifact for a CT designer to deal with is the ring and/or band artifacts due to inter-channel (and inter-module) variation in the detector's gain, as illustrated in Figure 3.8a. It has been well investigated and concluded that even a 0.1%~0.2% inter-channel variation in the gain may cause subtle but visible ring artifacts, and a 0.3% variation definitely induces apparent ring and/or band artifacts. In practice, these ring artifacts can be removed by the process called air calibration, as shown in Figure 3.8b, which is actually a normalization using a flat-field image acquired without any object in the X-ray beam. Notably, the air calibration can be very complicated, since the flat-field image may vary azimuthally while the CT gantry is rotating during the scan.

3.5.2 ARTIFACTS CAUSED BY BEAM HARDENING OF POLYCHROMATIC X-RAYS

Thus far, only polychromatic X-ray sources are available for CT to be viable for routine diagnostic imaging tasks in the clinic. Among all the X-ray photons penetrating an object to be imaged, the ones with lower energy are more likely to be removed from the beam by the object. Thus, if a circular object is placed in an MDCT without a bowtie, the effective energy of X-ray photons in the beam passing the phantom's center is higher than that at the peripheral. In other words, the material, water in this case, at the center of the phantom is effectively less attenuating that those at the peripheral. Hence, the CT number at the center of the water phantom should be lower than that at the peripheral, i.e., shading (cupping) artifact occurs. However, if a bowtie is in placement (see Figure 3.5a), the shading (cupping) artifact becomes glaring (capping) artifact, as illustrated in Figure 3.8b. Measures based on data fitting have been developed to effectively eliminate the glaring (capping) artifacts caused by beam hardening in an MDCT, as demonstrated in Figure 3.8c.

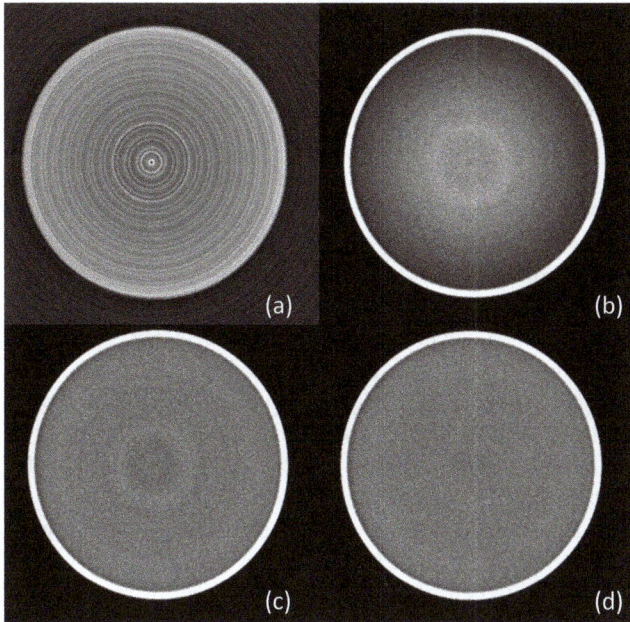

FIGURE 3.8   Artifacts in the CT image of a water phantom caused by (a) the detector's inter-cell gain variation, (b) beam hardening, (c) the detector's inter-cell spectral response variation, and (d) their removal.

3.5.3 ARTIFACTS CAUSED BY INTER-CHANNEL INCONSISTENCE IN DETECTOR'S SPECTRAL RESPONSE

Even after the ring and glaring/capping artifacts have been removed, an MDCT image may still be left with residual and subtle ring/band artifacts, especially in the central area, as shown in Figure 3.8c. The root cause behind this phenomenon, which is the most challenging issue for an MDCT designer to deliver image quality acceptable for diagnostic imaging in the clinic, is the inter-cell variation in the MDCT detector's spectral response to incident X-ray photons. It should be noted that, even though the X-ray photons emanating from the source possess identical spectra, each X-ray photon travels different routes and thus, unfortunately, has varying energy, which leads to subtle and variable ring/band artifacts, as illustrated in Figure 3.8c, because of the variation in the detector cells' spectral response. Empirical measures can be utilized to remove those subtle artifacts or reduce them to an invisible extent, as demonstrated in Figure 3.8d.

3.6 DISCUSSION

CT is a large and complicated imaging system, and its design and development demands extensive expertise and experience in physics, electrical engineering, electromechanical engineering, electronics and computer engineering. A concise introduction on the essential physics of MDCT – including generation of subject contrast, detection of X-rays via energy integration or photon counting, and the concept of ideal monochromatic CT and realistic polychromatic CT – is provided in this chapter. The chapter reviews CT system architecture, imaging chain and data acquisition schemes, followed by coverage on the major loops of the CT imaging chain. Also shown are the common artifacts in CT induced by the imperfections in X-ray sources such as the beam-hardening effect due to X-ray polychromatism and that in the imaging chain such as the inter-channel inconsistence in the detector's spectral response. In state-of-the-art MDCT with 256 detector rows, there may be 256,000 ($1000 \times 256 = 256{,}000$) detector elements, if each detector row comprises roughly 1000 detector elements, which may lead to many imperfections in the MDCT imaging chain, as so many detector elements are assembled together and rotating with the gantry at a relatively high speed of 5 rotation/sec.

In practice, these imperfections and resultant artifacts have to be dealt with case by case, e.g., being specific to each individual peak voltage (kVp) of the X-ray tube used in MDCT. Due to space limitations, comprehensive coverage on each of them is beyond the scope of this book. Prior to turning our attention to image formation in MDCT in the next two chapters, following is a brief list of imperfections in the MDCT imaging chain that may degrade imaging performance or cause artifacts in tomographic images.

- **Off-focal spot radiation in X-ray tube**: Ideally, X-ray photons emanating from an X-ray tube in MDCT should only come from the focal spot, with its dimension depending on the settings of the tube current. In reality, however, off-focal spot radiation commonly exists in MDCT, though suppression techniques are in place, which may lead to strong artifacts at the interface between two areas of abrupt variation in attenuation, e.g., the wall of a 20 cm water phantom against the air.
- **Variation in the location of the X-ray tube focal spot**: Ideally, the focal spot of an X-ray tube should stay at a fixed location, but, unfortunately, the anode's shape alters as a function of the anode's temperature, especially in the case of MDCT in which the X-ray tube is of high power and thus the variation in temperature can be wide. Owing to the 1D or 2D ASG, especially the latter, installed in front of the detector array, such a temperature-induced variation in the focal spot's location may worsen the artifacts that are usually manifested as subtle arc artifacts or central smudge, due to the drifted inter-channel inconsistence in the detector's gain and spectral response over the hundreds of thousands of detector elements.
- **Mechanical displacement associated with gantry rotation**: Ideally, there should exist no mechanical displacement, called "sagging" in the CT industry, while the tube-and-detector assembly, including the 1D or 2D ASG, is rotating along with the CT gantry at a relatively high speed. However, in reality, the mechanical integrity of the tube-and-detector assembly may be compromised due to faults in the assembly's installation and/or weighting

balance, which may lead to subtle artifacts manifested as thick and/or thin arcs in tomographic images.

- **Latitudinal inter-modular inconsistence in the X-ray detector**: In MDCT, the hundreds of thousands of detector elements are fabricated in modules, e.g., 16×16, 32×16 or 64×16 dimensions, and those modules are assembled together into a 2D cylindrical detector array. In addition to the previously mentioned inter-channel inconsistence, there may exist inter-modular inconsistence in the detector elements' gain, spectral response or cross-talking. The inconsistence occurring along the latitudinal direction may incur strong or subtle spoke-like artifacts in tomographic images at the interface between two areas of abrupt variation in attenuation, e.g., the lateral edges of the liver in the abdominal cavity.

- **Inter-modular misalignment in the X-ray detector**: Inter-modular misalignment may be one-dimensional along the longitudinal direction only or three-dimensional if each module does not focus at the X-ray tube's focal spot. If the misalignment occurs in the longitudinal direction only, thick ring or bright smudge artifacts may occur at the location where steep variation in X-ray attenuation occurs along the longitudinal direction. More and subtle artifacts may appear if the inter-modular misalignment in the 2D X-ray detector in MDCT is three-dimensional.

4 Image Formation via Analytic Reconstruction Algorithms

The image reconstruction for image formation plays a central role in X-ray computed tomography (CT) (Kak and Slaney 1988). As indicated in Chapter 3, Section 3.1.2, the algorithms in the fashion of filtered back-projection (FBP) have been preferably adopted by all major CT vendors, mainly because of its efficiency in data flow and capability of getting the first tomographic image as fast as possible. It also should be noted that the algorithms in the fashion of FBP may reach the most achievable spatial resolution, since it makes use of interpolation, which may degrade the spatial resolution in reconstructed images, as little as possible. Starting from the most fundamental image reconstruction solutions for image formation in single-detector row CT, we go over 4-detector, 16-detector, 64-detector and beyond, and provide a concise introductory description of the typical FBP reconstruction solutions used in multi-detector CT for diagnostic imaging over clinical applications.

4.1 IMAGE RECONSTRUCTION SOLUTIONS IN SINGLE-DETECTOR CT

4.1.1 AXIAL SCAN

The classic FBP algorithm for image reconstruction starts at the parallel beam geometry and can be expressed as (Kak and Slaney 1988; Buzug 2008)

$$f(x,y) = \int\limits_{0}^{\pi} \int\limits_{-\infty}^{\infty} F(\omega, \gamma) e^{2\pi j \omega (x \cos(\gamma) + y \sin(\gamma))} |\omega| \, d\omega \, d\gamma \qquad (4.1)$$

In reality, however, the third-generation geometry for data acquisition is the fan beam, as shown in Figure 4.1a (also see Chapter 1, Figure 1.1c and Figure 1.3a). Hence, the projection data in the fan beam have to be converted into the parallel beam via fan-to-parallel rebinning for image reconstruction, even though the spatial resolution may be slightly compromised due to the interpolation that is an indispensable step in fan-to-parallel rebinning. Later on, the FBP algorithm for image reconstruction directly from the data in fan-beam geometry is derived, making image reconstruction much more efficient, while the spatial resolution reaches its highest potential. It is interesting to note that, around the year 2000, almost all major CT vendors turned

DOI: 10.1201/9780429028465-4

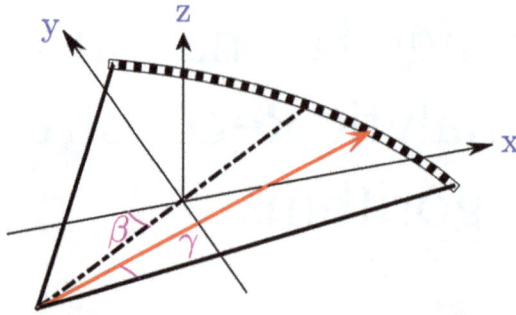

FIGURE 4.1   Schematic showing fan-beam geometry for data acquisition and image reconstruction in single-detector CT.

back to the FBP algorithm in parallel beam geometry for image reconstruction at the expense of slightly degraded in-plane spatial resolution (Besson 1998), in which the scheme of fan-to-parallel rebinning was reused, mainly for removing the so-called zebra artifacts caused by the distance-dependent weighting on the noise in the multi-planner reformatted (MPR) view of MDCT images.

4.1.2 SPIRAL/HELICAL SCAN

A brief review of image reconstruction in the spiral/helical single-detector (SDCT) would be beneficial to understand the spiral/helical image reconstruction algorithms employed in MDCT. In a spiral/helical SDCT scan, the artifact is mainly owing to the data inconsistency caused by movement of the patient table, because, given an image at a specified location, image projection can only be recorded with full fidelity by the 1D detector array when the spiral/helical source trajectory exactly intercepts the plane at which the image slice (namely, mid-way) locates. At any other angular location the image slice does not intercept the source trajectory, and thus, interpolation, either in the 180° or 360° fashion, has to be carried out to obtain the needed projection (Kalender et al. 1989, 1990; Crawford and King 1990). In geometry, this is to obtain the desired projection via view-wise (360°; Figure 4.2a) or ray-wise (180°; Figure 4.2b) interpolation of two corresponding projections based on their longitudinal distance. Apparently, only the projection at the mid-way is identical to or consistent with the true projection of the image slice, but all other projections obtained by interpolation are just approximations. Such inconsistency causes inaccuracies in reconstructed images, which is the underlying reason why spiral/helical artifacts have been termed *inconsistency artifacts* (Larson 1998; Kachelrieβ 2000; Bruder 2000; Heuscher 2002; Tang 2003). Note that the slice sensitivity profile (SSP) of an SDCT is dependent on the interpolation method that is used. In addition, the SSP is also dependent on the spiral/helical pitch that is usually defined as the ratio of the distance proceeded by the patient table within one spiral/helical turn over the beam aperture of the X-ray detector along the craniocaudal direction.

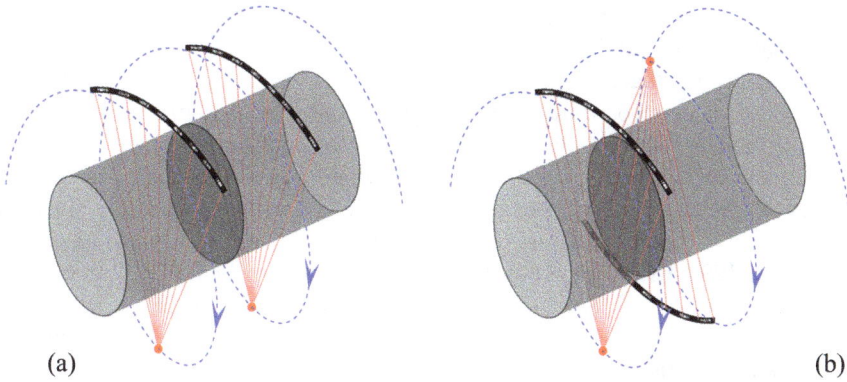

FIGURE 4.2 Schematic diagrams showing the (a) view-wise (360°) and (b) ray-wise (180°) interpolation algorithms used in an SDCT to synthesize the projection data for image reconstruction.

4.2 IMAGE RECONSTRUCTION SOLUTIONS IN FOUR-DETECTOR CT

4.2.1 AXIAL SCAN

The geometry for image reconstruction in a four-detector CT scanner is assumed as 2D or fan beam, though the scan is in fact carried out in 3D or cone beam (CB) (Figure 1.3b). In an axial scan, the mismatch between the data acquisition and image reconstruction geometries may result in inaccuracies in the reconstructed images. However, corresponding to the typical 20 mm longitudinal beam aperture in four-detector CT scanners in 5 mm × 4 or 10 mm × 2 mode, the cone angle of the outmost image slice is $\frac{1}{2}\alpha_m = {\sim}0.79°$ or $\frac{1}{2}\alpha_m = {\sim}0.53°$, respectively, which is quite small. The resultant inaccuracy (artifacts) in reconstructed images is almost undetectable when the cone beam at such a small cone angle is assumed as four fan beams stacked parallel to each other along the longitudinal direction. This means that each image slice in the four-detector CT scanner in axial scan mode is treated exactly the same as that in SDCT. Moreover, note that the back-projector used by all the major CT vendors in four-detector CT for image reconstruction is 1D, i.e., in fan beam, exactly the same as those used in SDCT (Tang et al. 2018).

4.2.2 SPIRAL/HELICAL SCAN

In the spiral/helical MDCT scan, we are no longer bothered by the data inconsistency problem, since, in principle, the wider longitudinal dimension of the 2D detector array keeps intercepting the X-ray flux that has penetrated the image slice at the mid-way position, i.e., recording the projection, as long as the orthogonal distance between the X-ray focal spot to the image slice at the mid-way position is within a reasonable range. Thus, resorting to adequate ray tracking and view weighting techniques, the projection data over the angular positions of the image slice at a specified position can be obtained via cross-detector row interpolation (Hu 1998; Taguchi and Aradate 1998) that is totally different from that in the spiral/helical SDCT. This can be better understood if the reader imagines that the interpolation in MDCT can be eliminated if the longitudinal sampling rate of the multi-row detector is sufficient and the detector is aligned perfectly to record the projection at each angular position, whereas the interpolation in the spiral/helical SDCT is always necessary. Since the interpolation is conducted across detector rows, rather than across views (Kalender et al. 1989, 1990; Crawford and King 1990) in the spiral/helical SDCT, the SSP of an MDCT in principle is just slightly dependent on the spiral/helical pitch. Once the projection data are obtained, the ramp filtering and 1D back-projection are employed to generate tomographic images.

The most remarkable benefit brought about by the four-detector MDCT to clinics is the speeding of scan (Rydberg 2000). In the step-and-shoot axial scan mode of four-detector CT, it is intuitive to understand that each step of patient table proceeding is equal to four times that of an SDCT. Figure 4.3a shows the case of spiral/helical SDCT scan at pitch 1:1. If the scan speed needs to be increased by a factor of four, the SDCT may increase either the pitch or slice thickness by four times (see Figure 4.3b and 4.3c), which results in a substantial inter-helix gap or degradation in the longitudinal spatial resolution, respectively. Note that a spiral/helical scan at a pitch larger than 1:1 does exist in practice, but a pitch as large as 4:1 definitely rules out the possibility of image reconstruction at high quality. However, if there

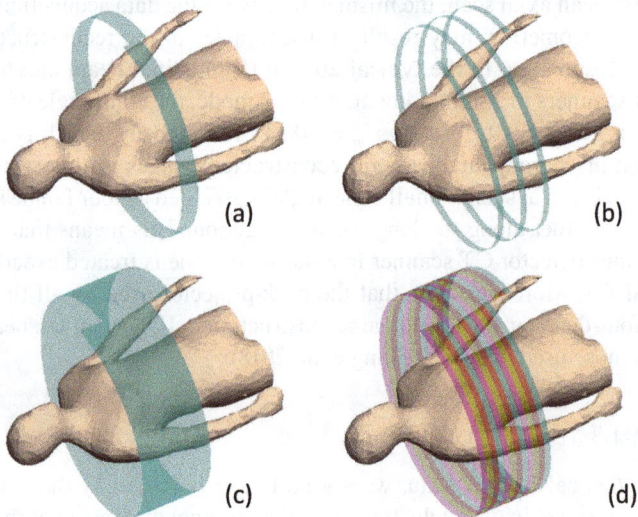

FIGURE 4.3 Schematic diagrams showing the scanning of (a) SDCT at helical pitch 1:1, (b) SDCT at helical pitch 4:1, (c) SDCT at helical pitch 1:1 but four times thicker image and (c) four-detector MDCT at helical pitch 1:1.

are four-detector rows in the scanner, a spiral/helical scan at pitch 1:1 can scan the patient four times faster without an inter-helix gap while thin slices can be maintained (Figure 4.3d). In general, with recourse to the multi-detector row technology, the upper limit of spiral/helical pitch is approximately up to 1.5:1, depending on the gantry geometry and field of view (FOV) of the scan and image reconstruction (Kachelrieβ 2000; Bruder 2000; Heuscher 2002; Tang 2003). Notably, an increase in the pitch of the spiral/helical scan reduces the radiation dose to the patient proportionally, while the noise index in the CT image deteriorates in a manner that is inversely proportional to the square root of the increment in pitch.

4.3 IMAGE RECONSTRUCTION SOLUTIONS IN 16-DETECTOR MDCT

4.3.1 AXIAL SCAN

Although other numbers of detector rows, such as 8, 10 or 12, exist in MDCT, every major CT vendor positioned its 16-detector MDCT scanner as the flagship product in the early 2000s. Despite the number of detector rows increasing fourfold, the typical longitudinal beam aperture is still 20 mm in a 16-detector MDCT, which can be implemented via adequate combination in 1.25 mm × 16, 2.5 mm × 8, 5 mm × 4 and 10 mm × 2. The maximum half cone angle corresponding to the outmost slice in 1.25 × 16 mm mode is $\frac{1}{2}\alpha_m \cong 0.99°$, while that of the outmost slice in 5 mm × 4 mode in a four-detector MDCT scanner is $\frac{1}{2}\alpha_m \cong 0.79°$. Obviously, the maximum full cone angle in 16-detector MDCT is approximately the same as that of 4-detector MDCT. Consequently, the geometry of stacked fan beams is still assumed for image reconstruction in the axial scan of 16-detector MDCT (Tang et al. 2018).

4.3.2 SPIRAL/HELICAL SCAN

The leap from 4 to 16 detector rows has provided the opportunity to implement image reconstruction in 3D geometry wherein a 2D detector is utilized. However, rather than taking this opportunity, the image reconstruction solution developers of almost all the major CT vendors constrained themselves to what they had done in single-detector CT or four-detector MDCT: converting the 3D geometry into 2D geometry wherein the 1D back-projector could still be utilized. The main reason behind this choice is for cost savings, since the 1D back-projector implemented with a specially designed array processor is still fast enough to fulfill the requirements of image-generation speed. This constraint makes the spiral/helical image reconstruction in 16-detector MDCT extremely difficult.

Presented in Figure 4.4a′ are the projections of an orthogonal disc with its height equal to that of a detector row (Figure 4.4a) when the X-ray source focal spot is at view angle $\beta = -90°, -45°, 0°, 45°$ and $90°$. It is observed that, except at the mid-way position ($\beta = 0°$), the projection of a thin disc occupies a variable number of detector rows in the multi-row detector. The larger the magnitude of the viewing angle, the

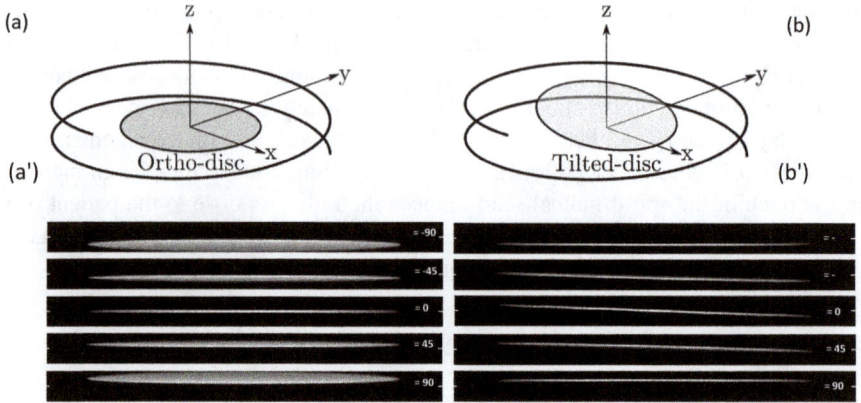

FIGURE 4.4 The scan geometry in MDCT with a disc (a) orthogonal and (b) tilted to its rotation axis, and the projection at view angle β = –90°, –45°, 0°, 45° and 90° of the (a') orthogonal and (b') tilted discs.

greater the number of detector rows that are intercepted by projection of the thin disc. It is not hard to imagine that, if a 1D back-projector is used, all the projection data must fit into one detector row. Consequently, data loss occurs with increasing view angle β. On the other hand, if the thin disc is tilted to conform to the spiral/ helical source trajectory as illustrated in Figure 4.4b, its projection at various angular positions (Figure 4.4b') can fit into an oblique 1D detector. Then, the loss of projection data can be substantially mitigated in comparison to the case of the orthogonal thin disc (Larson 1998; Kachelrieß 2000; Bruder 2000; Heuscher 2002; Tang 2003). In reality, no oblique 1D detector is needed, because the projection of the tilted thin disc can be obtained via cross-row interpolation. As such, the tilted thin disc can be well reconstructed using a 1D back-projector, and the entire 3D Cartesian coordinate system can be covered by nutating tilted thin discs. Any image corresponding to the orthogonal thin disc in the Cartesian coordinate system can be readily obtained via 1D interpolation along the z-axis.

An inspection of the images in Figure 4.5a and Figure 4.5b shows that the image reconstruction via a nutation of tilted thin discs outperforms the one with orthogonal thin discs in reducing the artifacts caused by the spiral/helical inconsistency. However, three undesirable side effects can be attributed to the nutation of tilted thin discs: (i) the spatial sampling by tilted thin discs is not uniform, (ii) the 1D interpolation along the z-axis may slightly broaden SSP, and (iii) a larger beam over-range at the starting and finishing ends of the spiral/helical scan (Tzedakis 2005; Molen and Geleijns 2006) compared to that without tilting the thin disc, given an identical imaging zone.

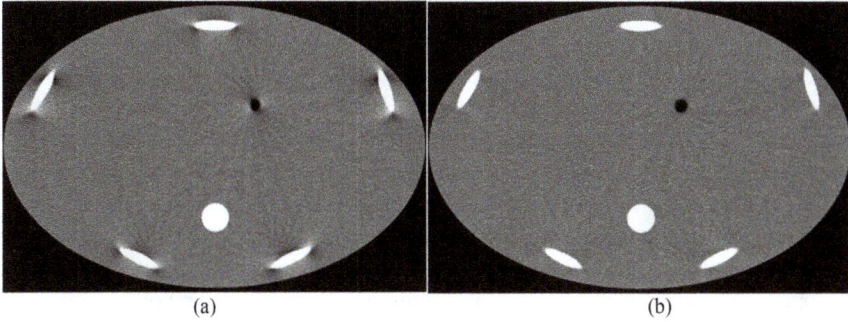

(a) (b)

FIGURE 4.5 Transverse images of the helical body phantom reconstructed from simulated projection data in a 16-detector CT at the spiral/helical pitch 25/16:1 = 1.5265:1, using (a) an orthogonal image slice with view weighting and (b) tilted image slice without view weighting.

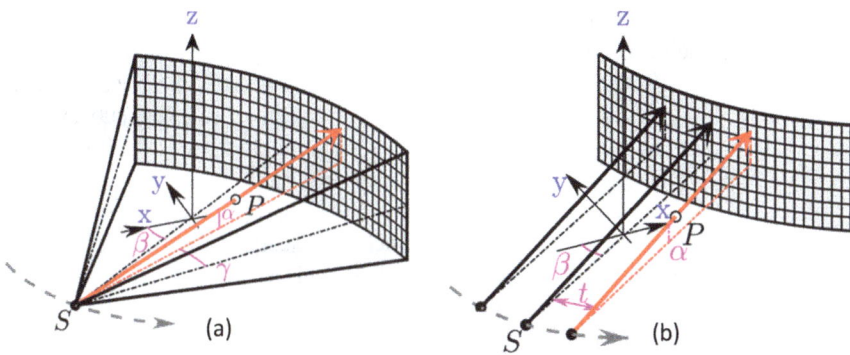

FIGURE 4.6 The schematic diagram showing (a) the native cone-beam geometry and (b) the cone parallel geometry obtained from the native cone beam geometry via row wise fan to-parallel rebinning.

4.4 IMAGE RECONSTRUCTION SOLUTIONS IN 64-DETECTOR MDCT

4.4.1 AXIAL SCAN

In a 64-detector MDCT, the half cone angle $\frac{1}{2}\alpha_m$ typically becomes larger than 2°. Then, no matter how the projection data is cleverly manipulated, there is no choice but to use a 2D detector and 3D cone-beam geometry for image reconstruction (Figure 4.6a), and thus there is no geometric mismatch between image reconstruction and data acquisition (Tang et al. 2005, 2006). In order to have uniform noise distribution in reconstructed images, the image reconstruction needs to be carried out in the so-called cone-parallel geometry (Figure 4.6b) that is obtained from the native CB geometry via row-wise fan-to-parallel rebinning. As we know, the root cause of CB artifacts is violation of the data sufficiency condition in the Radon space, as covered in Chapter 2. However, this problem may be studied equivalently in a straightforward manner in the spatial domain.

In a full axial scan, the data redundancy of the vast majority of voxels in the volume to be reconstructed is one or two, and a redundancy of one is sufficient for image reconstruction. Assuming 250 mm FOV, shown in Figure 4.7 is the redundancy in the three outmost image slices in 64-detetor MDCT. Almost all the voxels in the third outmost image slice are of data redundancy two and thus can be reconstructed appropriately. Actually, as observed in Figure 4.7a, almost all the voxels in the outmost image slice are of data redundancy larger than one, while those in the central region are of redundancy two. This means that, in the 64 image slices corresponding to each detector row, all image slices, including the outmost slices at the upper and lower ends, have sufficient projection data, though the projection data suffer from the cone-angle-induced contamination, for reconstruction of an image at 250 mm FOV, as long as the data redundancy is adequately handled (Tang et al 2005, 2006).

The preceding reasoning can continue by taking a sagittal view of the axial data acquisition geometry as illustrated in Figure 4.8a, whereby 64 slices of images are to be reconstructed from the data acquired in a 64-detector MDCT. Due to the cone angle, the image zone corresponding to a data redundancy of two gets substantially indented to be just roughly 55% of the detector's longitudinal dimension, if the original Feldkamp–Davis–Kress (FDK) reconstruction algorithm (Feldkamp et al 1984) is utilized. Using an anthropomorphic humanoid head phantom, the images displayed in Figure 4.9 are examples to illustrate the efficacy of adequate handling of the data redundancy and data inconsistency (see details later). It is a common practice in image formation (or 3D back-projection) to use heuristic data extensions for handling of data redundancy, which can be either a replication of the data acquired at the outmost detector row, or an average of the data at the outmost and second outmost detector rows. In general, such a heuristic approach may work well at the boundary where no abrupt variation exists, as demonstrated in the case of Figure 4.9a and Figure 4.9a′,

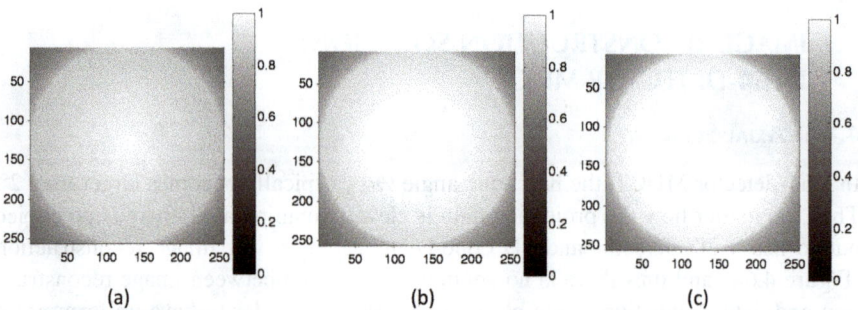

FIGURE 4.7 The counting of data redundancy in the (a) outmost, (b) second outmost and (c) third outmost image slices in the axial scan of a 64-detector MDCT (detector dimension: 64×0.625 mm; SID: 541 mm; FOV: 250 mm).

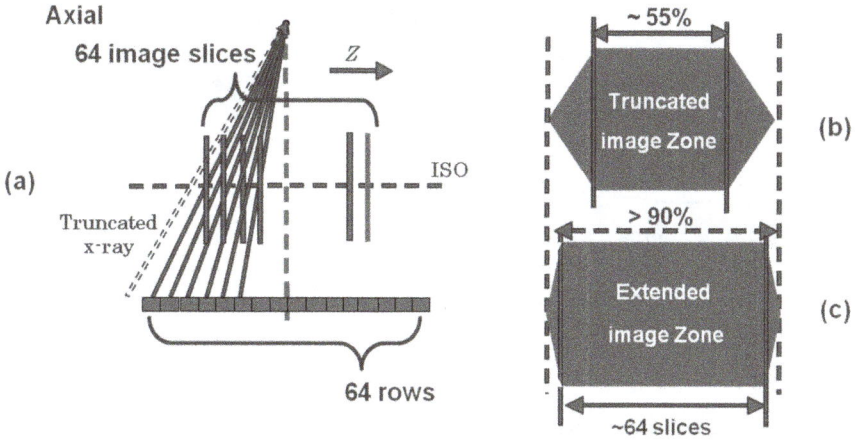

FIGURE 4.8 Schematic diagrams showing (a) data acquisition in the axial scan, (b) the indented image zone due to cone angle and (c) the extension of the image zone by cone-angle-dependent weighting.

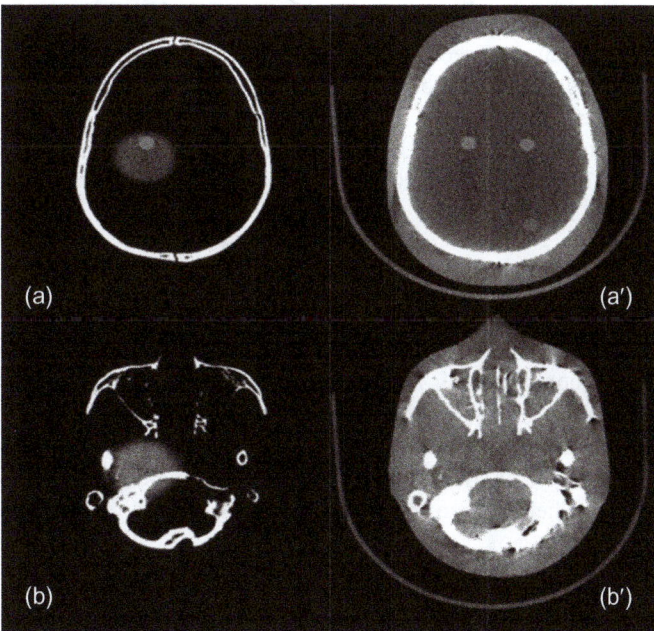

FIGURE 4.9 Transaxial images of anthropomorphic head phantom reconstructed at the outmost slice (cone angle 2.08°) in a 64-detector MDCT (64 × 0.625 mm) by the 3D weighted CB–FBP algorithm (Tang et al. 2005) (a and b) without and (a′ and b′) with redundancy handling (DW/DL: 200/75).

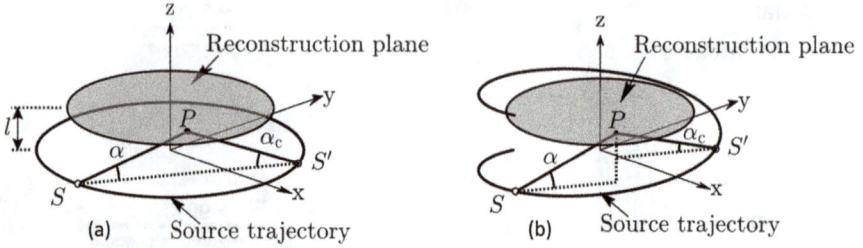

FIGURE 4.10 Schematic diagram showing the rationale of cone-angle-dependent weighting to deal with the data redundancy in an (a) axial and (b) spiral/helical scan.

but there is no guarantee if the structures to be reconstructed vary abruptly around the outer detector rows, as shown in the case presented in Figure 4.9b and Figure 4.9b′.

An approach to handle the data inconsistency is shown in Figure 4.10a. Given a voxel P with data redundancy two, there exists a pair of conjugate rays SP and $S'P$ that may contribute to image formation. Intuitively, the contribution from the ray with a smaller cone angle, e.g., ray SP with cone angle α , should be more accurate (Tang et al. 2005, 2008b; Taguchi et al 2004) than that with a larger cone angle, e.g., ray $S'P$ with cone angle α', for image formation. Hence, a cone-angle-dependent weighting scheme can be used to suppress the artifacts due to data inconsistency. Figure 4.11 shows performance of the cone-angle-dependent weighting scheme (termed as 3D weighted CB-FBP algorithm in the literature), whereby the artifacts in the head phantom (a and a′) and humanoid thoracic phantom (b and b′) are significantly reduced (Tang et al. 2005, 2006).

4.4.2 SPIRAL/HELICAL SCAN

As shown in Figure 4.10b, the cone-angle-dependent weighting scheme can also be employed in a spiral/helical scan, whereby the calculation of the cone angle corresponding to each conjugate pair is a little bit more complicated, because movement of the patient table during a scan has to be taken into account (Taguchi et al. 2004; Tang et al. 2006; Tang and Hsieh 2007; Heuscher 2002; Stierstorfer 2004). Presented in Figure 4.12 are typical clinical images in which the superior image quality provided by the spiral/helical scan in 64-detector row CT for clinical applications can be appreciated.

4.5 IMAGE RECONSTRUCTION BEYOND 64-DETECTOR MDCT

4.5.1 AXIAL SCAN

Inspection of images reconstructed by the FDK algorithm (the Defrise phantom in Chapter 2, Figure 2.8) shows that CB artifacts manifest as shading/glaring and/or streak artifacts surrounding structures of extremely high or low attenuation compared

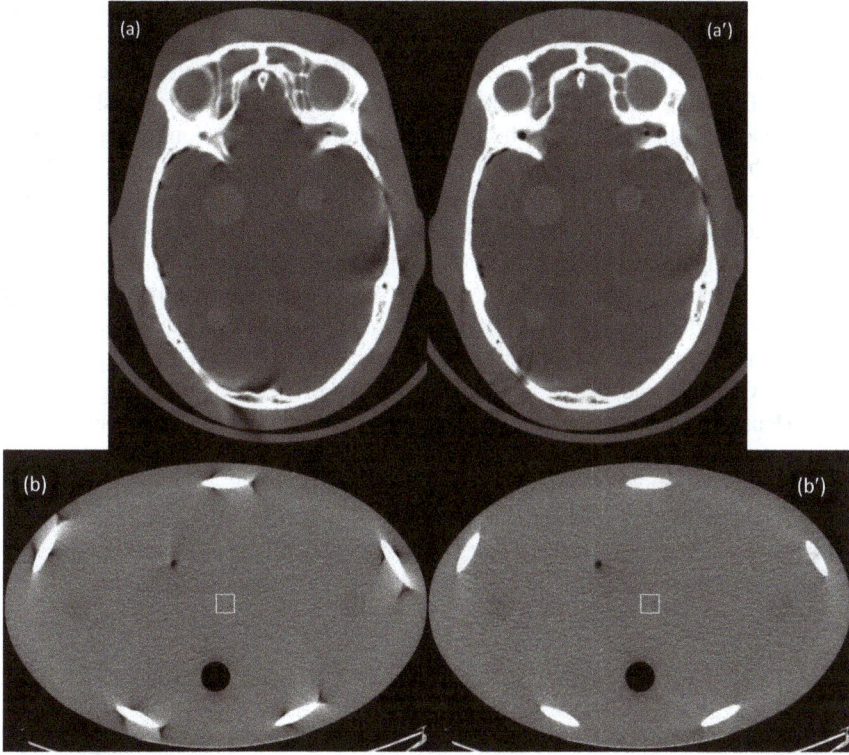

FIGURE 4.11 Images of the head phantom reconstructed by the FDK algorithm (a) without and (a′) with the cone-angle-dependent weighting, and (b and b′) corresponding images of humanoid thoracic phantom.

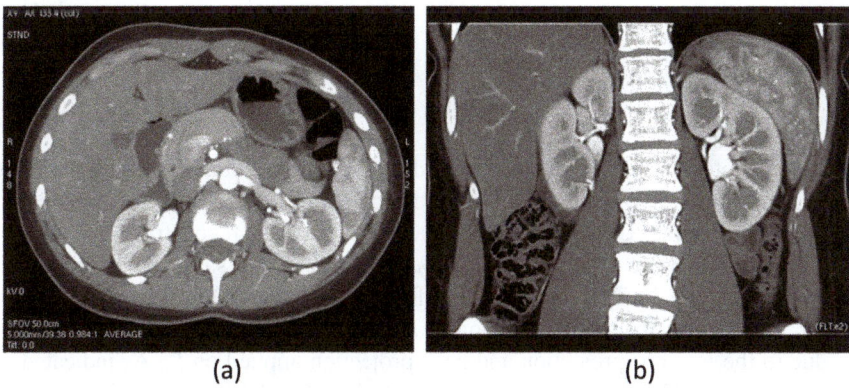

FIGURE 4.12 Typical transverse images (a) reconstructed from the projection data of a 64-detector spiral/helical MDCT scan using cone-angle-dependent weighting and (b) the coronal view of a multi-planner reformatted image.

to soft tissues (e.g., bony structures or airy cavities). Notably, those shading/glaring and/or streaking artifacts can be suppressed or eliminated if the aforementioned 3D weighted CB-FBP algorithm (Tang et al. 2005, 2006) is reformatted into 3D weighted CB-BPF/DBPF (Tang and Tang 2016). Further inspection shows they are morphologically similar to the beam-hardening artifacts commonly observed between the petrous bones in MDCT/CBCT images of the head (Joseph and Spital 1978; Joseph and Ruth 1997; Hsieh 2000a; Kyriakou 2010). Intuitively, the iterative bone operation (IBO), which is popularly used in MDCT for suppression of artifacts caused by X-ray spectral polychromatism (i.e., beam hardening), should be useful to suppress CB artifacts. It turns out that this is indeed the case with the two-pass CB reconstruction algorithm (Hsieh 2000b; Forthmann et al. 2009). As its name implies, the two-pass algorithm comprises the first pass that is FDK (Feldkamp 1984) or any other CB–FBP reconstruction algorithm (Tang et al. 2005, 2006; Taguchi et al. 2004; Heuscher 2002; Stierstorfer et al. 2004), and the second pass goes through forward-projection and back-projection after the structures at extremely high and/or low attenuation are adequately segmented from soft tissues.

In principle, the two-pass reconstruction is a type of FBP. Supposing the first-pass FDK-reconstructed image as f and the segmented (modified) one as f_m, the algorithmic steps in the second pass can be (Hsieh 2000b; Forthmann et al. 2009)

$$f_m = S(f) \tag{4.2}$$

$$g_m = P(f_m) \tag{4.3}$$

$$f'_m = B(g_m) \tag{4.4}$$

$$f_a = f'_m - F_1(f_m) \tag{4.5}$$

$$f_c = f - F_2(f_a) \tag{4.6}$$

where S denotes the segmentation operated on the image reconstructed by the FDK algorithm in the first pass, P is the forward-projection in the CB geometry identical to that in the original CB data acquisition and B is the FDK reconstruction. Notably, Equations 4.2–4.6 are a paraphrase of (but not exactly the same as) the two-pass CB reconstruction implemented in the references (Hsieh 2000b; Forthmann et al. 2009). F_1 accounts for the degradation of spatial resolution in f'_m in comparison to f_m, due to the forward-projection and back-projection applied on f_m. As indicated in Forthmann et al. (2009), F_1 can be carried out via either detector row-wise forward-projection and back-projection in the fan-beam geometry, or adaptive filtering in the image domain. As implemented in Forthmann et al. (2009), F_2 is a filter to remove the high-frequency artifacts that might exist in f_a, since the F_1 implemented in image domain (Hsieh 2000b) may not be able to mimic the cascaded fan-beam forward-projection and FBP. For more detail, readers are referred to the references (Hsieh 2000b; Forthmann et al. 2009). Illustrated in Figure 4.13 are results obtained using the two-pass algorithm, showing the two-pass reconstruction (i) is effective in reducing streak artifacts surrounding the discs, (ii) is less effective in reducing the distortion in shape and drop in the Hounsfield unit (HU) of outer discs, and (iii) the threshold in segmentation plays a significant role in artifact suppression and can even alter the shape of the outer discs. Hence, it should be fair to say that the two-pass CB reconstruction is good at reducing CB artifacts in axial MDCT, but still cannot eradicate the artifacts.

As illustrated in Figure 4.14a, decomposition of the reconstruction zone may be informative to understanding the efficacy and limitation of the two-pass CB reconstruction in suppressing CB artifacts in axial MDCT. Given the projection data

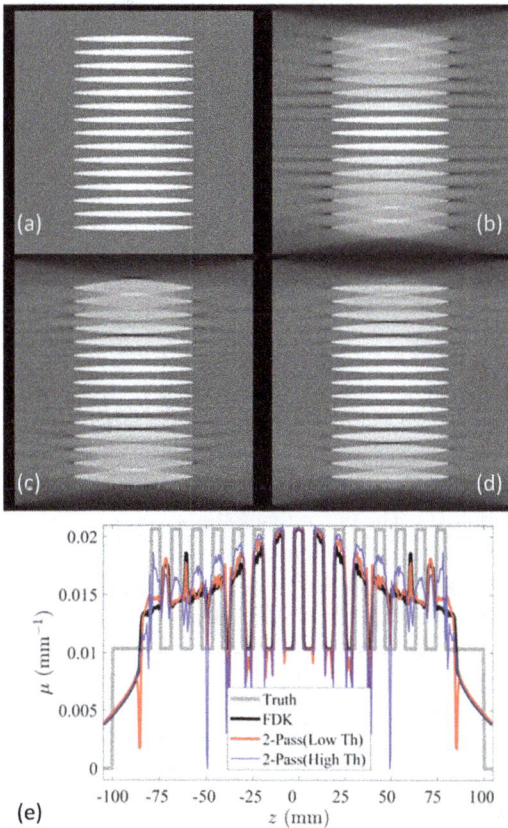

FIGURE 4.13 (a) The Defrise phantom at linear attenuation coefficient equivalent to water and (b) reconstruction by the original FDK, the two-pass CB reconstruction at relatively (c) low and (d) high thresholding in segmentation, and (e) corresponding central profiles (DW/DL: 1000/500).

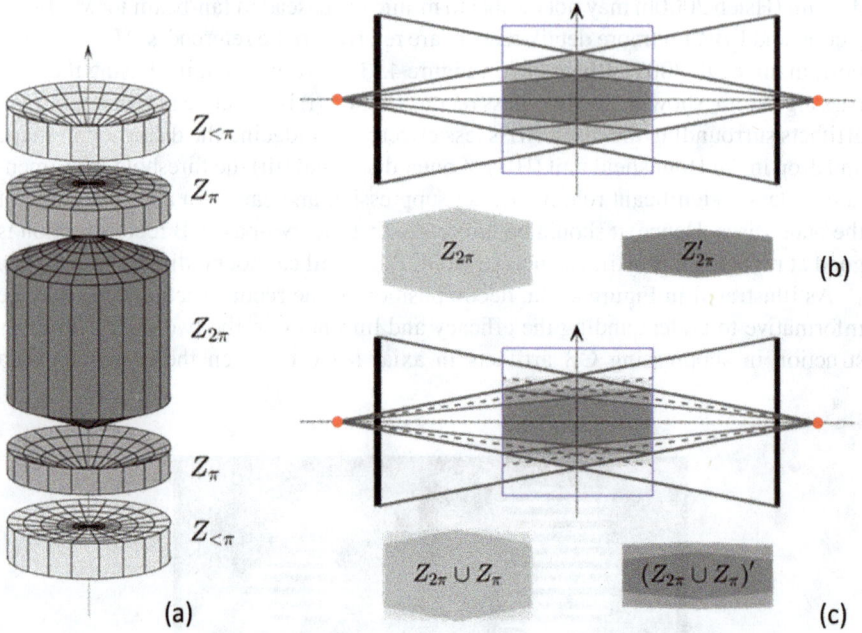

FIGURE 4.14 (a) Schematic showing the decomposed zone corresponding to a redundancy of two, between one and two and smaller than one. The zones that can be reconstructed by the two-pass CB reconstruction from a (b) short and (c) full scan corresponding to $180° + \gamma_m$ and $360°$ scan range, respectively. (Drawings adopted from Reference 70 with modification).

acquired in a full (360°) axial scan with the X-ray source collimated to the detector, the cylindrical volume with its axis concurrent to the CT axis of rotation can be decomposed into three sandwiched zones (Forthmann et al. 2009; Tang et al. 2018). The central zone (dark gray) is denoted as $Z_{2\pi}$, in which each voxel is always irradiated over angular range 2π. The outer zones (light gray) are denoted as Z_π, in which each voxel is irradiated over an angular range smaller than π. The zones in between (mid-gray) are $Z_{\pi/2\pi}$, in which each voxel is irradiated over an angular range between π and 2π. Thus, with or without a weighting scheme, zone $Z_{2\pi}$ can be reconstructed exactly to the first-order approximation, and so can zone Z_π, even though a weighting scheme is mandatory for adequate handling of data redundancy. However, because of longitudinal data truncation, there is no guarantee that zone $Z_{<\pi}$ can be accurately reconstructed to the first-order approximation, though the heuristic data extension in Section 4.4.1 may help.

The key to the two-pass CB reconstruction lies in the second pass, in which CB artifacts are reproduced at relatively high fidelity, via forward-projection cascaded by FBP reconstruction that is exactly the same as that in the first pass. For the second pass to work, the structures that induce CB artifacts should have been accurately reconstructed in the first pass to the first-order approximation (Hsieh 2000b). Hence, as shown in Figure 4.14b, if the projection data are acquired in a short scan, only the

CB artifacts generated by the artifacts-inducing structures within zone $Z'_{2\pi}$, which is defined by the thin solid lines, can be suppressed by the second-pass CB reconstruction, i.e., indention occurs in the imaged zone compared to zone $Z_{2\pi}$. If the projection data are acquired in a full scan, the counterpart of $Z_{2\pi}$ is $Z_{2\pi} \cup Z_\pi$, if adequate weighting schemes are adopted (see Figure 4.14c). Then, the counterpart of $Z'_{2\pi}$ becomes $(Z_{2\pi} \cup Z_\pi)'$, which is defined by the dotted lines, i.e., indention occurs again in the imaged zone in comparison to zone $Z_{2\pi} \cup Z_\pi$. Note that $Z'_{2\pi}$ is a subset of $Z_{2\pi}$, while $(Z_{2\pi} \cup Z_\pi)'$ is a subset of $Z_{2\pi} \cup Z_\pi$. In practice, the indention in the imaged zone should be tolerable, as the majority of organs/tissues that may contain pathology are within zone $Z'_{2\pi}$ or $(Z_{2\pi} \cup Z_\pi)'$. However, it may not be optimal from the standpoint of radiation dose efficiency, as the imaged zone is smaller than the irradiated zone. If projection data are acquired over a short scan (i.e., angular range is between $\pi + \gamma_m$ and 2π, where γ_m is the X-ray beam's fan angle), the imaged zone further indents to $Z'_{2\pi}$ (Figure 4.14b).

To improve radiation dose efficiency, an axial MDCT scan with dual-source–single-detector for preservation of the scan field of view has been proposed (Forthmann et al. 2009). This axial MDCT scan is physically a circle-plus-circle source trajectory, but can actually be counted as a circular one because the X-ray source and detector assembly rotate only one turn. The results of simulation studies using a digital head phantom (Figure 4.15) show that the axial MDCT in this special scan geometry with two-pass CB reconstruction can have image quality that may be potentially sufficient for diagnostic imaging, though further and thorough evaluation and verification are warranted. Note that the CB artifacts are relatively stronger at the middle in Figure 4.15a2–b2, as it is at the mid-way between the circle-plus-circle trajectory.

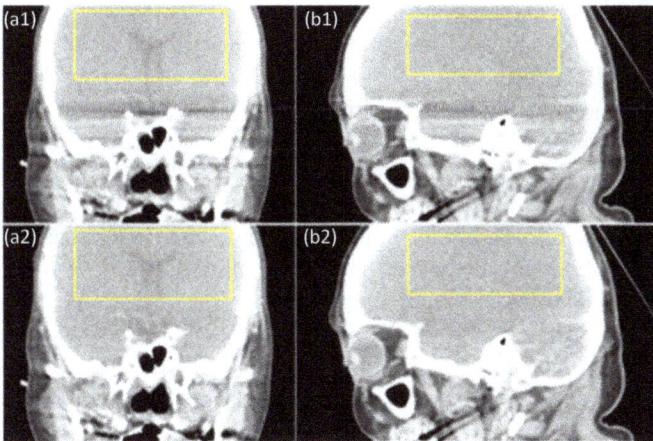

FIGURE 4.15 Coronal and sagittal views of a digital head phantom (a1 and b1) reconstructed by the FDK algorithm and (a2 and b2) the two-pass CB reconstruction from the projection data acquired in an axial scan with the dual-source–single-detector configuration (DW/DL: 300/0). (Images adopted with permission from Forthmann et al. 2009.)

Since additional forward- and back-projection are required, the computational cost of the two-pass CB reconstruction is substantially higher than that of the original FDK (Feldkamp et al. 1984) algorithm or other weighted CB–FBP algorithms (Tang et al. 2005, 2006; Taguchi et al. 2004; Heuscher 2002; Stierstorfer et al. 2004). However, recognizing its potential for significantly improving reconstruction accuracy in axial MDCT/CBCT, including both inaccuracy in CT number and distortion in geometry, the extra computational effort required by the two-pass CB reconstruction should be acceptable, especially in light of the fact that the power of computation engines (e.g., GPU) is increasingly affordable.

4.5.2 SPIRAL/HELICAL SCAN

Though it continues to increase, the number of detector rows used for spiral/helical scanning in MDCT in the clinic may not exceed 64 or 128, i.e., the increase in number of detector rows is mainly to benefit the axial scan for coverage of a large organ in one gantry rotation. Notably, at a given spiral/helical pitch, detector row width and gantry rotation speed, e.g., 1:1, 0.625 mm and 0.5 s/r, respectively, an X-ray beam aperture larger than 128×0.625 mm = 80 mm results in patient table motion at speed 160 mm/sec, which may cause unacceptable discomfort to patients due to the acceleration or deceleration when the scan starts or ends. Moreover, a patient table proceeding at such a high speed may substantially run ahead of the contrast agent, making the bolus chasing in clinical settings not feasible due to unexpected involuntary visceral motion.

The spiral/helical scan of MSCT actually meets the data sufficiency condition (DSC) (Tuy 1983; Smith 1985, 1990), as long as the effective spiral/helical pitch is within a reasonable range. For instance, the allowable spiral/helical pitch in an MDCT scan is dependent on the gantry geometry and detector deployment, and a reasonable spiral/helical pitch up to 1.5:1 is routinely utilized in the clinic (Tang et al. 2005, 2006, 2007, 2008b; Taguchi et al. 2004; Heuscher 2004; Stierstorfer et al. 2004). However, no theoretically accurate image reconstruction has so far been used in this scan mode in MDCT, even though Katsevich published his breakthrough accurate reconstruction algorithm for the spiral/helical scan in 2001 (Katsevich 2002a, 2002b), right prior to the launching of 16-detector row CT in the marketplace by all major CT vendors. The most distinct feature of Katsevich's algorithm and its derivatives is the operation of filtering along the white curves shown in Figure 4.16. Another important feature is the handling of data redundancy via the Tam–Danielsson window (Tam 1995; Danielsson et al. 1997), which is also shown in Figure 4.16 by the curves in red color (indicated by red solid arrows). The DSC is satisfied, as long as the boundary of the Tam–Danielsson window is within the detector dimension of MDCT, which is equivalent to a spiral/helical pitch around 1:1. It has been experimentally evaluated and verified that, at a cone angle up to 4.5°, which roughly corresponds to that spanned in 64-detector row CT, there is no dominant advantage in reconstruction accuracy by Katsevich's algorithm over the approximate solutions that employ various weighing schemes to suppress the

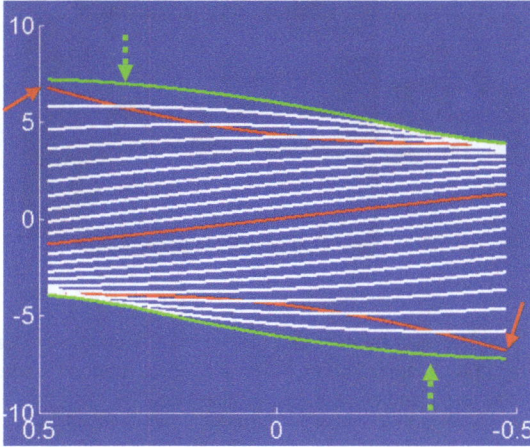

FIGURE 4.16 Schematic diagram showing the curves (white, no arrow) along which the filtering required by Katsevich-type algorithms is carried out, the Tam–Danielsson window indicated by the two red curves (solid arrows) and the boundary of data detection indicated by the outmost green curves (dashed arrow).

artifacts caused by data inconsistency and inadequate handling of the data redundancy (Tang et al. 2005, 2008b). According to evaluation and verification results, those approximate solutions, such as the one using the cone-angle-dependent weighting as delineated earlier, are anticipated to work well for the spiral/helical scan in 128-detector MDCT.

4.6 DISCUSSION

As already indicated in Chapter 1, the ultimate goal, most likely, of MDCT is to cover the entire heart in one gantry rotation, so the inter-slab discontinuity caused by the inconsistency in cardiac motion or contrast agent circulation can be avoided. Theoretically speaking, only the image reconstruction in an SDCT at the axial scan is accurate. All other reconstruction solutions, starting from the spiral/helical scan in SDCT and the axial scan in MDCT with the number of detector rows more than one, are only approximate. This fact may be surprising, but is what has been happening so far in SDCT and MDCT, and most likely will continue in the future. One may have to be cautious about the reconstruction accuracy that can be achieved by upcoming state-of-the-art CT scanners with an increasing number of detector rows.

In an axial scan, owing to the cone angle spanned by detector rows that are not located at the central plane determined by the source trajectory, even an MDCT with only two detector rows in principle does not satisfy the DSC (Tuy 1983; Smith 1985, 1990; Tang et al. 2018). The greater the number of detector rows, the more severe the cone-beam artifact, as demonstrated in Figure 4.17, wherein a phantom consisting

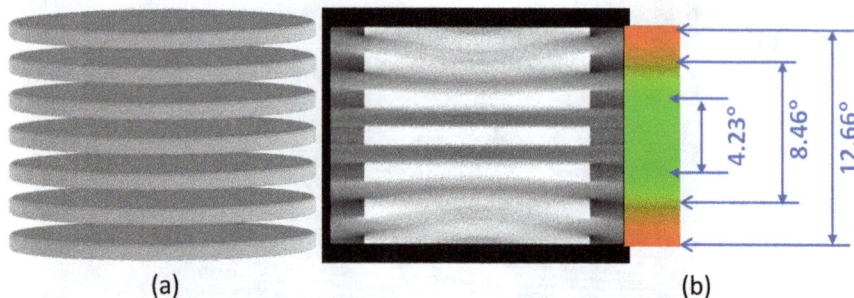

FIGURE 4.17 (a) The Defrise phantom and (b) the MDCT images in coronal view reconstructed from the projection acquired along a circular source trajectory, whereby the relationship between artifact severity and cone angle is illustrated.

of seven identical discs stacked parallel to each other along the craniocaudal direction is used to highlight the cone-beam artifacts. The root cause of the cone-beam artifacts is of course the violation of DSC, which may manifest itself as (i) streak-like shading or glaring adjacent to high-contrast structures, (ii) dropping of CT number (or Hounsfield unit) at the pixels that are not located within the central plane, and (iii) geometric distortion. The first two artifacts may be correctable with empirical approaches, but the geometric distortion artifact may result in distorted organ shapes and is much more difficult, if not impossible, to correct. It may be argued that no anatomic structure like the discs shown in Figure 4.17 exists in the human body, but the cone angle and resultant artifacts are indeed an open problem to be answered by scientists and researchers in the field.

Another argument that can be made is that the image formed by the X-ray beam in radiography is actually in cone-beam geometry, which is different from what is seen by a radiologist in the physical world. A radiologist is trained to detect and identify lesions that are 2D representations of the physical world. Therefore, even though residual CB artifacts (i.e., geometry distortion or intensity drop, or both) may still exist in axial MDCT images, the radiologists should still be able to detect and characterize lesions at high sensitivity and specificity, similar to what has been achieved in 2D radiography. However, this is subject to a thorough validation study with engagement of experts in image quality assessment and radiological physicians on a large cohort of patients with pathology in the head, thorax, abdomen, pelvis and extremities, and healthy people as the control group, via well-designed and well-implemented data collection and statistical analysis.

5 Image Formation via Iterative Reconstruction Algorithms

Computed tomography (CT) has been among the most popular imaging modalities in clinics to support healthcare providers by saving human lives or improving patients' quality of life. However, CT is an imaging modality that uses X-rays, the most common form of ionizing radiation, for signal detection (data acquisition). Consequently, its risk of inducing malignance in a patient, though the risk is low in light of its clinical benefits, cannot be ignored. The continuously increasing utilization of CT worldwide has drawn concern about the risks to patients and healthcare providers introduced by CT radiation (Brenner and Hall 2007). Furthermore, to meet the challenges posed by cardiovascular, neurovascular and oncological applications, researchers have never stopped advancing CT technology. For example, following the evolvement of the CT detector element aperture from centimeter to submillimeter (Flohr et al. 2003), the cross-plane spatial resolution (slice thickness) of all state-of-the-art multi-detector CT (MDCT) reached the submillimeter level at the turn of the new millennium. Since then, the improvement in MDCT cross-plane spatial resolution has continued and presently MDCT with image slices thinner than 0.5 mm is available in the marketplace. To maintain clinically acceptable noise in CT images acquired with thinner slices, the associated radiation dose has to be increased in squared proportion, which has been drawing further public concerns about CT's long-term consequences on patients' health.

In response to the public concerns associated with ionizing X-ray radiation, the CT industry and academic scientific community have recently come up with a paradigm shift in image reconstruction using the iterative image reconstruction (IIR) algorithm that differs fundamentally from filtered back-projection (FBP) algorithms. In fact, CT was invented with IIR, termed the algebraic reconstruction technique (ART), but gave way to FBP, due to IIR's daunting requirements on computation speed and data access. In the past decade, IIR has resurged as an appealing alternative for image formation in MDCT for clinical applications (Thibault et al. 2007; Han et al. 2011; Xu et al. 2012; La Rivière 2006; Fessler 2009; Pan et al. 2009; Lauzier 2012; Figueiredo et al. 2007; Sidky et al. 2011; Tang and Tang 2012) at reduced radiation dose, since it brings the tight trade-off between spatial resolution and noise (hopefully low contrast detectability) in the FBP reconstruction to a lesser extent, and the requirement on computation and data access is no longer as daunting as before, mainly due to the unbelievable advancement in computation power made by the semiconductor industry (Moore's law) in computer engineering.

DOI: 10.1201/9780429028465-5

5.1 CLASSIC ITERATIVE IMAGE RECONSTRUCTION

In IIR, the data acquisition of MDCT is modeled as an observation of a linear system of equations (Equation 5.1) and the reconstruction of the image is to find a solution of the linear system

$$M_{N \times P}^{+} g_{P \times 1} = M_{P \times N} \cdot f_{N \times 1} \tag{5.1}$$

where $N = n \times n$ is the number of pixels in the image to be reconstructed, P is the number of observations made in data acquisition, $M_{P \times N}$ is the system matrix, $g_{P \times 1}$ denotes the observed (acquired) projection data and $f_{N \times 1}$ is a representation of the image to be reconstructed. In a routine MDCT scan, P is significantly larger than N, and thus the linear system of equations in Equation 5.1 is overdetermined and can be mathematically perceived as the solution to a minimization problem, i.e.,

$$f_{N \times 1}^{*} = \arg\min_{f_{N \times 1} \in \Omega} | M_{P \times N} \cdot f_{N \times 1} - g_{P \times 1} |^{2}, \tag{5.2}$$

where Ω represents the set of potential solutions. Equation 5.2 can be solved using the approach of least squares (or minimized norm)

$$f_{N \times 1}^{*} = (M_{P \times N}^{T} M_{P \times N})^{-1} M_{P \times N}^{T} g_{P \times 1} \equiv M_{N \times P}^{+} g_{P \times 1} \tag{5.3}$$

where $M_{N \times P}^{+}$ is the Moore–Penrose matrix. In theory, Equation 5.3 can be solved using singular value decomposition (SVD). However, N is usually on the order of $\sim O(10^{6})$ and a direct inversion of the matrix in Equation 5.3 is formidable. Hence, iterative algorithms have to be adopted to solve the problem (Buzug 2008).

Compared to FBP image reconstruction, the modeling of an MDCT system and its noise can be embedded into the system matrix $M_{P \times N}$ to make (i) the image reconstruction more tolerable to imperfection or even data missing in data acquisition, (ii) the iterative process more tractable in convergence and (iii) the reconstructed image optimal in terms of the trade-off between spatial resolution and noise.

The earliest IIR solution ART implemented in the first commercially available CT scanner was in the fashion of beam-wise pixel updating (Buzug 2008). For better image quality, the ART was superseded by the simultaneous iterative reconstruction technique (SIRT), which is in the fashion of image-wise pixel updating though it converges slower than the ART (Buzug 2008). Later, it was found that the slowness in the convergence of SIRT can be remedied by the scheme called ordered subset, in which the projection data are sorted and fed into the iterative process in a specially designed order. Such a combination has been called ordered-subset SIRT (OS-SIRT) in the community. Presented in Figure 5.1 are images of an MDCT quality assurance (QA) phantom, as the examples to show the intermediate results at the 1st, 3rd, 5th, 10th, 25th and 50th iterations when the OS-SIRT is used for image reconstruction. It is observed that, with an increasing number of iterations, the intermediate image becomes increasingly better in terms of image fidelity, and arrives at an excellent

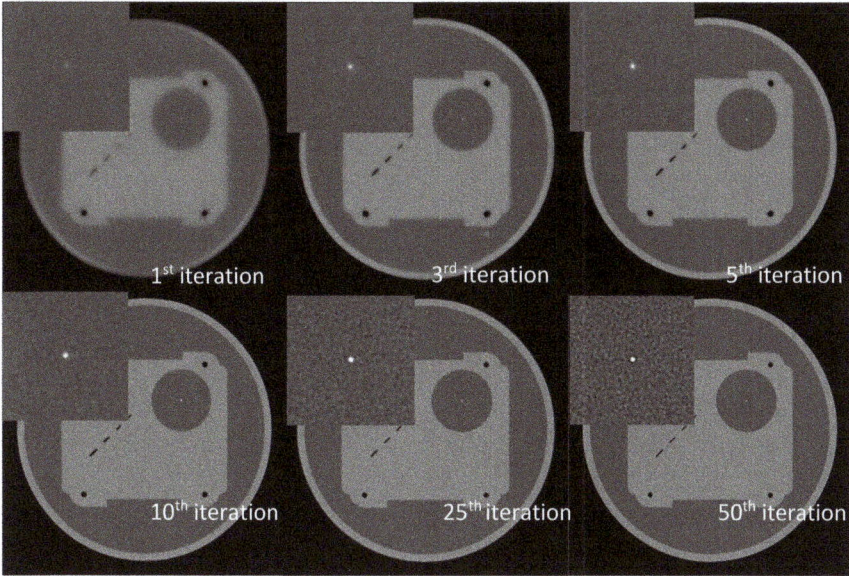

FIGURE 5.1   Intermediate images of a QA phantom reconstructed by the OS-SIRT algorithm without regularization, from the data acquired by an MDCT, in which the area enclosing the metal wire is zoomed.

status around the 50th iteration. Simultaneously, however, the intermediate images become increasingly noisy (see the zoomed region enclosing the tungsten wire), while the edges at the interface between structures that differ significantly in attenuation becomes increasingly sharper.

5.2 ITERATIVE IMAGE RECONSTRUCTION WITH REGULARIZATION

The convergence of SIRT has not been mathematically proven yet. In fact, the noise in the images presented in Figure 5.1 continues to grow with increasing iterations after the 50th iteration. Moreover, as we know, similar to other optimization problems, the minimization problem of Equation 5.2 is usually ill-posed, i.e., some relatively small noise or data inconsistency in the observation (projection data) may lead to severe artifacts (anomalies or oscillation) in reconstructed image (Buzug 2008). It has been well studied that the instability of the solution to an optimization problem can be mitigated by regularization (or *a priori*), which is a functional added to the objective function and dramatically improves the conditioning (or preconditioning) of a linear system of equations (Fessler and Booth 1999; Buzug 2008; Fessler 2009; Barber et al. 2016). Numerous functionals, e.g., the Gibbs distribution of the generalized Gaussian Markov random field (GGMRF) (Bouman and Sauer 1993; Saquib et al. 1996), have been proposed in the literature. It has been reported that, as one of the regularization strategies for system preconditioning, the functional called total variation (TV), which is the magnitude of the first-order gradient of an image, is very effective in noise reduction while simultaneously maintaining the spatial resolution (image sharpness) (Sidky et al. 2006b). By incorporating TV into the minimization problem, Equation 5.2 becomes (Sidky and Pan 2008; Pan et al. 2009; Sidky et al. 2011; Han et al. 2011)

$$f^*_{N\times1} = \underset{f_{N\times1} \in \Omega}{\arg\min} \left(|\, M_{P\times N} \cdot f_{N\times1} - g_{P\times1}\,|^2 + \lambda \,\|\, f_{N\times1}\,\|_{TV} \right). \qquad (5.4)$$

The images reconstructed by the OS-SIRT with TV regularization are correspondingly presented in Figure 5.2, which demonstrates that the structures and edges of the phantom become increasingly sharper, with almost no increment in noise. Apparently, the IIR with regularization behaves more tractable than that without regularization in the trade-off between spatial resolution and noise. However, it should be noted that, though the adoption of regularization (or objective functions that are usually defined as statistical norms) makes the iteration process convergent, it may still have to run up to hundreds or thousands of times (Sidky 2009). Moreover, readers are advised to keep in mind that the likelihood for the regularization in IIR to compromise the spatial resolution of a reconstructed image cannot be ignored, and also sometimes it is even unpredictable, since the regularization may be not only non-linear but also shift variant, e.g., it may alter the variation in local contrast. Meanwhile, notably, the parameter λ in Equation 5.4 plays a critical role in

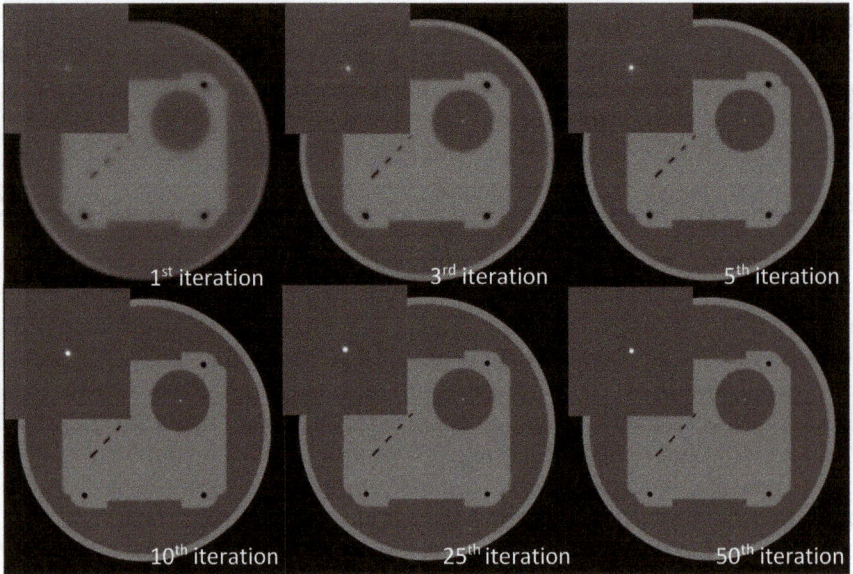

FIGURE 5.2 Intermediate images of a QA phantom reconstructed by the OS-SIRT algorithm with TV regularization, from the data acquired by an MDCT, in which the area enclosing the metal wire is zoomed.

controlling the compromise between the spatial resolution and noise, in addition to its role in controlling the convergence speed.

5.3 OPTIMIZATION-BASED ITERATIVE IMAGE RECONSTRUCTION FROM INSUFFICIENT DATA

The TV, which is the magnitude of the first-order gradient of an image (Sidky and Pan 2008; Sidky et al 2011), based on algorithms as defined next, have been recognized as a very effective solution for image reconstruction under the framework of compressed sensing

$$f_{N\times 1}^{*} = \arg\min_{f_{N\times 1}\in\Omega} \| f_{N\times 1} \|_{TV} \tag{5.5.1}$$

subject to

$$| M_{P\times N} \cdot f_{N\times 1} - g_{P\times 1} | \leq \varepsilon \tag{5.5.2}$$

$$f_{N\times 1} \geq 0 \tag{5.5.3}$$

As demonstrated by simulation in the reference (Sidky and Pan 2008), if the image reconstruction from the data acquired in axial MDCT is treated as a solution to an optimization problem (Equations 5.5.1–5.5.3), and the projection data of an object, which is discretely defined on 3D voxels, is generated via an "idealized" manner, i.e., Equation 5.1, the Defrise phantom can be reconstructed by the ASD-POCS (adaptive steepest descending–projection onto convex sets) algorithm (also termed the TV algorithm by its inventors) quite accurately in both Hounsfield unit (HU) and shape, by setting a perfect constraint on fidelity (i.e., $\varepsilon = 0$ in Equation 5.5.2). Nevertheless, as shown in Figure 5.3, if noise is added or inconsistency between the projection data and system modeling exists (e.g., the projection data is analytically generated, the case in reality), the TV reconstruction of the Defrise phantom becomes inaccurate, as manifested by the noise and distortion in shape (Figure 5.3d–f) (Sidky and Pan 2008), even though the TV algorithm outperforms the POCS algorithm considerably, since the fidelity can no longer be set as $\varepsilon = 0$ in Equation 5.5.2. It is very interesting and important to note that, as illustrated in Figure 5.3, with increasing tolerance in the fidelity, the noise is mitigated in the TV reconstruction, while the distortion in shape worsens.

Moreover, it has been reported (Choi and Baek 2015) that, with the step size λ determined by the Barzilai–Borwein gradient-projection algorithm, Equation 5.4 was utilized as a TV-constrained algorithm for iterative cone-beam reconstruction in axial cone-beam CT (CBCT) that is different from the MDCT only in the geometry of the 2D detector array. Using a downsized Defrise phantom from the projection data acquired in a full CBCT scan, the TV-constrained iterative image reconstruction outperforms the two-pass reconstruction. The preliminary results encourage speculation that the constrained iterative image reconstruction or iterative image

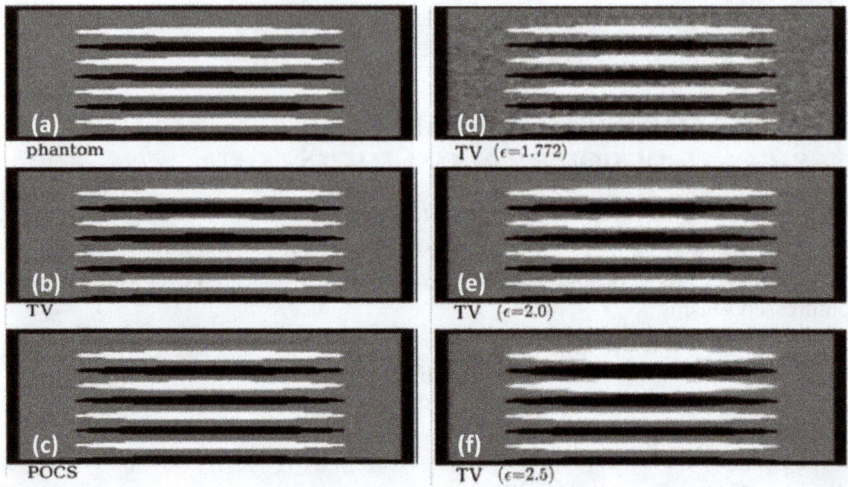

FIGURE 5.3   (a) Central coronal view of the Defrise phantom, (b) the images reconstructed via ASD-POCS (TV) by setting $\varepsilon = 0$ in Equation 5.5.2, (c) POCS from noiseless projection data, and the ASD-POCS (TV) algorithm by setting (d) $\varepsilon = 1.772$, (e) $\varepsilon = 2.0$ and (f) $\varepsilon = 2.5$ from noisy projection data acquired at 128 angular positions (DW/DL for panels a–c: –100/100; DW/DL for panels d–f: –50/50). (Images adopted with permission from Sidky and Pan 2008.)

reconstruction with regularization may bring about innovative solutions (Sidky and Pan 2008; Pan et al. 2009) to deal with the cone-beam artifacts that have been hunted in axial MDCT for a long while, although further and thorough evaluation and verification by reconstruction of more realistic structures are warranted.

5.4   DE-NOISING IN IMAGE DOMAIN VIA ITERATIVE ALGORITHMS

Recently, a number of non-linear shift-variant approaches in image domain to significantly reduce noise while maintaining spatial resolution have been proposed and implemented in MDCT for neurological, body and cardiovascular applications. These image domain-based methods vary in implementation, but have the following features in common: (i) noise reduction via forward anisotropic diffusion (Black et al. 1998; Perona and Malik 1990; Gerig et al. 1992), (ii) preservation and even boosting of edges via backward anisotropic diffusion and (iii) blending of the non-linear processed image with the original image reconstructed by the FBP algorithm to make the appearance of the finally obtained images similar to that of conventional CT images. Presented on the right of Figure 5.4 is an MDCT image of an anthropomorphic head phantom with de-noising based on anisotropic diffusion, and that of the original image is on the left for comparison. It is interesting to note that, because the anisotropic diffusion is usually carried out via iteration, these non-linear approaches may have been claimed as iterative image reconstruction by MDCT vendors, even

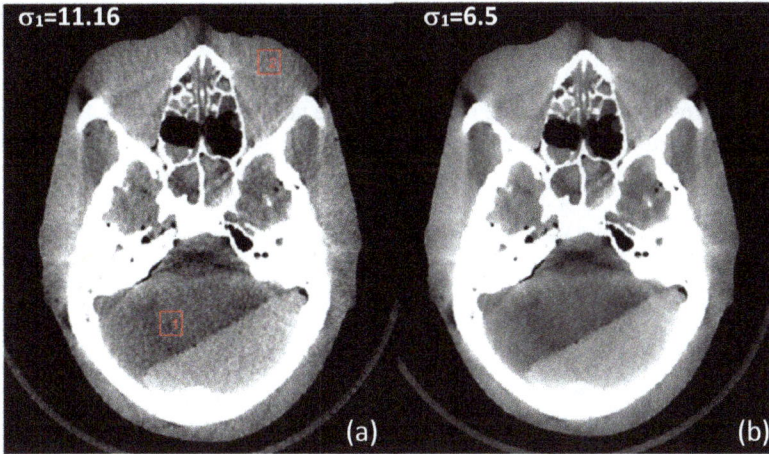

$\sigma_1 = 11.16$ $\sigma_1 = 6.5$

(a)   (b)

FIGURE 5.4   (a) The original FBP image of an anthropomorphic head phantom and (b) that with noise reduced by anisotropic diffusion.

though all these non-linear approaches are confined to be carried out in image domain only. In light of the widely accepted concept of iterative image reconstruction wherein the back-and-forth operations between the projection and image domains are essential (see Section 5.1) (Shepp and Vardi 1982; Lange and Carson 1984; Lange and Fessler (1995); Bouman and Sauer (1996); Fessler 2009; Xu et al. 2009), these controversial claims have triggered debate in the CT imaging community. This is the reason why this section is titled "de-noising in the image domain via iterative algorithms", rather than "de-noising via iterative reconstruction algorithms".

5.5 DISCUSSION

One may intuitively think that a reduction of noise in an MDCT image can result in saving of radiation dose by observing the "square-root" rule, i.e., a k-folds reduction in noise results in an k^2-folds saving of radiation dose, and vice versa. Nevertheless, it is important to clarify that this intuitive logic only works in the case wherein linear de-noising algorithms are employed. If non-linear algorithms are utilized, this square-root rule in general may no longer hold. Various regularization schemes have been adopted in IIR, and these non-linear approaches are usually shift variant and thus one has to be cautious about the appealing claims made by MDCT vendors on the efficacy of radiation dose saving in their products whenever non-linear shift-variant approaches are used to support such claims.

With respect to the trade-off between spatial resolution and noise, the iterative image reconstruction with regularization significantly outperforms the one with no regularization, which in turn outperforms the analytic image reconstruction algorithms such as filtered back-projection. Even though, however, it is still likely that the iterative image reconstruction algorithms with regularization may compromise the spatial resolution of a reconstructed image while the noise is being reduced. Hence, the image quality should be assessed objectively and quantitatively using comprehensive figures of merits, as to be presented in the next chapter (Vaishnav et al. 2014; McCollough et al. 2015a).

6 Assessment of Image Quality in MDCT under Theory of Signal Detection and Statistical Decision

Owing to its revolutionary utility as a novel modality in the clinic for diagnostic imaging in the early 1970s, computed tomography (CT) led to a paradigm shift in the practice of contemporary medicine and thus was acclaimed by the medical community worldwide. Coincident to CT's advent, scientists in the field of medical imaging were starting to apply the theory of signal detection and statistical decision in radiography and fluoroscopy for assessment of imaging system performance and image quality, based on a fundamental assumption that in principle there exists no inter-element correlation in the noise of the X-ray detector used for data acquisition. However, though there also is no inter-element correlation in the noise of an X-ray detector used for data acquisition in CT, an inter-pixel correlation is induced in the noise of tomographic images due to the essential ramp filter and additional apodization filters to make the image reconstruction tractable in computation. It is a consensus that the noise behavior of CT can only be fully characterized by its noise power spectrum (or Weiner spectrum) – the distribution of noise power over spatial frequencies – no matter if it is a single-detector (SDCT) in the early days or a state-of-the-art multi-detector (MDCT) (Barret et al. 1976; Riederer et al. 1978; Wagner et al. 1979; Hanson 1979, 1980, 1981; Barrett and Swindell 1981; Faulkner and Moores 1984; Kijewski and Judy 1987; Bushberg et al. 2012; Siewerdsen et al. 2002; Tward and Siewerdsen 2009; Boedeker et al. 2007, Boedeker and McNitt-Gray 2007; Baek and Pelc 2010, 2011, 2013).

Across all modalities in general and specifically in CT, research in assessment of imaging system performance and image quality under the frameworks of signal detection and information theory hit its stride in the 1980s and 1990s (Wagner 1977; Wagner et al. 1979; Wagner and Brown 1985). Since an image is formed by an imaging system, the assessment of image quality is equivalent to assessing the imaging system's performance. Hence, from now on, I make no distinction between image quality and imaging system performance, unless such a differentiation is deemed necessary. By treating CT as a linear and shift-invariant system and assuming stationarity and ergodicity in its noise, the squared signal-to-noise ratio (SNR) or

DOI: 10.1201/9780429028465-6

detectability index is defined as the major figure of merit (FOM) to assess the image quality (Hanson 1979; Metz et al. 1995; ICRU 1996; Myers 2000). Resorting to the theory of statistical decision, the receiver operating characteristic (ROC) approach (Metz 2000; Tourassi 2019) and its derivatives have established themselves as the methods of choice for image quality assessment under the assumption that both the signal and background under study are exactly known (SKE/BKE) or at least statistically known (ICRU 1996). By adopting psychophysical principles (Myers 2000), a number of model observers with the capability of mimicking the ideal or human observer in image quality assessment, such as the pre-whitening matched filter observer, non-prewhitening matched filter observer, non-prewhitening matched filter with eye filter, Hotelling model observer and channelized Hotelling model observer, have been proposed for applications in CT (Abbey and Bochud 2000; Abbey and Barrett 2001; Abbey and Eckstein 2007, 2019), including the emerging novel imaging methods (e.g., differential phase contrast CT (Tang and Yang 2014)) and the latest developments in CT (Leng et al. 2013; Yu et al. 2013, 2017), such as the state-of-the-art spectral (dual energy) CT (Fan et al. 2023).

Even though the aforementioned FOM has existed since the early 1990s, the pixel-wise noise (gross variance) defined as the root mean square (RMS) or the standard deviation (SD) of image pixels within a region of interest (ROI) is still commonly employed in literature as the FOM for noise analysis or image quality assessment. There may exist at least four reasons behind this phenomenon: (i) the aforementioned ROC approaches and FOMs are costly and tedious in implementation, (ii) the pixel-wise noise and SNR are convenient to use in practice, (iii) the inconsistency in the nomenclature used in dispersive publications makes the learning curve of those approaches and associated FOMs rather long, and (iv), most important, with CT's increasing maturity in technology and clinical applications as an established imaging modality, the pixel-wise SNR is effective and seems sufficient as the rule-of-thumb metric (Burgess 1999) for routine quality assurance and protocol optimization. On a daily basis, the pixel-wise noise and SNR are utilized to analyze the gross variance in MDCT images as a function of tube current (radiation dose), image slice thickness and spiral/helical pitch. Nevertheless, as has been well understood from the very beginning (and see more later for clarification), the pixel-wise noise cannot adequately characterize CT's noise property (and other imaging modalities as well) (Burgess 1999).

As pointed out in Chapter 5, an iteration of mere forward and backward projections is linear, but the embedding of regularization may make the iterative image reconstruction (IIR) no longer linear. Moreover, the regularization is in general contrast dependent and thus makes the iteration process no longer shift invariant. Together, they invalidate the linearity, spatial shift invariance and noise stationarity that are the key prerequisites in defining the stochastic linear shift-invariant FOMs, e.g., the noise power spectrum (NPS) and modulation transfer function (MTF), that are the fundamental FOMs for assessment of system performance and image quality in CT with images reconstructed by filtered back-projection (FBP) algorithms. To cope with the loss of linearity, shift invariance and noise stationarity, due to the variation in contrast, dose and algorithmic parameters over locations in images formed by the IIR algorithms, alternative task-based (or getting-around) approaches have recently been proposed in the literature (Richard et al. 2012; Wilson et al. 2013). The basic idea underlying these getting-around strategies is to define the image quality FOM at various preset operating conditions over the entire dynamic range, i.e., piecewise linearization. For example, the MTF can be specified over a range of specific contrasts, while the NPS is defined in a region of interest at specific locations. There is no doubt that such compromises make it possible to reuse all the existing approaches under the stochastic linear shift-invariant assumption for quality assessment of the images formed by IIR. However, it may have to be acknowledged that the compromised solution can be exhaustive and thus ineffective and/or inefficient in its implementation and outcome interpretation.

Based on the preceding points, it is time for us to return to the basics and assess the image quality of MDCT under the framework of signal detection and statistical decision – the practice that has been established since the very beginning of CT and has been further refined over the years. Aimed at providing a tutorial for better interpretation and comprehension of image quality and its assessment, the fundamentals, including the concepts, approaches and FOMs, are presented in a way unified in the theory of signal detection and statistical decision, after a concise review of the FOMs that are routinely utilized in the MDCT product data sheet for communication among vendors, regulating or accrediting authorities, and customers.

6.1 SPECIFICATION OF IMAGING QUALITY IN MDCT

The major metrics to specify the image quality of an MDCT are the contrast, spatial and temporal resolution, with the recent addition of spectral (or energy) resolution implemented in state-of-the-art spectral (also called dual energy) MDCT.

6.1.1 CONTRAST RESOLUTION

Contrast resolution, also called low contrast detectability (LCD), is commonly defined as the ability to identify the low contrast (~0.1%–0.5%) targets at various dimensions (~1–5 mm), given a radiation dose quantified on the CT dose index (CTDI). The contrast resolution depends on the MDCT detector's absorption and conversion efficiency, in addition to its geometrical efficiency determined by the post-patient collimator and the active area of each detector element. The LCD is critical in detecting pathological lesions in soft tissues on the patient's body. For example, in scanning a large-size patient the noise level is usually high; high noise levels also occur when scanning pediatric patients, as the radiation dose has to be tuned down due to pediatric patients' tissue or organ sensitivity to radiation. Presented in Figure 6.1a is a drawing of the CTP515 LCD module in the CatPhan600 phantom (https://www.phantomlab.com/); the corresponding MDCT image is in Figure 6.1b, in which the LCD at a given radiation dose can be assessed. The contrast resolution is the differentiator between the CT for diagnostic imaging and that for other special purposes, such as cone-beam CT (CBCT) for image-guided radiation therapy and micro-CT for animal or specimen imaging in preclinical applications. Notably, to

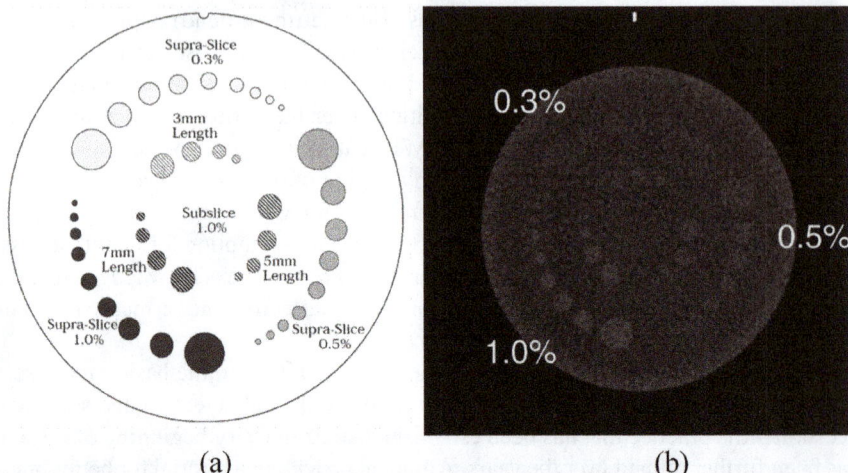

FIGURE 6.1   (a) Schematic diagram showing the CTP515 LCD module of the CatPhan-600 phantom and (b) an example of its transverse MDCT image. (With permissions, the drawing in panel a is adopted from The Phantom Laboratory (https://www.phantomlab.com/), while the image in panel b is from Thilander-Klang 2010.)

maximally make use of the X-ray photons that have penetrated a patient's body, the scintillator in a diagnostic MDCT detector is usually ~2.0–3.0 mm thick, which is substantially thicker than that of the flat panel used in CBCT (usually on the order of 0.5 mm).

6.1.2 Spatial Resolution

The spatial resolution, which is quantitatively defined by the MTF, indicates MDCT's capability of differentiating two high-contrast objects that stay close to each other. The spatial resolution of an MDCT is primarily determined by the dimension of its detector element, but can be boosted to approach twice the Nyquist frequency determined by the detector cell dimension (and thus the consequence of aliasing artifacts) (Flohr et al. 2007; Tang et al. 2010). The typical detector cell size in an MDCT is approximately 0.5 mm (projected at the isocenter), corresponding to a Nyquist frequency of 10.0 lp/cm. However, almost all MDCT offers the highest spatial resolution beyond 15.0 lp/cm. For example, presented in Figure 6.2a is the MTF of an MDCT scanner provided by a major vendor, in which the 10% cut-off frequency corresponding to the STAND reconstruction kernel is well below the Nyquist frequency. With sophisticated boosting techniques, the 10% cut-off frequency to the BONE+ kernel of the same MDCT can readily exceed the Nyquist frequency. A similar strategy is exercised by another major MDCT vendor in kernel optimization to fulfill the clinical requirements (Figure 6.2b). Aliasing artifacts may appear when the Nyquist frequency is exceeded, but the so-called quarter-offset technique (Tang et al. 2010) can effectively improve the sampling rate, if not double it, avoiding the occurrence of

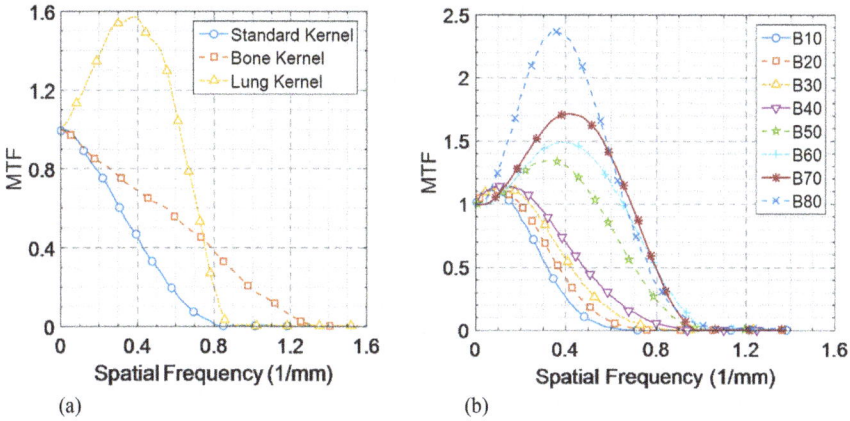

FIGURE 6.2   The MTF corresponding to the reconstruction kernels that are available in the MDCT scanners provided by two (a and b) vendors.

aliasing artifacts in clinical applications demanding high spatial resolution. Notably, in general, the aliasing artifacts in CT can be suppressed via advanced data acquisition techniques, e.g., interlacing of detector elements implemented in hardware or algorithms, using relatively sophisticated strategy under the theory of sampling on lattice (Xie and Tang 2017).

6.1.3 TEMPORAL RESOLUTION

The temporal resolution, determined by the period of time during which the projection data to form an MDCT image are acquired, aims to evaluate MDCT's capability of imaging the organ/tissue in motion, e.g., the heart or lung in cardiac or respiratory motion. In practice, given MDCT's gantry rotation speed, the short scan mode is used to achieve the best possible temporal resolution. The temporal resolution of a short scan is defined as $T \times (180° + \gamma_m)/360°$, where T is the time for CT gantry to rotate one turn. With an increasing number of detector rows, MDCT is routinely utilized in the clinic for cardiovascular imaging wherein the temporal resolution is of paramount importance.

6.1.4 SPECTRAL RESOLUTION

The spectral resolution implemented in spectral (dual energy) CT or photon-counting CT (to be presented in the next two chapters) is a new addition to MDCT's effectiveness in the clinic. In a single-energy (kVp) CT scan, the pixel intensity in a formed image is the linear attenuation coefficient that is jointly determined by the material's effective atomic number and mass density. Consequently, a material, e.g., iodine, with higher atomic number but lower mass density, may happen to have approximately the same linear attenuation coefficient, as that of other material, e.g., calcium, with lower atomic number but higher mass density. Meanwhile, the mass attenuation coefficient of a material varies over X-ray photon energy and that of various materials vary at different rates. It is apparent, as will be elucidated in the next two chapters, that such energy dependence can be utilized to differentiate materials that generate no contrast in a single-energy scan.

It should be pointed out that, though they are still being used for image quality evaluation in MDCT, almost all the phantoms used for such purpose, e.g., the LCD phantom displayed in Figure 6.1a, are designed for the SDCT working in fan-beam or single-detector row mode. The targets in these phantoms are cylindrical and required to be placed in parallel with the gantry's rotation axis, i.e., no variation along the craniocaudal direction. These cylindrical targets work well in SDCT and in principle work in MDCT with the fan-beam geometry for image reconstruction, but may result in at least two consequences in the MDCT that uses 3D CB geometry-based reconstruction algorithms for image formation. First, in general, a cylindrical target cannot detect the CB artifacts (see Chapter 4 for detail). Second, one may take advantage of the fact that there is no variation along the cylindrical targets to attain image quality that is not real. For instance, the LCD (Figure 6.1b) measured with the LCD phantom may falsely appear better than what it actually is, when certain filtering along the longitudinal direction is applied. Hence, new phantoms with adequate longitudinal variation to ensure the accuracy in image quality assessment are anticipated to be defined by regulatory and/or accrediting authorities.

6.2 FUNDAMENTALS OF SIGNAL DETECTION, STATISTICAL DECISION AND PSYCHOPHYSICS

Under the framework of signal detection and statistical decision, there exists a number of approaches and associated FOMs for assessment of image quality in MDCT. It is known that the assessment of image quality (including target, background and noise) needs to be task based, which implies that the approach and associated FOMs that are optimal to a task may not be optimal to another task (Myers 2000). At levels of fidelity, complexity and cost, these approaches and FOMs interact with one another and often lead to confusion as one is trying to have insightful understanding of the fundamentals that are usually presented in a manner jumping back and forth cross the spatial and frequency domains. Hence, to have an in-depth understanding of these approaches and FOMs, it is essential to grasp the basic concepts of signal detection, statistical decision and psychophysics, on which those approaches and FOMs are grounded.

6.2.1 Signal and Noise

In medicine, a signal is defined as pathophysiologic lesion(s) located in the biological environment inside the human body. The lesion(s) may be an anatomic abnormality that is focal or dispersive in tissues/organs (e.g., mass or stenosis) and/or malfunctions (e.g., cardiovascular ejection fraction and perfusion rates). In the realm of medical imaging, a signal is defined as the difference between a lesion and its healthy surroundings, characterized by its intensity (or contrast), shape, size and location. In the language of signal detection, a signal is usually defined as a function $s(x, t)$, where x and t, respectively, denote the location and time at which the signal is observed. In its simplest form, $s(x, t)$ may be approximated as a deterministic signal with known shape and size at a specified location, which is the case of the signal known exactly (SKE) and background known exactly (BKE) (ICRU 1996) Furthermore, as a result of the intra- and inter-patient variation in pathophysiology, we should be aware of that the signal $s(x, t)$ may be variable, e.g., the locations of lesions move over a number of specified spots, or more generally may vary statistically in other attributions, e.g., intensity. These two cases have been, respectively, termed as signal known exactly but variable (SKEV) and signal known statistically (SKS) in the literature, and their treatment in mathematics is much more complicated than the SKE/BKE case and is still an open area for research (ICRU 1996; Myers 2000). In any case, it makes more sense for us to treat the signal $s(x, t)$ as a random (stochastic) process.

It is basic understanding that the subject contrast of a pathophysiologic lesion (original signal) in CT is expressed by X-ray photons' interaction (mainly the photoelectric absorption and Compton scattering) with tissues and organs and its variation while the X-ray beam is penetrating the human body (Bushberg 2012; Johns and Cunningham 1983; Cody et al. 2005). Presented in Figure 6.3a is a schematic diagram showing the image formation process of CT (and other X-ray–related imaging modalities) (Myers 2000). The two Gaussian-shaped distributions (dotted profiles) above the first block in Figure 6.3a, which is reasonably assumed according to the central-limit theorem, denote the cases of signal present and absent (or signal and background), respectively. Let $s_1(x_1, t)$ and $s_0(x_0, t)$ be the cases of signal present and absent, respectively, associated with the uncertainty denoted by $\sigma_1(x_1, t)$ and $\sigma_0(x_0, t)$. The SNR at the subject contrast stage is (Myers 2000)

$$SNR_{ori} = \frac{(s_{1,ori}(x_1, t) - s_{0,ori}(x_0, t))}{\frac{1}{2}\left(\sigma_{1,ori}^2(x_1, t) + \sigma_{0,ori}^2(x_0, t)\right)^{\frac{1}{2}}} \tag{6.1}$$

which is actually the Euclidean distance between the means of the two populations corresponding to the two cases normalized by the averaged intra-population standard deviation. Usually, the signal is assumed small in magnitude (i.e., low signal) in assessment of image quality, i.e., $s_1(x_1, t) - s_0(x_0, t) \rightarrow 0$, and accordingly we have $\sigma_1(x_1, t) \approx \sigma_0(x_0, t)$ (Myers 2000).

The subject contrast (original signal) can be modulated (usually enhanced) by extrinsic factors, such as the enhancement by the iodinated contrast agent and lowered energy level in data acquisition. Notably, the extrinsic factors may inevitably increase the variation in expressed subject contrast, as illustrated by the two Gaussian distributions at larger standard deviation (dashed profiles above the second block in Figure 6.3a). Also, those extrinsic factors may favorably increase the intensity of the expressed signal, i.e., the two Gaussian distributions may shift horizontally (not shown in Figure 6.3). Hence, the SNR at the stage of the signal expressed is

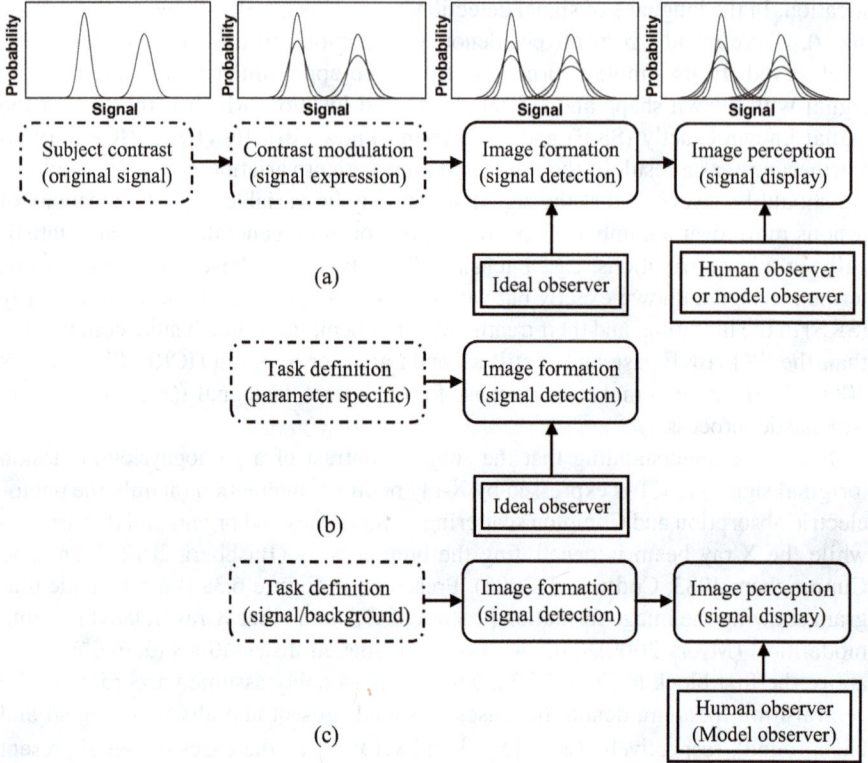

FIGURE 6.3 The schematic diagrams showing (a) the imaging chain of a medical imaging system, (b) assessment of the imaging system's performance and (c) the image quality perceived by an end user.

$$SNR_{exp} = \frac{(s_{1,exp}(x_1,t) - s_{0,exp}(x_0,t))}{\frac{1}{2}\left(\sigma_{1,exp}^2(x_1,t) + \sigma_{0,exp}^2(x_0,t)\right)^{1/2}} \qquad (6.2)$$

6.2.2 DETECTION OF SIGNAL IN NOISE

Noise is ubiquitous in medical imaging and can be characterized by a random (stochastic) process $n(x,t)$. In addition to the intra- and inter-patient pathophysiologic variation mentioned earlier, the quantum noise associated with X-ray photons' nature may enlarge the fluctuation in the formed image (detected signal). In signal detection theory, it is basic understanding that the conspicuity of the signal is determined by its intensity against the uncertainty in itself and the background, i.e., the SNR.

As will be elucidated later, the performance of an imaging system is jointly determined by its signal-transferring property and noise behavior. In general, the signal to be transferred in CT consists of the zero frequency (direct current) and non-zero frequency (detail) components, and their transferring depends jointly on the quantum efficiency of the X-ray detector used for data acquisition and the system's MTF. In reality, a CT is of limited system aperture (Hanson 1979, 1981; Wagner 1979; Wagner and Brown 1985) and thus not all the non-zero frequency details are equally transferred, leading to distortion or contamination in the signal, i.e., signals $s_{1,exp}(x_1,t)$ and $s_{0,exp}(x_0,t)$ at the stage of signal expression are converted into $s_{1,formed}(x_1,t)$ and $s_{0,formed}(x_0,t)$ at the stage of signal formation via a mapping that is assumed linear at this moment. There also exists electronic (thermal shot) noise in electronic systems, including CT that is basically a form of electronic systems, in addition to the quantum noise, which adds up to the uncertainties denoted by $\sigma_{1,exp}(x_1,t)$ and $\sigma_{0,exp}(x_0,t)$, leading to enlarged uncertainty $\sigma_{1,formed}(x_1,t)$ and $\sigma_{0,formed}(x_0,t)$ at the stage of image formation. Hence, at the stage of image formation, the signal in noise can be characterized by the two Gaussian distributions (thin solid profiles) above the third block in Figure 6.3a, and the resultant SNR turns into

$$SNR_{formed} = \frac{(s_{1,formed}(x_1,t) - s_{0,formed}(x_0,t))}{\frac{1}{2}\left(\sigma^2_{1,formed}(x_1,t) + \sigma^2_{0,formed}(x_0,t)\right)^{1/2}} \qquad (6.3)$$

Notably, in general, we have $SNR_{formed} < SNR_{expressed}$, since in reality an imaging system, including CT, cannot be perfect (at full fidelity) in transferring a signal over the entire spectrum, i.e., $(s_{1,formed}(x_1,t) - s_{0,formed}(x_0,t)) < (s_{1,exp}(x_1,t) - s_{0,exp}(x_0,t))$, in addition to the inevitable addition of quantum and electronic noise that implies $\sigma_{1,formed}(x_1,t) > \sigma_{1,exp}(x_1,t)$ and $\sigma_{0,formed}(x_1,t) > \sigma_{0,exp}(x_1,t)$. Also, consensus in the community is that the performance of an imaging system should be assessed at this stage by an ideal observer, which provides an upper bound in the imaging system's performance that is determined by the system's hardware. As such, the capability of an imaging system can be objectively assessed and optimized, though the upper bound in the imaging performance can never be reached by a human observer due to psychophysics factors (see Myers 2000 and more detail later in this chapter).

6.2.3 PERCEPTION OF SIGNAL IN NOISE

The end user of CT is usually a radiologist who searches for lesions in the images, interprets the findings based on his/her expertise and experience, and makes the final diagnostic decision for other clinicians to use to treat the patient. From the standpoint of psychophysics, a few factors, such as fidelity in image presentation, display window level and width, ambient lighting, fatigue, visual preference, confidence on landmarks and texture, and even internal noise, play critical or at least important roles in the visual process. Moreover, the inter-viewer variation may also play an important role in image quality assessment. Inclusively, all these factors add up and enlarge the variation at the stage of signal perception ($\sigma_{1,perceived}(x_1,t)$ and $\sigma_{0,perceived}(x_0,t)$) in the cases of signal present and absent, as shown in the two Gaussian distributions (thick solid profiles) above the fourth block in Figure 6.3a. As a result, the SNR at this stage becomes

$$SNR_{perceived} = \frac{(s_{1,perceived}(x_1,t) - s_{0,perceived}(x_0,t))}{\frac{1}{2}\left(\sigma_{1,perceived}^2(x_1,t) + \sigma_{0,perceived}^2(x_0,t)\right)^{1/2}} \qquad (6.4)$$

where $s_{1,perceived}(x_1,t)$ and $s_{0,perceived}(x_0,t)$ denote the signals perceived by a human observer.

Again, in general, we have $SNR_{perceived} < SNR_{formed} < SNR_{exp}$, since in reality we have $\left(s_{1,perceived}(x_1,t) - s_{0,perceived}(x_0,t)\right) < \left(s_{1,formed}(x_1,t) - s_{0,formed}(x_0,t)\right) < \left(s_{1,exp}(x_1,t) - s_{0,exp}(x_0,t)\right)$, and $\sigma_{1,perceived}(x_1,t) > \sigma_{1,formed}(x_1,t) > \sigma_{1,exp}(x_1,t)$ and $\sigma_{0,perceived}(x_0,t) > \sigma_{0,formed}(x_0,t) > \sigma_{0,exp}(x_0,t)$. At this stage the image quality should be assessed by a human observer (see more details later), which provides an assessment of the ultimate image quality that can be perceived by a radiologist or other professionals, e.g., clinicians and medical physicists.

In reality, except for being counted as the landmarks to assist physicians in making diagnostic decisions, the surrounding anatomy superimposed on the pathophysiological lesion(s) is essentially another source of noise. Apparently, the so-called structured noise violates the assumption the noise's wide-sense stationarity and ergodicity and thus makes the assessment of imaging performance and image quality extremely challenging in medical imaging (Myers 2000; Abbey and Barret 2001; Abbey and Eckstein 2007). Fortunately, however, this is not the case in CT since the anatomic superimposition is effectively removed or largely reduced by the tomographic process (Hanson 1979).

6.2.4 TASK SPECIFICATION

In general, a task is defined as a job to be accomplished in the relevant environment (ICRU 1996; Myers 2000). For example, in consumer electronic imaging, e.g., digital camera, the task is to ensure aesthetical visualization of subject(s) at vivid color and sharpness, while that in medical imaging is to make the fidelity of pathophysiological presentation from which the clinician can find the target at the highest sensitivity (true positivity) under a preset false positivity (or false alarm, as termed in the Pearson criteria (Wald 1942)) as the highest priority. The assessment of image quality in medical imaging needs to be task-based, and thus the identification and specification of a task is of prominent importance. Depending on the ultimate goal, a task in medical imaging may fall into two primary categories: classification and estimation (ICRU 1996; Myers 2000). The classification between the two cases of lesion present (positive) and absent (negative) at one single and/or multiple locations is called signal detection. Under estimation, the task is to get a quantitative characterization of pathophysiological parameters, e.g., tumor size and stage, vascular stenosis and calcification score, or the wash-in and wash-out of contrast agent. Conceptually, estimation is a superset of classification, if each value of the parameter(s) to be estimated is treated as a target to be classified (ICRU 1996; Myers 2000). Recognizing the fact that assessment of estimation performance is much more challenging than that of classification, we constrain our effort on classification in this chapter, in alignment with the practice that has been in the field for a long while.

Ideally, the identification of tasks for image quality assessment should be as objective as possible in representing clinical practice. For example, in the case of malignance detection, the size, shape, boundary, texture, infiltration to surrounding tissues/organs and intra-tumor inhomogeneity are of clinical relevance. In reality, however, the defining of tasks has to weigh the fidelity of clinical representation, feasibility of implementation and standardization for wide acceptance, which, in general, leads to simplification and abstraction of the pathophysiological signal in its shape, magnitude, size, boundary and location, and uniformity in the background (ICRU 1996; Myers 2000). The noise is usually assumed to observe the Gaussian distribution, though it may be white or colored, depending if there exists inter-pixel correlation (Myers 2000; Abbey and Barret 2001; Abbey and Eckstein 2007).

In the simplest implementation of image quality assessment, the signal is assumed to appear at a single specified location, which is usually not the case in the clinic. To make the assessment of image quality objective in representing clinical cases, especially in the situation when clumpy noise occurs, the signal should appear at one of the multiple locations. To be of sufficient statistical power, the signal's magnitude, which is jointly dependent on contrast and size, needs to be adequately low. Moreover, effort should be made to avoid the appearance of unintended visual features that may provide clues (and thus bias), along with the awareness that the noise and sharpness (spatial resolution) may actually change in a CT image, especially approaching the periphery of an image, though it is common for us to assume shift invariance in spatial resolution and stationarity in noise (ICRU 1996; Myers 2000).

6.2.5 TASK-BASED ASSESSMENT OF IMAGE QUALITY

Having defined the signal, noise and the task of detecting a signal in noise, it is now time for us to go through the cascaded medical imaging process illustrated in Figure 6.3a. Basically, it is identical to what has been proposed in the literature as two primary stages (ICRU 1996; Myers 2000): image formation (data acquisition/record) and image perception (image display/presentation). Such a separation is straightforward in digital imaging modalities, e.g., CT, but quite intricate in the early day analog imaging modalities, e.g., X-ray screen-film radiography. To be a bit more instructive, I added two pre-stages – subject contrast and contrast modulation – to the process. Given a specific task, the assessment of an imaging system's performance is carried out by an ideal observer (Figure 6.3b), while that of image quality is by a human observer (Figure 6.3c). Prior to delving into the details of assessing image quality, we need to get further prepared by exposing ourselves to more fundamental concepts, presented next.

6.2.6 IDEAL OBSERVER AND STATISTICAL DECISION-MAKING

In general, the assessment of imaging system performance and image quality consists of three major elements (Myers 2000): (i) a specific task (as introduced earlier), (ii) an observer who is assigned to the task and (iii) an FOM to quantitatively rate the observer's performance. As we'll see later in this chapter, there are a number of observers in reality, and the most omnipotent one is the ideal observer. Intuitively, an ideal observer refers to someone who fully knows the signal (intensity, shape, size and location), background and noise, and looks for the signal's appearance at a specified location. In statistical decision theory, the ideal observer is a decision maker who possesses all the needed information regarding the signal/background and noise (statistical property). Hence, he/she can make a decision on the signal's presence while minimizing the associated error or cost, such as the Bayesian risk (Berger 1985) or those by other criterion, e.g., the Pearson criterion for detecting a signal at the highest sensitivity under specified false alarm.

Let's have a relatively formal definition of the ideal observer here in the statistical decision theory, in which the noise is assumed as uncorrelated (i.e., white noise), wide-sense stationary and ergodic (Wagner 1979; ICRU 1996). We first denote the pixels in the CT image as a one-dimensional vector $\boldsymbol{g} = \left[g_1, \ldots, g_m, \ldots, g_M \right]^T_{1 \times M}$ and then suppose the noise in the image is additive and observes the Gaussian distribution. Under hypotheses H_0 and H_1 corresponding to the cases of a signal absent and present (s_0 and s_1 by stripping off the spatial and temporal dependence x and t from the notations used earlier for simplicity in expression), we have

$$\begin{cases} H_0: & g_m = \bar{g}_{m0} + n_{m0} & m = 1,2,\ldots,M \\ H_1: & g_m = \bar{g}_{m1} + n_{m1} & m = 1,2,\ldots,M \end{cases} \tag{6.5}$$

In the task of low signal detection, we have $n_{m0} = n_{m1} = n_m$, and thus Equation 6.5 can be rewritten into

$$\begin{cases} H_0: & g_m = \bar{g}_{m0} + n_m & m = 1,2,\ldots,M \\ H_1: & g_m = \bar{g}_{m1} + n_m & m = 1,2,\ldots,M \end{cases} \tag{6.6}$$

Under the assumption of additive Gaussian noise, we have

$$\begin{cases} H_0: & Prob(\boldsymbol{g}|H_0) = \prod_{m=1}^{M} \dfrac{1}{\sqrt{2\pi}\sigma} \exp\left(\dfrac{-\left(g_m - \bar{g}_{m0}\right)^2}{2\sigma^2} \right) \\[4mm] H_1: & Prob(\boldsymbol{g}|H_1) = \prod_{m=1}^{M} \dfrac{1}{\sqrt{2\pi}\sigma} \exp\left(\dfrac{-\left(g_m - \bar{g}_{m1}\right)^2}{2\sigma^2} \right) \end{cases} \tag{6.7}$$

where $Prob(\boldsymbol{g} \mid H_0)$ and $Prob(\boldsymbol{g} \mid H_1)$ denote the likelihood (joint probability) of observing all the image pixels $\boldsymbol{g} = \left[g_1, \ldots, g_m, \ldots, g_M \right]^T_{1 \times M}$ under the two hypotheses. We can have the likelihood ratio defined as

$$(\boldsymbol{g}) = \frac{Prob(\boldsymbol{g}|H_1)}{Prob(\boldsymbol{g}|H_0)} = \frac{\displaystyle\prod_{m=1}^{M} \dfrac{1}{\sqrt{2\pi}\sigma} \exp\left(\dfrac{-\left(g_m - \bar{g}_{m1}\right)^2}{2\sigma^2} \right)}{\displaystyle\prod_{m=1}^{M} \dfrac{1}{\sqrt{2\pi}\sigma} \exp\left(\dfrac{-\left(g_m - \bar{g}_{m0}\right)^2}{2\sigma^2} \right)} \tag{6.8}$$

A decision that accepts the hypothesis H_1 can be made if the likelihood ratio is larger than a threshold Λ_c, i.e., $\Lambda(g) \geq \Lambda_c$, or accepts the null hypothesis H_0 if $\Lambda(g) < \Lambda_c$. It has been shown that the likelihood ratio is an ideal observer who compares the likelihood ratio with an optimum threshold that is set to minimize the decision errors or average cost (Berger 1985).

In statistical decision theory, the observer is also called a decision variable or test statistic. For convenience in calculation, the decision variable or test statistic corresponding to the likelihood ratio can be simplified by incurring the monotonic logarithmic transformation (Myers 2000)

$$
\begin{aligned}
(g) = \log((g)) &= \sum_{m=1}^{M} \frac{-(g_m - \bar{g}_{m1})^2}{2\sigma^2} + \frac{(g_m - \bar{g}_{m0})^2}{2\sigma^2} \\
&= \sum_{m=1}^{M} \left(\frac{(\bar{g}_{m1} - \bar{g}_{m0})g_m}{\sigma^2} - \frac{\bar{g}_{m1}^2 - \bar{g}_{m0}^2}{2\sigma^2} \right) \cong \sum_{m=1}^{M} \left(\frac{(\bar{g}_{m1} - \bar{g}_{m0})g_m}{\sigma^2} \right)
\end{aligned}
\tag{6.9}
$$

As it has no influence on the decision-making, the constant term is removed from Equation 6.9 at the last step. Notably, the log-likelihood ratio is still an ideal observer if the decision rule is updated as: accepts the hypothesis H_1 if $\lambda(g) \geq \lambda_c$, otherwise accepts hypothesis H_0 if $\lambda(g) < \lambda_c$, where $\lambda_c = \log(\Lambda_c)$.

Without losing generality, Equation 6.9 can be reformatted into matrix form as

$$
\lambda(g) = \Delta\bar{g}^T (\sigma^2 I)^{-1} g
\tag{6.10}
$$

where the superscript T denotes matrix transpose. It is interesting and important to note that the production of σ^2 and unity diagonal matrix I ($\sigma^2 I$) is actually the covariance matrix under the assumption of white noise. Moreover, as shown in Equation 6.10, the Bayesian ideal observer is actually a linear cross-correlation operation $\Delta\bar{g}^T g$ (also called matched filter; see more in Section 6.4). According to the central-limit theorem in statistics, the log-likelihood decision variable (test statistics) obeys the bi-normal distribution, as shown in one of the examples illustrated in Figure 6.4b.

In the case of colored noise, Equation 6.10 becomes

$$
\lambda(g) = \Delta\bar{g}^T (K_n)^{-1} g
\tag{6.11}
$$

where K_n denotes the covariance matrix that is no longer diagonal because of the noise's color. In fact, the Bayesian ideal observer under colored noise is essentially the pre-whitening matched filter (see more in Section 6.6.1) that was derived by North in 1943 (North 1943) in the frequency domain, in which the Schwarz inequality in the integral form was used in a very clever manner. North's original derivation was for signal detection in radar, and it influenced generations of engineers and graduate students in the field of electrical and electronic engineering (Burgess 1999). The functional form of the ideal observer under other situations, such as Poisson

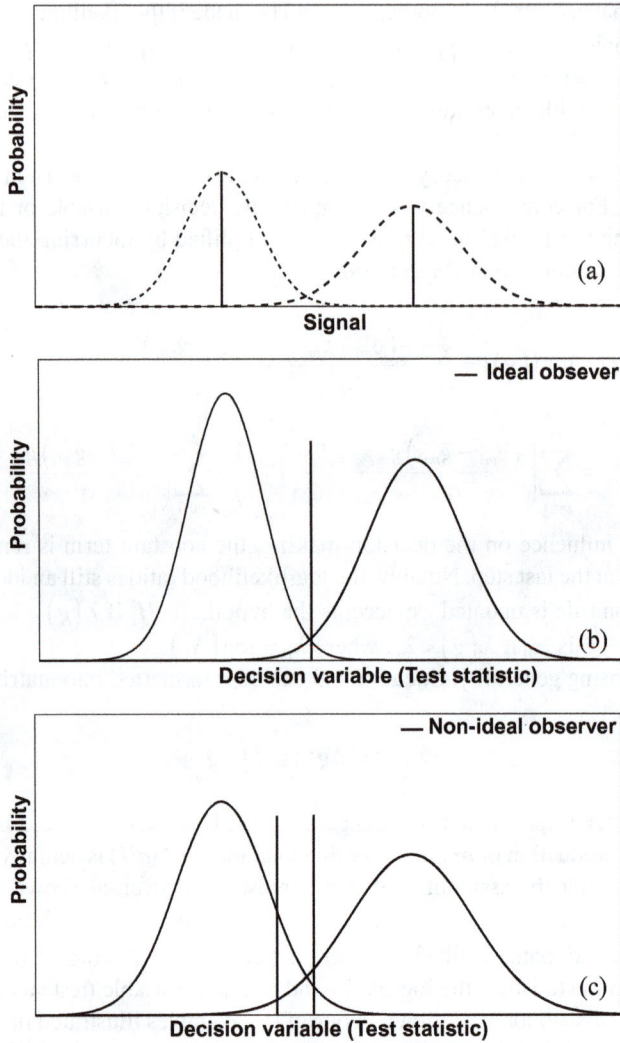

FIGURE 6.4 Schematic diagrams showing the probability distribution of (a) the signal, the process of decision-making by an ideal (b) or non-ideal (c) observer.

noise and the SKS case, is more complicated and readers interested in the details are referred to references in the literature (ICRU 1996; Myers 2000).

6.2.7 Ideal Observer and Associated Figures of Merit

Given the decision variable corresponding to the ideal observer defined in Equation 6.10, its performance can be quantitatively characterized by the detectability index defined as

$$d' = \frac{\left(\overline{\lambda_1}(g) - \overline{\lambda_1}(g)\right)}{\frac{1}{2}\left(\sigma_{\lambda_1}^2(g) + \sigma_{\lambda_0}^2(g)\right)^{1/2}} \tag{6.12}$$

which is also the Euclidean distance between the peaks of the bi-normal distribution (Tong 1990) normalized by the averaged variance. However, it should be noted that Equation 6.12 is valid only under the condition that the decision variable obeys or asymptotically obeys the Gaussian distribution, which, fortunately is the case in reality, according to the central-limit theorem in statistics (Durrett 2019). Therefore, given an ideal observer at the stage of image formation (Figure 6.4a), we have $d' = SNR_{formed}$.

By definition, the ideal observer knows exactly how to set the threshold for decision-making, i.e., it should be close to but not exactly in the middle of the bi-normal distribution, as exemplified in Figure 6.4b. In reality, no one is as wise as the ideal observer who sets the threshold exactly between the twin peaks of the bi-normal distribution, but an alternative strategy is to move the threshold cross the entire range as illustrated in Figure 6.4c. As such, given each threshold, there is a set of quantitative entities (Myers 2000):

$$TPF = \int_{\lambda_c}^{\infty} Prob(g \mid H_1) dg \tag{6.13}$$

$$FPF = \int_{\lambda_c}^{\infty} Prob(g \mid H_0) dg \tag{6.14}$$

$$TNF = \int_{-\infty}^{c} Prob(g \mid H_0) dg \tag{6.15}$$

$$FPF = \int_{-\infty}^{c} Prob(g \mid H_1) dg \tag{6.16}$$

in which TPF, FPF, TNF and FPF stand for the fraction corresponding to true positive, false positive, true negative and false positive, respectively. The TPF is termed Sensitivity, while the FPF is (1 – Specificity). By sweeping the threshold cross the entire range, the ROC curve can be formed with Sensitivity as the coordinate and (1 – Specificity) the abscess. Two examples of ROC curve are given in Figure 6.5, wherein the two circles on the ROC curves denote the operating condition of each observer. By definition, the area under the ROC curve (AUC) is an FOM that characterizes the observer performance. In the examples displayed in Figure 6.5, $AUC_A > AUC_B$, meaning that observer A outperforms observer B. Notably, the AUC of an ideal observer is maximized, but not perfect (i.e., AUC ≠ 1.0), unless there exists

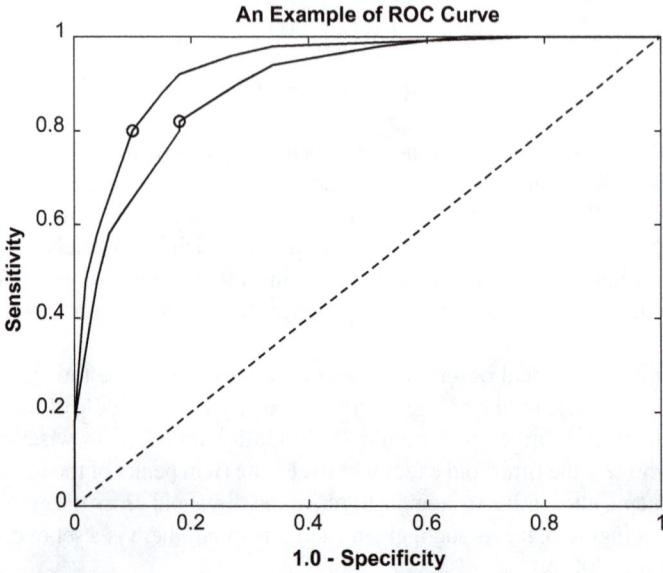

FIGURE 6.5 Diagram showing an example of two ROC curves, where the two circles indicate the operating conditions in each ROC curve.

no overlap between the two populations in the bi-normal distribution. Moreover, if someone makes the decision by taking chance, their performance is along the 45° diagonal dashed line (AUC = 0.5) (Metz 2000; Tourassi 2019).

An inspection of Equations 6.9–6.11 tells us that in general the decision variable is a linear summation of image pixels (random variables) and thus it is reasonable for us to assume that the decision variable obeys Gaussian distribution, which leads to the equality (Myers 2000)

$$AUC_A = \frac{1}{2} + \frac{1}{2} erf\left(\frac{d_A}{2}\right)$$ (6.17)

where $erf(\cdot)$ is the error function defined by

$$erf(z) = \frac{\pi}{\sqrt{2}} \int_0^z e^{-y^2} dy$$ (6.18)

Reversely, from AUC, we may get d_A defined next as a surrogate of the detectability d'

$$d_A = 2erf^{-1}(2AUC_A - 1)$$ (6.19)

Note that the equality $d_A = d'$ holds only under the condition that the decision variable observes Gaussian distribution.

6.2.8 HUMAN OBSERVER AND THEIR EFFICIENCY

As stated earlier, the performance of an ideal observer is the upper bound that cannot be reached by other observers. Due to the following reasons, the performance of a human observer is inferior to that of the ideal observer, as it would be very difficult, if not impossible, for a human observer to know the exact bi-normal distribution and set the threshold right according to the criterion. Additionally, a human observer may suffer from imperfect viewing conditions (ambient lighting, viewing distance, extra-large spatial extent occupied by the signal or even artifacts), fatigue, visual preference, lack of landmark and even internal noise, which are tantamount to broadened variance and thus increase the overlapping between the two populations in the bi-normal distribution (Figure 6.4c). As a result, the performance of a human observer is inferior to that of the ideal observer, i.e., $AUC_{Human} < AUC_{Ideal}$.

In practice, there are two ways – forced choice and rating scale – to conduct a human observer study, and following is a brief introduction to them and their associated pros and cons (Myers 2000; Abbey and Eckstein 2019).

- **Yes/no experiment**: Formally, this is called the two-alternative forced-choice (2AFC) approach, the simpler of the forced-choice category, in which a human observer is presented with a group of paired images corresponding to a signal present and absent. The observer is asked to choose the image in which the signal is present at a specified location, and the observer's score (percentage) of making the correct decision (P_C) is taken as the FOM that is a surrogate of AUC_A. The major pros of 2AFC are simplicity in implementation, as the observer is required to make a decision between a pair of images, and ease in analysis, but its cons include (i) a relatively large number of paired images is required and thus is suitable in situations when images are relatively easy to obtain, (ii) the magnitude of the signal has to be very low (weak), which may be quite demanding in practice, and (iii) the AUC_A obtained from the percentage correct P_C is only a summary FOM.
- **Multi-alternative forced choice (MAFC)**: This is a generation of 2AFC, in which an observer is presented with a number of grouped images and each group consists of M ($M > 2$) images (or M sub-images from one single image), and the observer is asked to choose the image (or sub-image) in which the signal is present. Again, the score (percentage) of the observer making the correct decision (P_C) is taken as a surrogate of AUC_A. Compared to 2AFC, the MAFC requires fewer images for an observer to work with, while the requirement of low signal magnitude can be adequately relaxed, and thus making implementation less demanding in practice. The MAFC experiment is especially suitable in situations when the availability or commitment of the human observer (radiological clinician) is limited. However, with increasing M, the analysis in MAFC becomes difficult, in addition to the disadvantage that, similar to 2AFC, this approach just provides only one single summary FOM.

- **Rating scale**: In comparison to 2AFC and MAFC, the human observer in a rating-scale experiment needs to be more attentive, because the observer is requested to rate their confidence on the possibility of the signal present and absent, usually via a five-point scale, e.g., signal definitely present (5), signal probably present (4), neutral (3), signal probably absent (2) and signal definitely absent (1). In practice, only seven samples, including the extremity at (0, 0) and (1, 1), are acquired over the entire range, and a smooth ROC curve can be obtained by either parametric (e.g., histogram fitting and ROC smoothing) or non-parametric (e.g., increasing monotonic transformation to get bi-normal distribution) data fitting (Metz 2000; Tourassi 2019). The forte of the rating-scale scheme lies at its capability of providing a whole picture of the ROC curve, rather than just one summary AUC_A. Additionally, roughly half of the number of images are needed in the rating-scale scheme, compared to that needed in 2AFC, which should be counted as a pro in situations in which the accessibility to images is limited.

In practice, the performance of a human observer in image quality assessment is evaluated using the metric called observer efficiency (Burgess 1999; Myers 2000)

$$\eta = \left(\frac{d_A^{human}}{d_A^{ideal}} \right)^2 \tag{6.20}$$

where d_A^{human} is obtained using Equation 6.19. Based on extensive experimental studies, it has been found that (i) under white noise, human observer performance is relatively stable ($\eta = 30\%\text{--}50\%$); (ii) under colored noise, human observer performance quickly drops to approximately 20%; (iii) a human observer is not sensitive to low-frequency noise, but their performance degrades dramatically if the noise's spectrum at low frequency is in the form f^n (Abbey and Eckstein 2007), where n is an integer; (iv) the performance of a human observer is poor over band noise, probably due to the fact that the human visual system works under a mechanism of channelization, leading to dramatic performance drop if the noise's spectral band mismatches that of the human visual system; (v) the human observer's performance in the SKS task does not drop too much compared to the ideal observer, i.e., it holds at ~50%. For more details, interested readers are referred to the literature (Burgess 1999; Myers 2000).

6.2.9 MODEL OBSERVERS

Usually, a radiologist is the end user of CT images for clinical diagnosis and thus it is certainly justified that the human observer study is the method of choice for image quality assessment. However, as one knows, the implementation of a human observer study is laborious and time-consuming, especially when in most cases a CT designer may only be interested in adjustment or optimization of a couple of parameters among the many parameters that affect the image quality. Moreover, a human observer may be under the influence of inadequate viewing conditions, fatigue, biased preference, and inter-case and inter-observer inconsistency, among others, which may further degrade their performance. Together, these factors may make a model observer (also called a machine or algorithmic observer) more appealing in terms of cost, objectiveness and consistency.

In recent years, extensive effort has been invested on exploring model observers' utility in carrying out objective image quality assessment in a cost-effective and consistent manner. Quite a few outcomes have made the model observers implemented in algorithms successful surrogates for human observers (Barret et al. 1993; Eckstein et al. 2000). Thus far, the most well-studied models include non-prewhitening (NPW) matched filter, non-prewhitening matched filter with eye filter (NPWE), Hotelling (pre-whitening matched filter) observer and channelized Hotelling observer (CHO). These models are linear and implemented in the spatial domain, with the channelized Hotelling model as the most successful (Barret et al. 1993; ICRU 1996; Abbey and Bochud 2000; Abbey and Eckstein, 2001, 2007, 2019; Kupinski 2019).

6.3 ASSESSMENT OF IMAGE QUALITY VIA FIGURE OF MERIT IN SPATIAL DOMAIN

Historically, all the approaches and FOMs for assessing imaging system performance and image quality initiate in the spatial domain, and accordingly we do so in this subsection.

6.3.1 PIXEL-WISE SIGNAL, CONTRAST AND SNR

Given the humanoid phantom displayed in Figure 6.6, suppose we want to measure the signal and contrast between the target and background. It is common to draw an ROI (dashed circle) within the target and another ROI (circle in dotted and dashed line) in the background (bkg). Then, the pixel-wise signal, contrast and SNR can be gauged using the following formulae:

$$signal = \bar{m}_{target} - \bar{m}_{bkg} \tag{6.21}$$

$$contrast = \frac{\bar{m}_{target} - \bar{m}_{bkg}}{\frac{1}{2}\left(\bar{m}_{target} + \bar{m}_{bkg}\right)} \tag{6.22}$$

$$SNR = \frac{\bar{m}_{target} - \bar{m}_{bkg}}{\frac{1}{2}\left(\sigma_{target}^2 + \sigma_{bkg}^2\right)^{1/2}} \tag{6.23}$$

where $\bar{m}_{target}$ and $\bar{m}_{bkg}$ are the means gauged in ROI$_{target}$ and ROI$_{bkg}$, respectively, while σ_{target} and σ_{bkg} are the associated standard deviation. Given a pixel in an image, its noise, in theory, should be gauged as the standard deviation over an ensemble of pixels that are at that location over a statistically sufficient number of images. The assumption of ergodicity in noise ensures that the noise can be estimated by

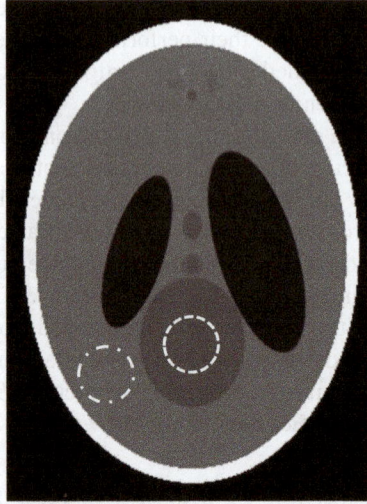

FIGURE 6.6 Schematic illustration of gauging pixel-wise signal, contrast, and signal-to-noise (SNR) ratio.

the standard deviation gauged in an ROI centered at the pixel, while that of wide-sense stationary ensures that the noise is statistically constant over the entire image. However, we have to be aware of that we have actually made an assumption that the FOMs defined in Equations 6.21–6.23 are pixel-wise defined and thus flawed in at least two aspects: (i) the signal's size (or dimension) is not taken into account, but usually the signal's size is substantially larger than a pixel; (ii) the noise's morphology (correlation) is ignored, but the morphology of noise in CT may dramatically affect perception of the signal. For example, the two CT images displayed in Figure 6.7 are of identical pixel-wise SNR, but, apparently, they differ substantially in visual conspicuity. Thus, though those pixel-wise FOMs may be sufficient for day-to-day quality assurance and/or protocol optimization, they may be misleading in situations when the tasks under study are complicated (Burgess 1999).

6.3.2 ROSE MODEL

In mid-20th century (1946–1948), Rose published three consecutive papers on human's visual detection of signals and its application in performance evaluation of electronic imaging systems (Rose 1946, 1948a, 1948b, 1953). The model bearing his name is based on an insightful understanding that fluctuations in the photons that form a scene play a fundamental role in limiting human's visual capability. A retrospective reviewing of this model shows that Rose is indisputably one of the most brilliant scientists in psychophysics, not only because of the prominent significance of his model but also the fact that he derived it prior to the birth of signal detection and statistical decision theory (Burgess 1999). By treating light as a flux of photons (particles) and exercising Poisson statistics, Rose obtained the result that is essentially an

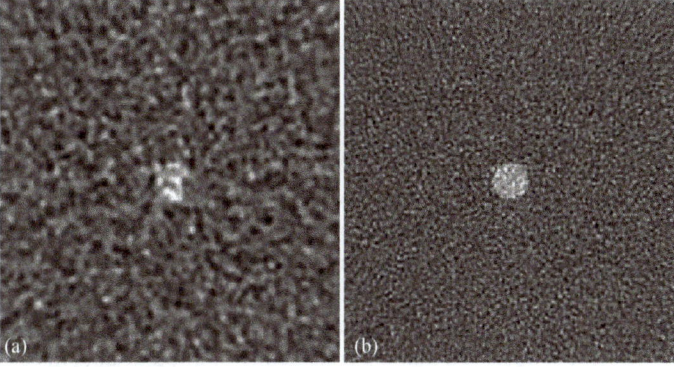

FIGURE 6.7 Presentation of two (a and b) CT images that are at quantitative identical pixel-wise SNR but differ substantially in visual appearance. (Adopted with permission from Boedeker and McNitt-Gray 2007).

approximation of the ideal observer for a SKE/BKE task under assumption of white noise. Basically, the Rose model states

$$SNR_{Rose} = \frac{A(\bar{q}_b - \bar{q}_o)}{\sqrt{A\bar{q}_b}} = C\sqrt{A\bar{q}_b} \qquad (6.24)$$

where A denotes the area (dimension) of the signal (assumed as a box function in Rose's original work), and $\bar{q}_o$ and $\bar{q}_b$ are the mean number of photons in the signal and background areas, respectively. Via extensive experimentation, Rose determined that for a signal to be readily detected by the human visual system, the SNR_{Rose} should be around 5 (actually in the range 3–7) (Rose 1948a; Burgess 1999; Cunningham and Shaw 1999). Setting the parameter k as the critical value of Rose's SNR, from Equation 6.24, we have

$$C_T = \frac{k}{\sqrt{A\bar{q}_b}} \qquad (6.25)$$

which is consistent with our experience in daily life that the larger a signal's dimension, the dimmer the signal can be allowed for the signal to be discernible.

The original Rose model was derived in spatial domain for continuous signal, which, in fact, can be paraphrased into its discrete form that is actually a revision of the pixel-wise SNR specified in Equation 6.23:

$$SNR = \frac{\sum_{i=1}^{I}(x_i - \bar{m}_{bkg})}{\frac{1}{2}(\sigma_{ROI1}^2 + \sigma_{ROI2}^2)^{1/2}} \qquad (6.26)$$

Notably, Equation 6.26 can be used only as a "back-of-the-envelope" approach for daily quality assurance or protocol optimization, since it does not take the noise correlation into account (Burgess 1999).

6.3.3 CONTRAST-DETAIL (C-D) APPROACH

Inspired by Rose's work, Sturm and Morgan proposed the contrast-detail (C-D) phantom for assessing imaging system performance and image quality in radiography and fluoroscopy (Sturm and Morgan 1948). The C-D phantom consists of an array of circular dots at various contrast (horizontally) and dimension (vertically) and presented in Figure 6.8 are two CT images of the C-D phantom acquired at different X-ray dose. It is observed that the conspicuity of circular dots in each column, though they are at identical contrast, drops with decreasing dimension, and so does the signal's conspicuity with decreasing contrast in each row. It seems that the C-D phantom can serve well for assessing image quality in CT too. However, the C-D phantom is not an objective approach for assessing imaging system performance and image quality, due to two fundamental issues: (i) an observer knows the existence of circular dots (signal is always present) and (ii) no statistics can be provided by just one single image. Hence, again, the C-D phantom may be used as a daily quality checking tool, but, for objective assessment of imaging system performance and image quality under the framework of signal detection and statistical decision, more sophisticated approaches and FOMs that take noise statistics (correlation) and human observer psychophysics into account should be adopted.

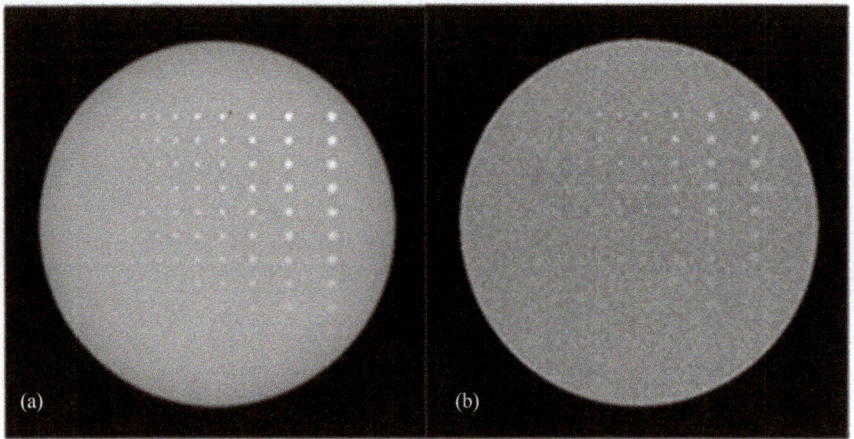

FIGURE 6.8 Simulated CT images of the contrast-detail phantom acquired at a relatively (a) high and (b) low X-ray dose.

6.4 ASSESSMENT OF IMAGE QUALITY IN MDCT VIA FIGURES OF MERIT IN FREQUENCY DOMAIN

The signal transfer property of a linear shift-invariant system can be well character-ized by its impulse response function that is usually termed the point spread func-tion (PSF), as well as in CT as it can be assumed as a linear shift-invariant system if certain assumptions are made. In CT, the PSF is conventionally characterized separately in the in-plane and cross-plane modes. Usually, a metal (e.g., tungsten) wire at high contrast and orthogonal to an image slice serves as the input impulse for in-plane PSF measurement, while a metal (e.g., molybdenum) foil is used for cross-plane measurement. Recently, the geometry for image reconstruction in state-of-the-art MDCT has evolved from 2D into 3D, while the 3D geometry has been utilized from the beginning in CBCT that uses a flat panel for data acquisition. It is becoming increasingly common in the community that the 3D PSF is used in CT for assessment of the signal transferring property (ICRU 1996; Cunningham and Shaw 1999; Cunningham 2000). As in any other linear shift-invariant systems in which the signal transferring property is preferably characterized in the frequency domain, we study CT's signal transferring property, which is jointly determined by CT's noise property and spatial resolution, in the frequency domain in this section.

6.4.1 POINT SPREAD FUNCTION AND OPTICAL TRANSFER FUNCTION

As shown in Figure 6.9a, suppose we have a one-dimensional rectangular pulse function in the spatial domain:

$$PSF(x) = \begin{cases} A & |x| \leq \dfrac{1}{2T} \\ 0 & other \end{cases} \tag{6.27}$$

As illustrated in Figure 6.9b, its Fourier transform is a $sinc(\cdot)$ function in the spatial frequency domain:

$$FT\big(PSF(x)\big) = AT \cdot \frac{\sin(\pi kT)}{\pi kT} \tag{6.28}$$

In general, the Fourier transform of PSF is called the optical transfer function (OTF) (Cunningham 2000), which can be of phase if it is not an even function in the spatial domain (note that k denotes 1D spatial frequency in Equations (6.28) and (6.29), which differs from that in Equation (6.25)).

6.4.2 MODULATION TRANSFER FUNCTION

The modulation transfer function (MTF) is defined as the modular of OTF (Cunningham 2000), i.e.,

$$MTF_{total}(k) = \frac{\big|OTF(k)\big|}{\big|OTF(0)\big|}. \tag{6.29}$$

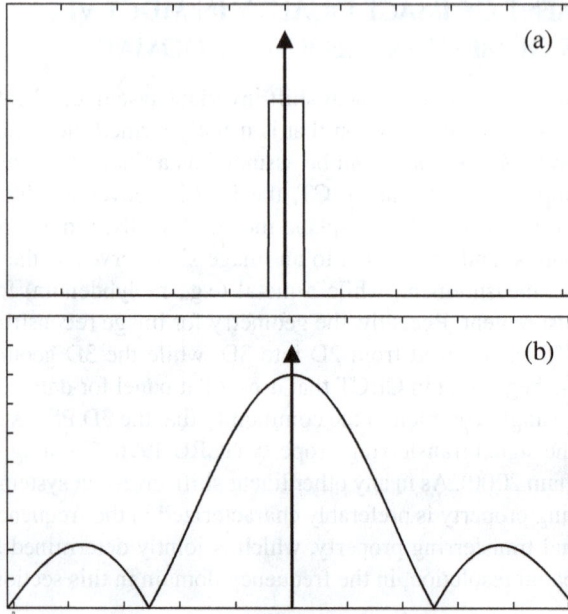

FIGURE 6.9 Schematic profile plots showing (a) a rectangular (impulse) function in spatial domain and (b) its Fourier transform in spatial frequency domain.

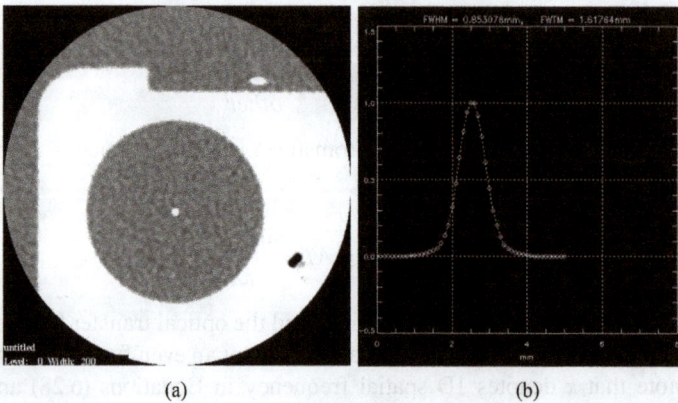

FIGURE 6.10 (a) A CT image of the spatial resolution phantom, in which the tungsten wire is used for the (b) MTF measurement.

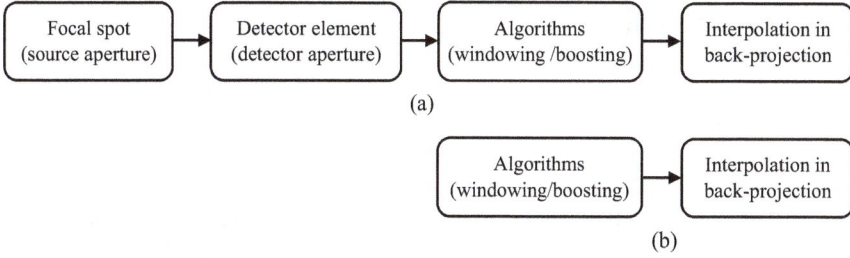

FIGURE 6.11   Schematic diagrams showing (a) the primary loops in the imaging chain that determine the signal transferring (MTF) and (b) noise property (NPS) in a CT.

Displayed in Figure 6.10a is a CT image of a thin tungsten wire, i.e., the in-plane point spread function of CT, along with the plotting of its $MTF_{total}(k)$ in Figure 6.10b. Notably, in addition to characterizing an imaging system's signal (detail) transfer property, the $MTF_{total}(k)$ also serves as a descriptor of the system's spatial resolution. More important, as illustrated in Figure 6.11a, the transferring of signal in CT starts from the X-ray source focal spot – the first loop in the CT imaging chain – goes through the detector element's aperture, followed by the contributions from the algorithmic filter (windowing or other manipulation to obtain adequate trade-off between spatial resolution and noise) and the interpolation carried out in the back-projection for image reconstruction as well. This is the reason that we add "total" as the subscript in Equation 6.29.

6.4.3 NOISE POWER SPECTRUM

In the early days of CT, an observation of the morphologic difference in CT noise against white noise suggested that there was inter-pixel correlation. By analyzing the 2D distribution of noise power over spatial frequency k, i.e., the noise power spectrum $NPS(k)$, the inter-pixel correlation is confirmed, even though there is no inter-element correlation in noise of the detector used for data acquisition (Riederer et al. 1978; Wagner et al. 1979; Hanson 1979, 1980, 1981; Barrett and Swindell 1981; Faulkner and Moores 1984; Kijewski and Judy 1987). Since then, the groundwork of using $NPS(k)$ and spectrum of noise equivalent quanta $NEQ(k)$ to analyze CT signal transfer and noise behavior has been laid out. It has become consensus that the signal transfer property of an imaging system is dependent on its modulation transfer function $MTF(k)$, while the noise property can only be thoroughly characterized by $NPS(k)$ (Siewerdsen et al. 2002; Tward and Siewerdsen 2009; Boedeker et al. 2007; Boedeker and McNitt-Gray 2007; Baek and Pelc 2010). According to the Wiener–Khinchin theorem, the noise power spectrum is defined as the Fourier transform of an autocorrelation function in 2D images (Hanson 1979), i.e.,

$$NPS(k) = \frac{1}{A}\left\langle \left| \iint_A R(x)e^{-2\pi x \cdot k}dx \right| \right\rangle, \qquad (6.30)$$

where $R(x)$ is the autocorrelation and $\langle \cdot \rangle$ denotes the ensemble average. If there is inter-pixel correlation in noise $n(x, t)$ (i.e., colored noise), the scaler entity of noise defined as its pixel-wise standard deviation can no longer faithfully characterize the noise. If this is the case, one has to use the noise power spectrum (Wiener spectrum) defined in Equation 6.30 for noise characterization.

A number of strategies, e.g., the method proposed by Barret (Hanson 1979), the central slice theorem (Barrett and Swindell 1981), information theory (Hanson 1981) and statistical detection theory (Faulkner and Moores 1984), have been exercised to obtain the $NPS(k)$ in CT, and all lead to the same functional form:

$$NPS(k) = \frac{aA}{N_\theta \overline{N}} |k| \left| MTF_{alg}(k) \right|^2 = \frac{\pi}{bN_\theta \overline{N}} |k| \left| MTF_{alg}(k) \right|^2, \qquad (6.31)$$

where a is the detector pitch, b is the detector height and k is the radial frequency. N_θ is the number of angular locations at which the projection data are acquired, and $\overline{N}$ is the mean number of X-ray photons detected at each detector element. As no object should be placed in the X-ray beam in the investigation of noise property, $\overline{N}$ is assumed equal across all the detector elements. $MTF_{alg}(k)$ denotes the algorithmic contributions, including windowing and/or boosting in the frequency domain for optimization between noise and spatial resolution, to the modulation transfer function.

Shown on the left of Figure 6.12 is an example of a CT noise power spectrum, while that on the right is a display of the NPS radial profile, in which the influence (doughnut shape) by the ramp filtering is readily observable.

6.4.4 SPECTRUM OF NOISE EQUIVALENT QUANTA

In general, the spectrum of noise equivalent quanta of an imaging system is in the functional form (Swank 1973; Wagner et al. 1979; Hanson 1979; Wagner and Brown 1985; Metz et al. 1995; ICRU 1996; Barret 2009; Tanguay et al. 2010, 2013, 2015)

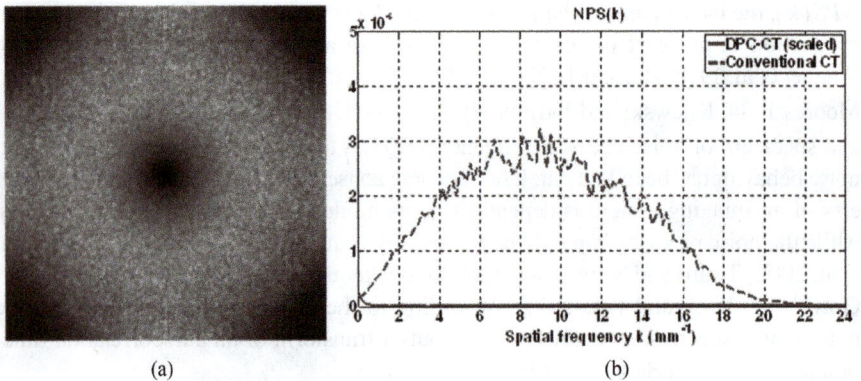

(a)   (b)

FIGURE 6.12 The noise power spectrum shown in (a) 2D distribution and (b) 1D radial profile.

$$NEQ(k) = G^2 \frac{MTF_{total}^2(k)}{NPS(k)}.$$ (6.32)

By definition, G, $MTF_{total}(k)$ and $NPS(k)$ denote the imaging system's large area gain, signal transfer characteristic and noise property, respectively. In various imaging modalities, Equation 6.32 can be in different expressions. For instance, the spectrum of noise equivalent quanta in radiography and fluoroscopy is expressed exactly the same way as in Equation 6.32, whereas that of CT is expressed as

$$NEQ(k) = \frac{\pi}{b} \frac{|k| MTF_{total}^2(k)}{NPS(k)}.$$ (6.33)

6.4.5 Signal-to-Noise Ratio

It should be noted that the NPS in the denominator of Equation 6.33 is measured at the stage of image formation, i.e., it is the NPS right at the imaging system's output. Therefore, if a signal is represented by $\Delta S(k)$ in the spatial frequency domain, its multiplication with the spectrum of noise equivalent quanta is

$$\Delta S(k) NEQ(k) = \frac{\pi}{b} \frac{\Delta S(k)|k| MTF_{total}^2(k)}{NPS(k)}.$$ (6.34)

Then, the signal-to-noise ratio of a CT system is given by the integral

$$SNR = \int_{-\infty}^{\infty} \Delta S(k) NEQ(k) dk$$ (6.35)

It has been proven that the SNR defined in Equation 6.35 is indeed the SNR of an imaging system under the framework of the ideal observer. Equation 6.35 is an integration of factorization and states that, given a specific task $\Delta S(k)$, the ideal observer performance of an imaging system can be optimized by maximizing its $NEQ(k)$. Usually, the task is to differentiate a lesion from the surrounding tissues or organs, or simply an object from its background. Therefore, the signal $\Delta S(k)$ in Equation 6.35 should be perceived as a difference or contrast between the object to be imaged and the background (Wagner et al. 1979; Wagner and Brown 1985; ICRU 1996; Myers 2000).

As pointed out by Wagner et al. (Wagner et al. 1979; Wagner and Brown 1985) and Hanson (Hanson 1979), a linear filter does not affect the $NEQ(k)$ of a CT system that uses FBP for image reconstruction, as long as the $MTF_{alg}(k)$ does not drop to zero ahead of the aperture. However, a linear filter may moderately affect the image quality, as the human observer is not an ideal observer and seems under the mechanism of visual channelization that may incur unrecoverable distortion or lost in signal component in the frequency domain (Myers and Barret 1987; Abbey and Barret 2001). Further, the iterative image reconstruction may totally invalidate the assumption of a linear shift-invariant and stationarity and ergodicity in noise. Thus, the assessment of CT image quality has to use either human or model observers, as introduced in the next sections.

6.4.6 PIECEWISE LINEARIZED SIGNAL TRANSFER PROPERTY AND NOISE BEHAVIOR

As indicated earlier, the assumption of a linear shift-invariant in signal transfer and stationary in noise is no longer valid in CT with iterative algorithms for image formation, due to the roles played by the regularization in IIR algorithms. The task-based MTF and NPS have been proposed in the literature (Richard et al. 2012; Wilson et al. 2013) to get around the invalidity in shift-invariant linearity and noise stationarity, which, as indicated at the beginning of this chapter, are compromised solutions by piecewise linearization of the ideal observer-based approach and FOMs in the spatial frequency domain. There is no doubt that those piecewise linearized solutions are of utilities in practice, but note that the piecewise linearization may not be able to exhaust all the situations in which the regularization in IIR behaves differently.

Prior to ending the introduction on assessing CT system performance via FOMs in the frequency domain, I want to make a point that, as indicated by Hanson (Hanson 1979), the SNR of CT under the ideal observer is actually not as good as that of radiography, as the noise in CT is colored while that in radiography is white. However, human's perceptual experience tells us that a lesion can be much more readily detected in CT than its detection in radiography, which, is mainly attributed to two factors: (i) an almost complete removal of anatomic structure's superposition (anatomic noise) by the tomographic reconstruction and (ii) an image can be displayed at an adequate display window level and width to overcome the minimum contrast threshold of the human observer.

6.5 ASSESSMENT OF IMAGE QUALITY BY HUMAN OBSERVER

We have learned in previous sections that, in addition to coming up with a single summary quantity, the ROC curve provides an entire picture on performance of the imaging system or method under study. As an FOM for image quality assessment, the ROC approach is independent of class prevalence and decision criteria, and applicable in the cases of both ordinal and continuous data (Tourassi 2019). It has been agreed on that the human observer study with ROC as the FOM is the gold standard for assessing system performance and image quality in medical imaging (Burgess 1999), especially in light of the fact that IIR with regularization or constraint for CT image formation is gaining acceptance in clinical applications (Yu et al. 2013, 2017; Leng et al. 2013; Fan et al. 2023). Earlier section in this chapter covered the basics in human observer studies; the following sections cover relatively advanced topics on ROC human observer study.

6.5.1 ROC HUMAN OBSERVER STUDY

Mathematically, each of the three ways to carry out the human observer study using ROC as the FOM can be specified as follows (Abbey and Eckstein 2019):

$$\textbf{2AFC}: Decision = \begin{cases} Target\ present & if\ \lambda > \lambda_c \\ Target\ absent & if\ \lambda \leq \lambda_c \end{cases} \quad (6.36)$$

where λ and λ_c are the decision variable and threshold, respectively.

$$\textbf{MAFC}: Decision = \begin{cases} Decision\ 1 & if\ \lambda_1 > \max(\lambda_2, \lambda_3, \ldots, \lambda_M) \\ Decision\ 2 & if\ \lambda_2 > \max(\lambda_1, \lambda_3, \ldots, \lambda_M) \\ \vdots & \vdots \\ Decision\ M & if\ \lambda_M > \max(\lambda_1, \lambda_2, \ldots, \lambda_{M-1}) \end{cases} \quad (6.37)$$

where $\lambda_1, \lambda_2, \ldots$ and λ_M are the decision variables.

$$\textbf{Rating-scale}: Decision = \begin{cases} Decision\ 1 & if\ \lambda \leq \lambda_1 \\ Decision\ 2 & if\ \lambda_1 < \lambda \leq \lambda_2 \\ \vdots & \vdots \\ Decision\ M & if\ \lambda_{M-1} < \lambda \leq \lambda_M \end{cases} \quad (6.38)$$

where λ is the decision variable, and $\lambda_1, \lambda_2, \ldots$ and λ_M are thresholds.

In ROC human observer study, the visual experiment should be carried out over all cases under study, such as target shape, size, various parameters in data acquisition and image formation, and associated radiation dose. Close attention should be given to determining the adequate magnitude of the signal, which is quite demanding in practice (especially in 2AFC), as illustrated by the examples displayed in Figure 6.13. In each disciplined experimental session carried out in a darkened room with adequate ambient lighting, images should be presented in a display window that is identical to clinical settings. The participant should view each image binocularly from ~40 cm, with no constraint on the time for the viewer to make a decision. To avoid fatigue, the time span of each session should be set appropriately, e.g., 2 hours per session.

6.5.2 PARTIAL ROC HUMAN OBSERVER STUDY

In its simplest form, all the thresholds (operating condition) in a human observer ROC study are assumed equally important, but this may not be the case in the clinic, as a specific operating condition may be more important than others. Also, as illustrated in Figure 6.5, it is quite easy for a system designer to make the judgment that imaging system A outperforms system B, as $AUC_A > AUC_B$ holds over the entire range. But, more challenging cases often occur in practice, as illustrated in Figure 6.14, in which the two ROC curves intersect each other, though their AUCs are roughly the same. Under such circumstances, an adoption of the partial ROC (pROC) makes more sense, in which, the AUC is only assessed within a specified (focused) interval, enabling a system designer to make the call on the imaging system performance or image quality in the neighborhood of a specific operating point. Only a brief introduction on the pROC is given here with an exemplification shown

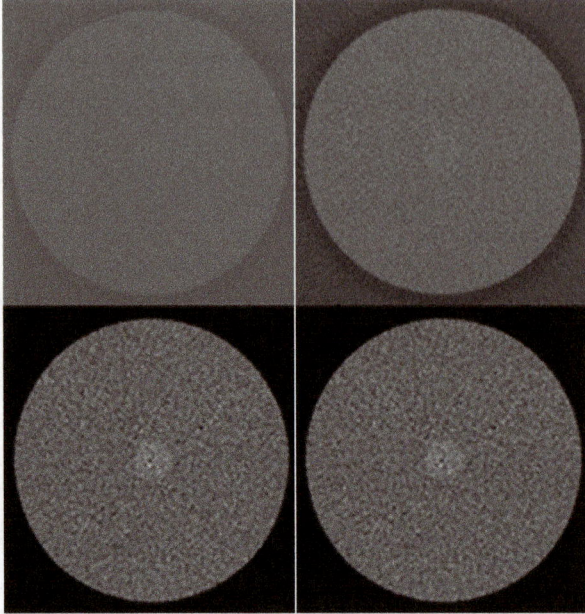

FIGURE 6.13   CT images showing the challenge in determining the adequate low contrast for a 2AFC ROC study.

in Figure 6.14 (Yang et al. 2019). Readers who are interested in more details are referred to the literature (Tourassi 2019).

6.5.3 Location ROC Human Observer Study

In addition to assuming that all the thresholds for decision-making are equally important, the location of the signal present in ROC human observer study is also fixed (SKE/BKE task), which again is not the case in the clinic in which the clinician is supposed to search for abnormality over the entire image. To make ROC study more truthful in predicting the performance of human observers under clinical settings, the location ROC (LROC) approach is proposed, in which the observer is asked to make decision on the signal's presence at one of the multi-locations (or ROIs as illustrated in Figure 6.15) that are known to the observer in advance (Vaishnav et al. 2014). In principle, this is the so-called task of signal known exactly but variable (SKEV). During testing, the observer can only score a "correct" if they detect the signal's presence at a spot that is within a preset distance away from the true location. Hence, the task in an LROC study is harder than that in an ROC study. Accordingly, the AUC in LROC is smaller than its counterpart in ROC, as exemplified in Figure 6.16 (Popescu and Myers 2013; Leng et al. 2013).

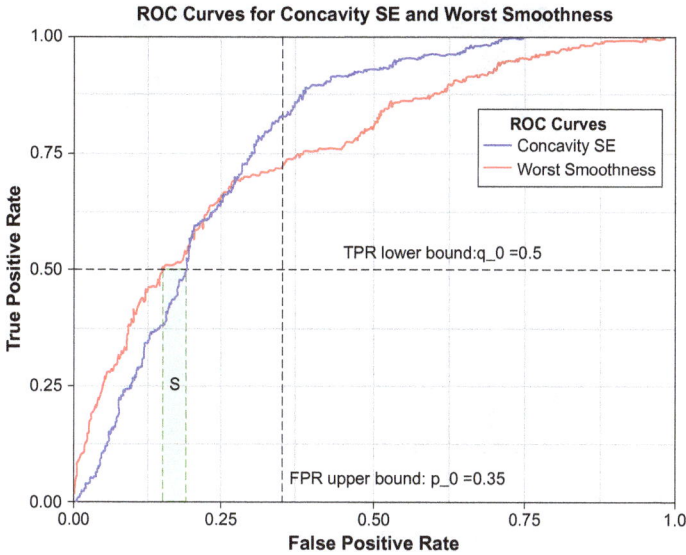

FIGURE 6.14   An example showing the case of intercepted ROC curves and the definition of a partial ROC study. (Adopted from Yang et al. 2019 with permission.)

6.5.4 EXPONENTIAL TRANSFORMATION OF FREE-RESPONSE EFROC HUMAN OBSERVER STUDY

The clinical task of identifying and localizing all the pathophysiological lesions in an image or a sequence of images (signal-at-unknown-location problem) is a formidable challenge from the psychophysical point of view. To meet this challenge, the free-response ROC (FROC) has been proposed and increasingly used in studies (Charkraborty 2013). Unlike the ROC and LROC, the AUC of FROC cannot be used as a summary index of imaging system performance or image quality, since the abscess in FROC goes to positive infinite. This issue can be solved by an exponential transformation ($1-e^{-v}$, where v is the abscess in the FROC plot) (Popescu 2011). Encouraging results have been reported in recent studies, showing that the EFROC outperforms LROC in assessment of image quality in CT with IIR for image formation, though both of them are of sufficient power (Popescu 2011). There are more advanced topics in FROC, such as AFROC1 and AFROC2, the two-alternative free-response ROC, and inferred ROC, and readers who are interested are referred to the literature (Charkraborty 2013; Popescu 2011).

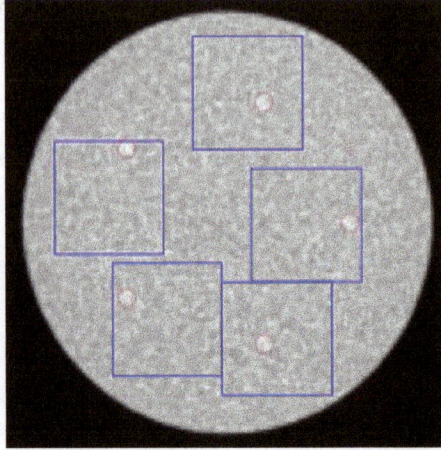

FIGURE 6.15 An example that schematically shows the experiment of LROC study in which the signal location may vary in each of the square ROIs. (Adopted from Vaishnav et al. 2014 with permission.)

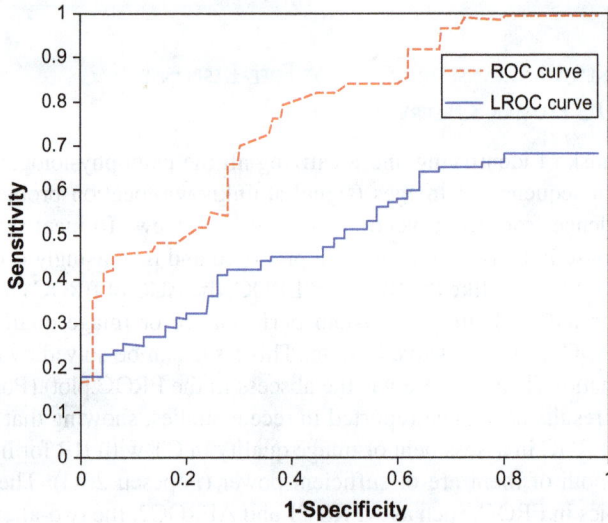

FIGURE 6.16 Examples of ROC and LROC curves, in which the performance of an ROC study is always better than that of an LROC study. (Adopted from Leng et al. 2013 with permission.)

6.6 ASSESSMENT OF IMAGE QUALITY BY MODEL OBSERVER

Ultimately, a human observer study for assessment of imaging system performance and image quality should be carried out via clinical trials in which a relatively large population of patients and observers (physicians) is essential. In practice, the recruitment of a large cohort of patients may not be feasible due to ethical considerations and costs (Barret 1993; Burgess 1999; Myers 2000). As an alternative, a human observer study can be conducted by assessing the ROC/AUC in a downsized cohort of patients and observers. However, even a downsized cohort of patients and observers may still be costly and time-consuming, especially when the imaging system under investigation is in its early stage, in which the design trade-offs have to be made in numerous system parameters. A more accessible and thus economic way to carry out an observer study is employing an algorithmic model observers. A number of model observers have thus far been developed, of which the channelized Hotelling observer (CHO) has found application in multiple imaging modalities, as it can well emulate the human observer behavior while both crispy (high frequency) and clumpy (low frequency) noise are in the background (Barret 1993; Abbey and Eckstein 2019). Hence, in the upcoming sections, following a concise introduction to all the model observers, there is in-depth coverage of the CHO.

6.6.1 OBSERVER MODELS WITH NO CHANNELIZATION

A model observer refers to a virtual observer who makes decisions based on the information offered by an algorithm or algorithms. As covered in Section 6.2.6, an observer, e.g., the ideal observer, can be abstracted as a decision variable (or test statistic) that is characterized by an analytic formula. As illustrated next, this strategy has been readily extended to each of the model observers.

In general, the functional form of a model observer can be written as

$$\lambda = \lambda\left(\boldsymbol{g}\right) + \varepsilon \tag{6.39}$$

where $\lambda\left(\cdot\right)$ is a function that may be non-linear, and ε denotes the so-called internal noise that is added to make the model observer's performance compatible to that of a human observer. If the function $\lambda\left(\cdot\right)$ can be assumed linear, the computation to get the decision variable becomes much more tractable. Then, Equation 6.39 can be rewritten in matrix form (Abbey and Eckstein 2019)

$$\lambda = \Lambda^{T}\boldsymbol{g} + \varepsilon \tag{6.40}$$

where Λ is called the observer template, and the superscript T denotes the matrix transpose. Given the decision variable of a model observer, its performance can be characterized via ROC by sweeping the threshold over the entire range, or, by the detectability index (Abbey and Eckstein 2019)

$$d' = \frac{\Lambda^{T}\left(\bar{\boldsymbol{g}}_{1} - \bar{\boldsymbol{g}}_{0}\right)}{\left(\dfrac{1}{2}\Lambda^{T}\left(\Sigma_{g_{1}} + \Sigma_{g_{0}}\right)\Lambda + \sigma_{\varepsilon}^{2}\right)^{\!{}^{1\!/_{2}}}} \tag{6.41}$$

where $\bar{g}_1$, $\bar{g}_0$, Σ_{g_1} and Σ_{g_0} are the means of observation and their covariance when the signal is present and absent, respectively. Under low signal assumption, we have $\Sigma_{g_1} = \Sigma_{g_0} = \Sigma_g$, and Equation 6.41 becomes

$$d' = \frac{\Lambda^T \left(\bar{g}_1 - \bar{g}_0 \right)}{\left(\Lambda^T \Sigma_g \Lambda + \sigma_\varepsilon^2 \right)^{1/2}} \tag{6.42}$$

- **Non-prewhitening observer**: The observer template of a non-prewhitening observer is (Abbey and Eckstein 2019)

$$\Lambda_{NPW} = \Delta \bar{g} \tag{6.43}$$

which is a linear cross-correlator (matched filter) and also an ideal observer under additive white Gaussian noise, as elucidated in Section 6.2.6. Further, under the white noise assumption, we have $\Sigma_g = \sigma_n^2 I$, and then the detectability index becomes (Abbey and Eckstein 2019)

$$d' = \frac{\sqrt{\left(\bar{g}_1 - \bar{g}_0 \right)^T \left(\bar{g}_1 - \bar{g}_0 \right)}}{\sigma_n} \tag{6.44}$$

- **Hotelling (prewhitening) observer**: Under colored noise, the so-called prewhitening matched filter is an ideal observer, as covered in Section 6.2.9. Its observer template and detectability index are, respectively, given by (Abbey and Eckstein 2019)

$$\Lambda_{PW} = \Sigma_g^{-1} \Delta \bar{g} \tag{6.45}$$

$$d' = \frac{\Lambda^T \left(\bar{g}_1 - \bar{g}_0 \right)}{\left(\Lambda^T \Sigma_g \Lambda + \sigma_\varepsilon^2 \right)^{1/2}} \tag{6.46}$$

- **Non-prewhitening observer with eye filter**: The human observer is not an ideal observer under colored noise. It was found that the performance of a non-prewhitening model observer can be made to approach the performance of a human observer in noise at low frequency by applying an eye filter in the functional form $E(k) = k^a e^{-bk}$ (Burgess 1994). Then, the observer template with the eye filter becomes (Abbey and Eckstein 2019)

$$\Lambda = E^T \Delta \bar{g} \tag{6.47}$$

where E denotes matrix corresponding to the eye filter, and the resultant detectability index is

$$d' = \frac{\sqrt{(\bar{g}_1 - \bar{g}_0)^T (\bar{g}_1 - \bar{g}_0)}}{\sigma_n} \tag{6.48}$$

Notably, under noise at mid- and high-frequency, the performance of a non-prewhitening observer with eye filter still substantially differs from that of a human observer.

6.6.2 CHANNELIZED HOTELLING OBSERVER

Letting T denote the matrix of a channel template, the channel output of a channelized linear model observer can be expressed as (Abbey and Barret 2001; Abbey and Eckstein 2007, 2019)

$$v = T^T g + z \tag{6.49}$$

where z denotes the internal noise in channel response. Specifically, the linear CHO decision variable is formed as (Abbey and Barret 2001)

$$\lambda_{CHO} = s^T T \left(T^T \Sigma_g T + \Sigma_z \right)^{-1} v \tag{6.50}$$

where g represents signal and s is the difference between the signals with a target present or absent, and Σ_g and Σ_z are their covariance matrix, respectively. It has been shown that the CHO observer template can be mathematically expressed as

$$w_{CHO} = T \left(T^T \Sigma_g T + \Sigma_z \right)^{-1} T^T s \tag{6.51}$$

and the detectability index d' assessed by the CHO model is

$$d'_{CHO} = \frac{w_{CHO}^T s}{\sqrt{w_{CHO}^T \Sigma_g w_{CHO} + \sigma_\varepsilon^2}} \tag{6.52}$$

where α_e is the variance of internal noise accounting for the psychophysical uncertainty in the human visual system (Barret and Myers 2004; Abbey and Barret 2001; Abbey and Eckstein 2019; Barret et al. 1993).

A number of channel response functions, which can be radially symmetric, e.g., the Laguerre–Gauss function and difference-of-Gaussian (DOG) function, or incorporate the orientation and phase, e.g., the Gabor function, have been proposed to make the channel template (Barret and Myers 2004; Yu et al. 2013; Leng et al. 2013). If the target is radially symmetric and located in the center of the field of view (FOV), the radially symmetric Laguerre–Gauss function or DOG channel template are preferable (Barret and Myers 2004; Tang and Yang 2014). The 1D analytic functional form of the DOG channel template is defined here as (Wunderlich and Noo 2008; Yu et al. 2013)

$$C_j(k) = exp\left(-\frac{1}{2}\left(\frac{k}{Q\sigma_j}\right)^2\right) - exp\left(-\frac{1}{2}\left(\frac{k}{\sigma_j}\right)^2\right) \qquad (6.53)$$

$$\sigma_j = \alpha^j \alpha_0, \quad j = 1, 2, \dots, 10 \qquad (6.54)$$

Note that the DOG channel template reaches zero response at zero frequency, which is consistent with the human eye that is not sensitive to noise at low spatial frequency, but this is not the case in the Laguerre–Gauss channel template. Hence, if the Laguerre–Gauss channel template is used in a model observer study, e.g., the channelized Hotelling observer, the outcome may not be consistent to that of a human observer study (Barre and Myers 2004).

In the case when the target is neither radially symmetric nor located in the center of the FOV, the Gabor channel template (Abbey and Barret 2001), as analytically defined in Equation 6.55, is more appropriate:

$$G(x, y) = exp\left(-4ln2\left((x - x_0)^2 + (y - y_0)^2\right) / \omega_s^2\right)$$

$$cos\left(2\pi k_c\left((x - x_0)\cos\theta + (y - y_0)\sin\theta\right) + \beta\right) \qquad (6.55)$$

An example of the Gabor channel template in the spatial domain corresponding to five scales and five orientations at one phase is presented in Figure 6.17 for illustration.

6.6.3 INTERNAL NOISE IN CHO AND ITS DETERMINATION

In practice, a model observer usually outperforms a human observer in performance assessment of a medical imaging method or system. To make a model observer behave compatibly with that of a human observer, internal noise has been introduced to account for the psychophysical uncertainty in human visual perception, in addition to the uncertainty caused by the (external) noise existing in an image (Zhang et al. 2007). Thus, the internal noise plays an important role in the model observer study of CT imaging performance (Yu et al. 2013; Leng et al. 2013).

In principle, the internal noise can be added to the response of each channel or the total decision variable that is formed from the output of all channels (Eckstein 2003; Zhang et al. 2007). It has been reported that, both of these internal noise addition approaches make the performance of a CHO consistent with that of a human observer (Zhang et al. 2007), though the behavior of channel-wise addition matches more closely with that of a human observer. Specifically, the magnitude of internal noise is determined according to

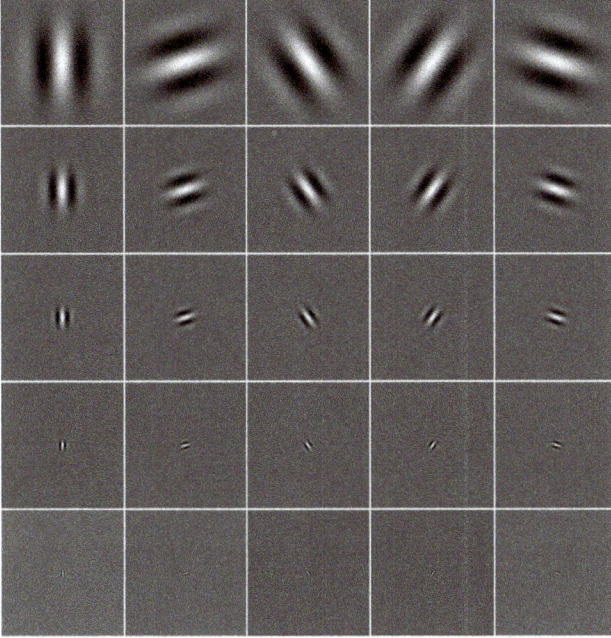

FIGURE 6.17 Display of Gabor channel response templates at five scales (top to bottom: 3/256, 3/128, 3/64, 3/32 and 3/16), five orientations (left to right: 0, $2\pi/5$, $4\pi/5$, $6\pi/5$ and $8\pi/5$) and one phase (0).

$$\sigma_{in} = \alpha\sigma_{\lambda\_bkg} \qquad\qquad (6.56)$$

where σ_{λ_bkg} is the standard deviation of decision variable λ_{CHO} when the signal is absent, i.e., background only. α is a weighting factor and can be determined via calibration such that the performance of the resultant linear CHO matches that of human observers (Zhang et all 2007; Abbey and Eckstein 2019). For example, using the percentage correct P_C as the FOM, the weighting factor α has been determined as $\alpha = 9.25$ to make 2AFC decisions in SKE scenarios (Yu et al. 2013), while that corresponding to the SKEV case has been determined as $\alpha = 6.0$ using AUC as the FOM (Figure 6.18) (Leng et al. 2013).

6.6.4 Assessment of Image Quality by CHO: An Example

Under the framework of model observer with signal and background exactly known (SKE/BKE) (Barret and Myers 2004), my team carried out an experiment to study the detectability of differential phase contrast CT compared with that of the conventional attenuation-based CT (Tang and Yang 2014). Using CHO and the DOG channel template (Abbey and Barret 2001), we investigated their detectability index over the dimension of object to be imaged and detector elements. In our quantitative study, it has been found that the number of DOG channels affects the

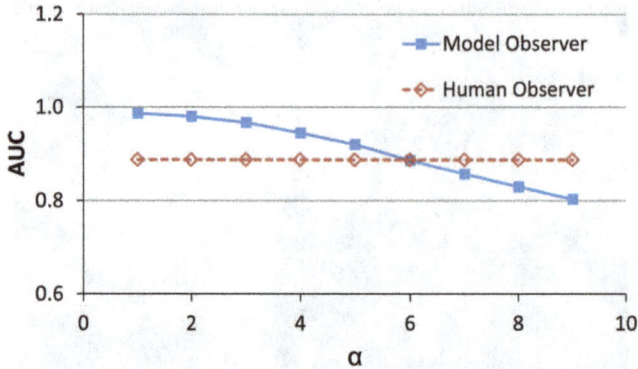

FIGURE 6.18 An example illustrating the determination of internal noise magnitude in an ROC model observer study via a calibration process with the engagement of human observers. (Adopted from Leng et al. 2013 with permission.)

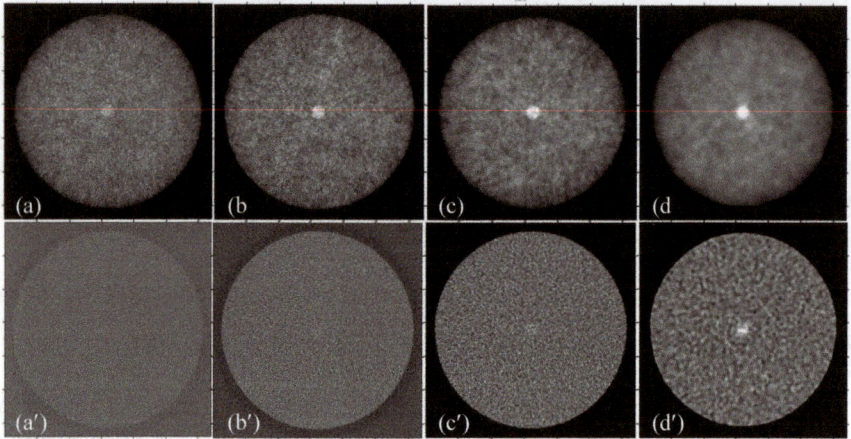

FIGURE 6.19 Transverse images of 2.5 mm target in a water phantom generated by a differential phase contrast CT (top) and conventional CT (bottom) from the projection data acquired at detector elements: (a) 64×64 μm^2, (b) 128×128 μm^2, (c) 256×256 μm^2 and (d) 512×512 μm^2.

results of the detectability index in the CHO study. With the channel parameters that are consistent with those reported in the literature (Abbey and Barret 2001; Wunderlich and Noo 2008, 2011), it has been determined that ten DOG channels are sufficient to make the results stable and consistent to human visual observation, along with the settings $\alpha = 1.4$, $\sigma_0 = 0.005$ cycles/pixel and $Q = 1.67$ (Barret and Myers 2004).

The decision to be made falls under the 2AFC, i.e., between the cases of signal present and signal absent. Typical images used in the experiments are displayed in

Figure 6.19 and Figure 6.20, in which the circular targets to be identified are at 3 mm and 5 mm in diameter, respectively. As already known, the FOM to quantify the performance of an observer in a 2AFC task is the proportion correct P_C, but the detectability index d' can serve the same purpose and thus is our choice here.

The internal noise is determined according to the results published in the literature, wherein the standard deviation of the decision variable λ in the case without the target, i.e., signal absent, is utilized (Abbey and Barret 2001; Wunderlich and Noo 2008; Leng et al. 2013). In the conventional attenuation-based CT, it has been determined through ROC study that factor α_{in} varies in a range between 2.5 and 9, and $\alpha_{in} = 5.5$ is an adequate choice (Wunderlich and Noo 2008; Leng et al. 2013). Hence, we set $\alpha_{in} = 5.5$ in this investigation in both the conventional attenuation-based CT and differential phase contrast CT, though it is believed that α_{in} should be smaller in the differential phase contrast CT than its counterpart in the attenuation-based CT as the differential phase contrast CT image is relatively rich in low spatial resolution noise (Tang et al. 2011; Raupach and Flohr 2011; Köhler and Roessl 2011; Tang et al. 2012) and human eyes are relatively insensitive to low frequency noise (Barret and Myers 2004; Barret et al. 1993). Recognizing the critical role played by internal noise in a model observer's performance, a further in-depth investigation into how to determine the internal noise via ROC study for the differential phase contrast CT is deemed necessary.

The detectability index assessed by the channelized Hotelling observer as a function of detector cell dimension corresponding to target size 1.0 mm and 2.5 mm are presented in Figure 6.21a and Figure 6.21b, respectively. As demonstrated, the differential phase contrast CT outperforms the conventional attenuation-based CT significantly in the scenarios where the target to be detected is small (1.0 mm). With the target size

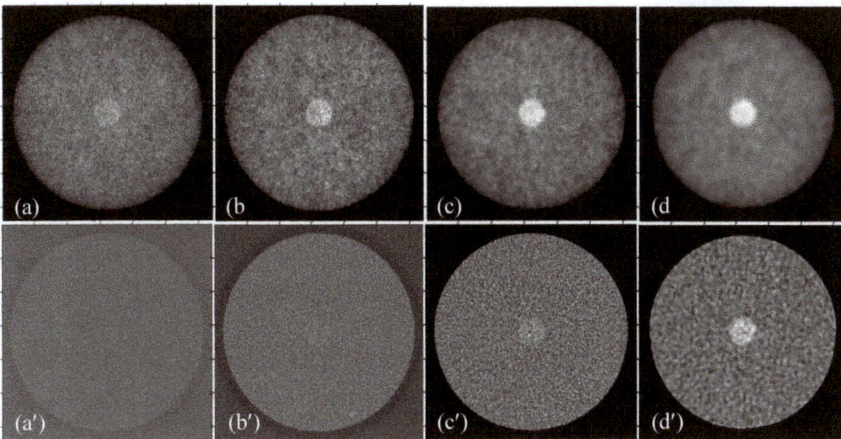

FIGURE 6.20 Transverse images of 5.0 mm target in water phantom generated by the differential phase contrast CT (top) and conventional CT from the projection data acquired at detector elements: (a) $64 \times 64 \ \mu m^2$, (b) $128 \times 128 \ \mu m^2$, (c) $256 \times 256 \ \mu m^2$ and (d) $512 \times 512 \ \mu m^2$.

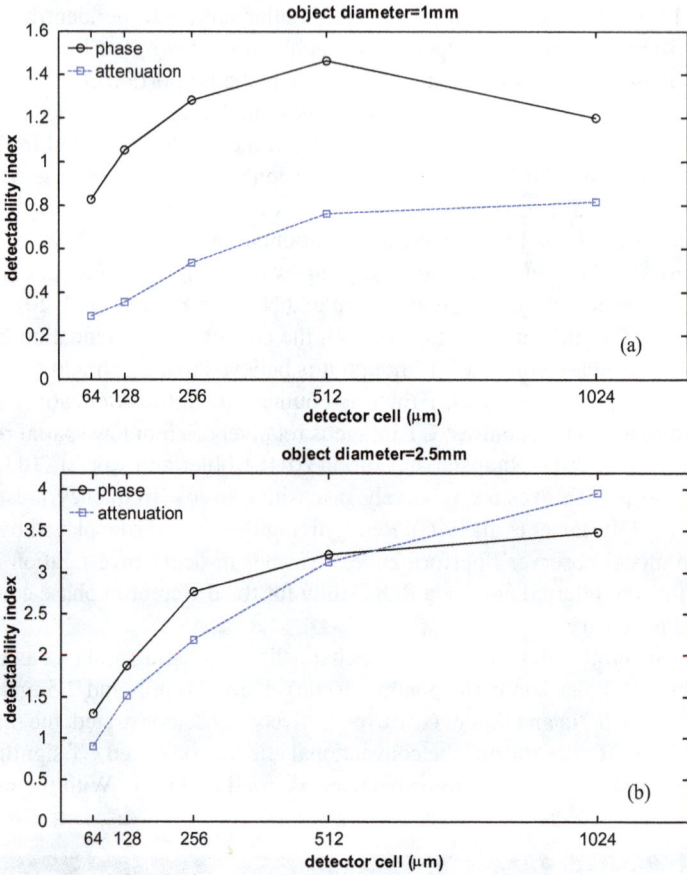

FIGURE 6.21 The detectability index assessed by a channelized Hotelling observer as a function of the detector element dimension at (a) 1.0 mm and (b) 2.5 mm target size.

increased to 2.5 mm, the differential phase contrast CT's dominance in the detectability index over the conventional attenuation-based CT diminishes. Notably, the differential phase contrast CT's dominance in the detectability index virtually disappear (or "make even") while the detector cell dimension is around 512 μm. It is interesting to note that the detectability index profiles plotted in Figure 6.21 are consistent with the visual observation by a human observer drawn from Figure 6.19 and Figure 6.20.

6.7 DISCUSSION

In response to increasing acceptance of IIR algorithm in state-of-the-art MDCT for image formation, research in the paradigms of assessing system performance and image quality based on the theory of signal detection and statistical decision is gaining momentum. Having gone through relatively lengthy coverage of the topic, we should be encouraged by the fact that there is a catalog of approaches and associated FOMs for us to choose. Meanwhile, we should have also learned that choosing the most appropriate paradigm to fulfill our goal is not trivial. The appropriateness of a choice can only be ultimately appraised by its utility and effectiveness in representing diagnostic imaging tasks under clinical circumstances, but other factors, such as statistical power, complexity and cost (either ethical or economic) may also play important roles. For example, either the pixel-wise noise and SNR or the Rose model should be sufficient for daily quality assurance, protocol optimization or incremental advancement in a clinically established imaging modality like CT. An observer study, via either model or human, should be employed as the paradigm if the advancement is a leap, like that in CT with image reconstruction evolving from FBP to IIR. However, as shown in Figure 6.22 (Wunderlich and Abbey 2013), even within the ROC paradigm, the decision to make under the possibility of multiple signals over locations is not easy. Prior to ending this chapter, below is a concise discussion of two more advanced topics.

6.7.1 TASK DEFINITION: CLINICAL RELEVANCE VS. PRACTICAL FEASIBILITY

Fairly speaking, all the tasks that have been considered so far are too simple to be of clinical fidelity, which may lead to overestimation of an imaging system's or

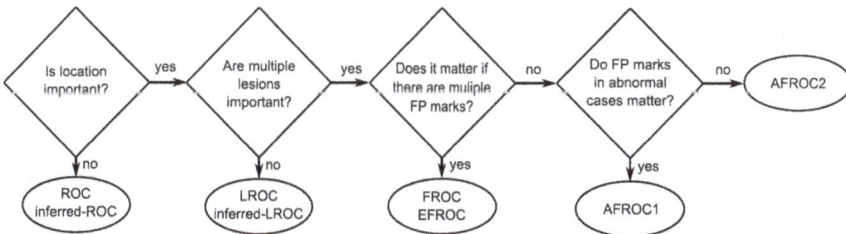

FIGURE 6.22 An example of the decision tree in choosing the approaches and associated figure of merit for assessment of image quality in CT via a free-response ROC study. (Adopted from Wunderlich and Abbey 2013 with permission.)

method's performance, or image quality. In the slightly more complicated case of the SKEV (signal known exactly but with variation) task, only the variation in location has thus far been studied. As such, the performance of either human or model observer can be obtained by averaging the FOMs obtained over specified locations. The SKS case is more complicated, but still only the variation in locations has been studied thus far. Actually, in the case of the SKS task, the statistical variation in signal can manifest itself in shape, size and location, which is essentially a wide-sense stationary random process that is characterized by its autocorrelation function in the spatial domain (or its power spectrum in the frequency domain).

In an SKE task, the performance of an ideal observer are depicted by Equations 6.34 and 6.35 in the frequency domain, and its counterpart in the SKS task becomes (ICRU 1996)

$$SNR = \int_{-\infty}^{\infty} \frac{\pi}{b} \frac{\Delta S(k)|k| MTF_{total}^2}{\Delta S(k)|k| MTF_{total}^2 + NPS(k)} dk, \tag{6.57}$$

which shows that the statistical variation in the signal is equivalent to noise in the SNR calculation.

The formation of a test statistic corresponding to a model observer under an SKS task becomes substantially more complicated (Abbey and Eckstein 2019). For example, given a state of the signal or parameter denoted by μ, let λ_μ be the corresponding decision variable with $\overline{\lambda}_\mu^+$ and $\overline{\lambda}_\mu^-$ as the mean values in the cases of the signal present and absent, respectively. If the associated variance can be assumed identical, i.e., $\sigma_\mu^+ = \sigma_\mu^- = \sigma_\mu$, a total decision variable is formed by summing all individual decision variables (Abbey and Eckstein 2019):

$$\lambda = \sum_\mu \pi_\mu exp\left(-\frac{1}{2}\left(\left(\frac{\lambda_\mu - \overline{\lambda}_\mu^+}{\sigma_\mu^2}\right)^2 - \left(\frac{\lambda_\mu - \overline{\lambda}_\mu^-}{\sigma_\mu^2}\right)^2\right)\right) \tag{6.58}$$

Notably, the total decision variable becomes much more complicated, and even its observation of the Gaussian distribution may be questionable. For more details on this topic, readers are referred to the references (Abbey and Eckstein 2019).

6.7.2 THE HORIZON: MODEL OBSERVER BASED ON MACHINE/DEEP LEARNING

The striking advancement made in machine/deep learning in recent years, especially the one implemented in the convolution neural network (CNN), is making ripples in almost every field, including image quality assessment. The kinship between the psychophysics underlying the methodology of observer study, either human or model, for image quality assessment, and the CNN's structure of emulating the human multilayer perceptual system, encourages belief that the progress in machine/deep learning is providing unprecedented opportunity for research and development in the paradigm of image quality assessment. In essence, the machine/deep learning-based approach is a non-linear discriminator with the capability of approaching any function (Nielson 2018). Therefore, with the preliminary but increasing data reported in the literature on CNN's application in CT image quality assessment (Han and Baek 2020), I optimistically anticipate that machine/deep learning-based model observers can outperform the existing model observers that are basically linear discriminators for assessment of MDCT image quality in challenging situations in which the task under study needs to be at high clinical fidelity, with variation in the signal's magnitude, shape and texture, and boundary regularity, and in a background that is full of noise that may be white, colored or even including anatomic noise.

7 Spectral MDCT (Part 1)
Physics, Data Acquisition and Image Formation

Enabled by advanced technologies, especially the multi-detector row and dual X-ray source, computed tomography (CT) has become one of the most potent imaging modalities in the clinic for diagnostic imaging of a variety of diseases. The new technologies synergized with novel image formation solutions have empowered state-of-the-art multi-detector CT (MDCT) with well-balanced image quality over the contrast, spatial, temporal and, very recently, spectral resolutions to overcome the challenges imposed by cardiovascular, neurovascular and oncological applications (Tang 2014). Unfortunately, despite enormous effort devoted by generations of scientists and researchers in the field, CT has still not been as potent as positron emission tomography (PET) and magnetic resonance imaging (MRI) in contrast resolution that is critical to early detection of cancer malignance and characterization of vulnerable plaques in vascular atherosclerosis. The following paragraphs are an analysis and comparison of the three primary diagnostic imaging modalities, to provide an insightful understanding of the motivation driving the community to push forward CT's capability in soft tissue differentiation via spectral CT and its potential and limitations, from the perspectives of science, technologies and clinical applications.

The first perspective of our analysis and comparison is in signal generation (also termed *subject contrast*). The major mechanism limiting CT's capability in soft tissue differentiation lies in the fact that only variation in a material's atomic number and density leads to variation in X-ray attenuation and thus generates the contrast via photoelectric absorption and Compton scattering (Bushberg et al. 2012; Huda 2016). This means that the mechanism of subject contrast generation in CT is at the atomic level. As we know, the bone generates high contrast against soft tissues in CT because the atomic number of calcium, a major constituent of bone, is $Z_{Ca} = 20$ and substantially larger than that of carbon ($Z_C = 6$), nitrogen ($Z_N = 7$), hydrogen ($Z_H = 1$) and oxygen ($Z_O = 8$), the four major constituents of soft tissues in human body. The mass density of soft tissues, except for adipose and muscle, in the human body is quite similar ($\rho_{soft\text{-}tissue} = 1.0$ g/ml). Accordingly, the contrast in CT images among the soft tissues is relatively low, except for adipose and muscle due to their relatively smaller ($\rho_{adipose} = 0.9$) and larger ($\rho_{soft\text{-}tissue} = 1.06$) mass density. However, variation at the molecular level (or molecular environments), especially in large molecules such as protein, generates variation in the magnetic resonance signal and thus the subject contrast in MRI, leading to the fact that MRI outperforms CT substantially in soft tissue differentiation.

DOI: 10.1201/9780429028465-7

The second perspective is in the mechanism of signal detection (or data acquisition). As an imaging method, CT works in transmission mode, in which the signal generated by pathologic lesions in CT are submerged in background signals (they are in fact noise) generated by all tissues/organs in the X-ray beam. However, PET/SPECT works in an emission mode that is similar to the concept of dark field imaging in microscopy, in which only the targeted pathologic lesions take up radiolabels and generate signals. Moreover, the radiation dose in CT is proportional to the time of data acquisition. Given a dose rate that is jointly determined by the peak voltage kVp and tube current, the data acquisition (scan) time in CT should be as short as possible in light of the radiation dose delivered to the patient that may induce malignance in the long run. However, once a dose of radiopharmaceuticals (and thus radiation dose) is administrated in PET/SPECT, the longer the time for data acquisition, the stronger the signal and the better the subject contrast. In clinical practice, one may be used to a relatively long scan time in PET/SPECT, but may want a CT scan to be completed at an ever fastest speed, which is an extra factor that is favorable to PET/SPECT in terms of subject contrast generation.

The third perspective is in the mechanism of contrast enhancement. In essence, the radiolabels utilized in PET/PET are forms of contrast agents consisting of small molecules that can be excreted by the renal circulation system. In fact, contrast agents, mainly iodine based and also in the form of small molecules, have been routinely used in CT for diagnostic imaging (ACR 2021). The contrast agent (radiolabel) in PET/SPECT is delivered specifically toward targeted pathologies at the molecular level, whereas the iodinated contrast in CT is delivered via vasculature and body compartments, which is significantly less effective in terms of pathology targeting (Lusic and Grinstaff 2013). As we know, the expression of malignant pathology at the molecular level is much earlier than angiogenesis and neovascularization that may coexist with malignant neoplasm. Hence, though it can substantially enhance the subject contrast in cardiovascular and parenchymal imaging (e.g., angiography and perfusion) (Bae 2010) and even in early detection of malignant tumors with angiogenesis and neovascularization, CT, aided by iodinated contrast agent for conspicuity enhancement, is still less sensitive compared to PET/SPECT and MRI in early detection, and characterization of cancer and vulnerable atherosclerosis – the two major life-threatening diseases.

The relatively low inter-soft tissue contrast in CT is attributed to all three aforementioned intrinsic shortcomings, and researchers in the field have long tried to improve the subject contrast of pathologic lesions in CT. Though it has been well-known that both photoelectric absorption and Compton scattering (and thus the attenuation) decrease with increasing energy of the X-ray beam, it was Alvarez and Macovski who showed that such an energy-dependent property can be utilized to improve the subject contrast in CT (Alvarez and Macovski 1976). Their milestone discovery proved that, within the 15–150 keV range for diagnostic imaging but above the K-edge, the photoelectric absorption and Compton scattering can approximately span a linear space in which the mass attenuation coefficient of a material can be quasi-accurately represented as a linear combination. This was a conceptual breakthrough and paved the way for material decomposition and virtual monochromatic imaging, the earliest forms of spectral imaging in CT. Inspired by this discovery, there was a surge in the research and development (R&D) of spectral CT, and its implementation (e.g., fast kV-switching and layered detector) and preclinical/clinical applications (even the concept of CT histogram was conceived) (Riederer and Mistretta 1977; Latchaw et al. 1978; Brody et al. 1981; Lehmann et al. 1981; Marshall et al. 1981). However, the enthusiasm subsided in the mid-1980s, and followed by a revisit in the late 1980s and early 1990s (Kalender et al. 1986; Vetter 1986; Chuang and Huang 1988;), mainly because the then technologies were not ready to support spectral CT, in which quite a few challenges, such as suppression of Compton scattering, overlapping of source spectra and motion-induced spatial mis-registration between data acquisition at high and low kVps, had to be addressed.

The recent renaissance in dual-energy CT started in the mid-2000s and was highlighted by the advent of dual-source–dual-detector (DSDD) CT launched by Siemens in 2005, enabling clinical researchers to explore its preclinical and especially clinical utilities, with quite fruitful outcomes in the most recent ten years. Actually, in history, dual-energy CT – the earliest prototype of spectral CT – was initially implemented in the image domain in EMI's CT scanner (Hounsfield 1973). Using sophisticated beam-hardening correction techniques, DSDD CT has reinforced the implementation of spectral CT in the image domain (Flohr et al. 2008). Following the preliminary success of DSDD-based spectral CT in clinics, the spectral CT implemented in the projection domain via fast kV-switching (Forghani et al. 2017a, 2017b, 2017c) and layered detectors (Duan et al. 2018) has been launched in the marketplace, providing the functionalities of attenuation decomposition, material decomposition, virtual monochromatic imaging, decomposition of atomic number and electron (and mass) density (Behrendt et al. 2009; Srinivasan et al. 2013; Forghani 2017c), and other linear (Schmidt 2009; Yu et al. 2009) and non-linear (Holms et al. 2008; Kim et al. 2010) combination-based image formation and presentation.

Thus far, all commercially available spectral CTs are based on X-ray detection via energy-integration (McCollough et al. 2015b; Ren et al. 2021). Recently, photon-counting-based detection of X-rays has been identified as a more effective way to implement spectral CT (Patino et al. 2016; Willemink et al. 2018; Leng et al. 2019; Flohr et al. 2020). A photon-counting detection-based spectral cone-beam CT (CBCT) has been prototyped in my laboratory, in addition to an energy-integration based one, in accordance with the extensive and fast-growing research in the field to advance spectral CT imaging performance and to extend its clinical utility. Based on my understanding of spectral CT and hands-on experience in implementing both energy-integration and photon-counting-based spectral CT, this chapter aims at updating the community with in-depth information on spectral CT physics, implementation technologies, noise analysis, imaging performance optimization and, especially, the potentials and limitations of its clinical/preclinical applications. With novelty, completeness and depth in coverage of current and future technologies, this chapter and the next chapter may distinguish themselves from others in the literature and may benefit researchers who are interested in R&D opportunities in spectral CT and/or clinicians who are interested in its physical fundamentals, and exploring its potentials and limitations in preclinical/clinical applications.

7.1 FUNDAMENTALS OF PHYSICS IN SPECTRAL CT

7.1.1 IDEAL SPECTRAL MDCT VIA DUAL-ENERGY SCANS

As demonstrated in Equations 3.1, 3.5 and 3.6 (see Chapter 3), the attenuation $\mu(x, y; E)$ is jointly dependent on atomic number and mass density. As a result, there exist situations in practice that two different materials become undifferentiable as the material with lower atomic number may possess higher mass density. In cardiovascular imaging, for example, dense calcification may not be differentiable from iodine contrast agent because of calcification's high density. In practice, it is hoped to image various materials regardless of the mass density, which can be achieved if another monochromatic energy is added to Equation 3.7, i.e.,

$$I_l = \int_L \alpha(x,y)dl \cdot f_c(E_l) + \int_L \beta(x,y)dl \cdot f_p(E_l)$$
$$\equiv A_\alpha \cdot f_c(E_l) + A_\beta \cdot f_p(E_l) \tag{7.1.1}$$

$$I_h = \int_L \alpha(x,y)dl \cdot f_c(E_h) + \int_L \beta(x,y)dl \cdot f_p(E_h)$$
$$\equiv A_\alpha \cdot f_c(E_h) + A_\beta \cdot f_p(E_h) \tag{7.1.2}$$

where E_l and E_h denote the monochromatic energy at high and low levels, respectively, and

$$A_\alpha \equiv \int_L \alpha(x,y)dl \tag{7.1.1'}$$

$$A_\beta \equiv \int_L \beta(x,y)dl \tag{7.1.2'}$$

Since both $f_c(E_l)$ and $f_p(E_h)$ can be calculated according to Equations 3.2 and 3.3, Equations 7.1.1 and 7.1.2 are a system of linear equations with two variables, and thus A_α and A_β can be analytically solved from measurements I_l and I_h. The spatial functions $\alpha(x, y)$ and $\beta(x, y)$, which are determined by atomic number and mass density, can be reconstructed from A_α and A_β via filtered back-projection (FBP) or iterative reconstruction algorithms. Such a process has been termed *interaction decomposition* in the literature (Tang and Ren 2021).

7.1.2 ENERGY-INTEGRATION SPECTRAL CT VIA SCANS AT DUAL KVP

Since only a polychromatic X-ray source is available in practice, dual-energy CT imaging has to be implemented via a dual-kVp CT scan. By adding another E_{kVp}, Equation 3.11 becomes

$$I_l = \int_{E_l} S_l(E) \int_L \alpha(x,y) dl f_c(E) dE + \int_{E_l} S_l(E) \int_L \beta(x,y) dl f_p(E) dE$$

$$\equiv \int_{E_l} S_l(E) A_\alpha f_c(E) dE + \int_{E_l} S_l(E) A_\beta f_p(E) dE$$

(7.2.1)

$$I_h = \int_{E_h} S_h(E) \int_L \alpha(x,y) dl f_c(E) dE + \int_{E_h} S_h(E) \int_L \beta(x,y) dl f_p(E) dE$$

$$\equiv \int_{E_h} S_h(E) A_\alpha f_c(E) dE + \int_{E_h} S_h(E) A_\beta f_p(E) dE$$

(7.2.2)

Apparently, Equations 7.2.1 and 7.2.2 are no longer a system of linear equations of variables A_α and A_β, and numerical approaches are needed to obtain A_α and A_β from I_l and I_h (see more detail in Section 7.3.2).

7.1.3 Material Decomposition in Energy-Integration Spectral CT

Interaction decomposition is a discovery made by Alvarez and Macovski (Alvarez and Macovski 1976), and the even more meaningful breakthrough brought about by dual-energy or dual-kVp spectral CT is the so-called material decomposition, as elaborated next (Alvarez 1976, 2013).

7.1.3.1 Two-Material Decomposition in Projection Domain

Suppose two materials are known and their attenuation functions can be represented as

$$\mu_1(x,y;E) = \alpha_1(x,y) f_c(E) + \beta_1(x,y) f_p(E)$$

(7.3.1)

$$\mu_2(x,y;E) = \alpha_2(x,y) f_c(E) + \beta_2(x,y) f_p(E)$$

(7.3.2)

Then, it should not be hard to obtain

$$f_c(E) = \frac{\mu_1(x,y;E)\beta_2(x,y) - \mu_2(x,y;E)\beta_1(x,y)}{\alpha_1(x,y)\beta_2(x,y) - \alpha_2(x,y)\beta_1(x,y)}$$

$$\equiv \frac{\beta_2(x,y)}{\alpha_1(x,y)\beta_2(x,y) - \alpha_2(x,y)\beta_1(x,y)} \mu_1(x,y;E)$$

(7.4.1)

$$- \frac{\beta_1(x,y)}{\alpha_1(x,y)\beta_2(x,y) - \alpha_2(x,y)\beta_1(x,y)} \mu_2(x,y;E)$$

$$f_p(E) = \frac{\mu_2(x,y;E)\alpha_1(x,y) - \mu_1(x,y;E)\alpha_2(x,y)}{\alpha_1(x,y)\beta_2(x,y) - \alpha_2(x,y)\beta_1(x,y)}$$

$$\equiv -\frac{\alpha_2(x,y)}{\alpha_1(x,y)\beta_2(x,y) - \alpha_2(x,y)\beta_1(x,y)}\mu_1(x,y;E) \tag{7.4.2}$$

$$+\frac{\alpha_1(x,y)}{\alpha_1(x,y)\beta_2(x,y) - \alpha_2(x,y)\beta_1(x,y)}\mu_2(x,y;E)$$

Subsequently, given any material, its attenuation can be expressed as

$$\mu(x,y;E) = \alpha(x,y)f_c(E) + \beta(x,y)f_p(E)$$

$$= \alpha(x,y)\frac{\mu_1(x,y;E)\beta_2(x,y) - \mu_2(x,y;E)\beta_1(x,y)}{\alpha_1(x,y)\beta_2(x,y) - \alpha_2(x,y)\beta_1(x,y)}$$

$$+\beta(x,y)\frac{\mu_2(x,y;E)\alpha_1(x,y) - \mu_1(x,y;E)\alpha_2(x,y)}{\alpha_1(x,y)\beta_2(x,y) - \alpha_2(x,y)\beta_1(x,y)} \tag{7.5}$$

$$\equiv a_1(x,y)\mu_1(x,y;E) + a_2(x,y)\mu_2(x,y;E)$$

where

$$a_1(x,y) = \frac{\alpha(x,y)\beta_2(x,y) - \beta(x,y)\alpha_2(x,y)}{\alpha_1(x,y)\beta_2(x,y) - \alpha_2(x,y)\beta_1(x,y)} \tag{7.6.1}$$

$$a_2(x,y) = \frac{\beta(x,y)\alpha_1(x,y) - \alpha(x,y)\beta_1(x,y)}{\alpha_1(x,y)\beta_2(x,y) - \alpha_2(x,y)\beta_1(x,y)} \tag{7.6.2}$$

Conceptually, Equation 3.1 states that the attenuation of a material is a function in the functional space spanned by the two base (interaction) functions $f_c(E)$ and $f_p(E)$, whereas Equation 7.5 states that it is a function in the functional space spanned by the two base (material) functions $\mu_1(x, y; E)$ and $\mu_2(x, y; E)$. Notably, $a_1(x, y)$ and $a_2(x, y)$ in Equation 7.5 have no dependence on energy, and Equation 7.5 governs how the variation of a material's attenuation over energy ($\mu(x, y; E)$) depends on the variation of two base materials' attenuation ($\mu_1(x, y; E)$ and $\mu_2(x, y; E)$) over energy. This means that any material can be decomposed into a linear combination of two basis materials (Alvarez 1976, 2013). From Equation 3.1 to Equation 7.5, we are not just playing with mathematics, but rather the conversion is of clinical relevance: one can have a detailed view of the interested material if the two basis materials are chosen appropriately, similar to the situation in which one adjusts the level and width of the display window in routine radiology (Tang and Ren 2021).

A human head phantom is employed to illustrate how material decomposition works in spectral CT, in which water and iodine are selected as the base materials, with the data being acquired at 80 kVp and 140 kVp. As shown in Figure 7.1, the head image is shown as water and iodine equivalent images. Notably, the skull's bony structure is mainly seen in the iodine equivalent image, while the soft tissues, including the soft tissues in the bone, are mainly visible in the water equivalent image.

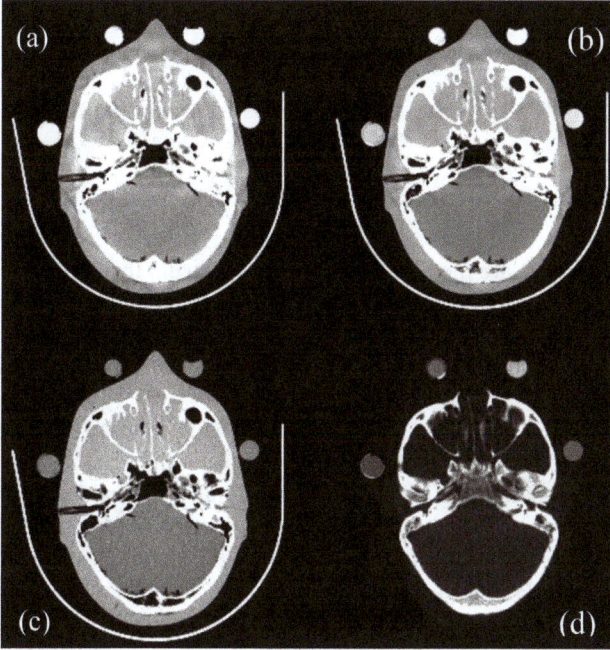

FIGURE 7.1 An illustration of material decomposition in spectral CT implemented via dual-kVp scan: (a) the image at 80 kVp, (b) the image at 140 kVp, and (c) the water equivalent and (d) iodine equivalent images.

7.1.3.2 Decomposition of Material into Atomic Number and Mass Density

In fact, in addition to being decomposed into the linear combination of photoelectric absorption and Compton scattering (Equation 3.1) or two basis materials (Equation 7.5), the attenuation of a material can be decomposed into its mass density and atomic number Z (termed ρZ *decomposition* henceforth) (Heismann et al. 2003).

$$\rho(x,y) = \frac{1}{\beta} \frac{g_h \mu_l(x,y) - g_l \mu_h(x,y)}{g_h - g_l} \tag{7.7.1}$$

$$Z(x,y) = \left(\beta \frac{\mu_h(x,y) - \mu_l(x,y)}{g_h \mu_l(x,y) - g_l \mu_h(x,y)} \right)^{1/3.8}$$

$$= \left(\beta \frac{1 - \mu_l(x,y)\big/\mu_h(x,y)}{g_h \mu_l(x,y)\big/\mu_h(x,y) - g_l} \right)^{1/3.8}, \tag{7.7.2}$$

where μ_l and μ_h are the reconstructed effective linear attenuation coefficients at low and high kVp settings, respectively. Furthermore,

$$g_l = \alpha \int_0^{kVp_l} \frac{S_l(E)}{E^{3.2}} dE \qquad (7.7.3)$$

$$g_h = \alpha \int_0^{kVp_h} \frac{S_h(E)}{E^{3.2}} dE \qquad (7.7.4)$$

where $S_l(E)$ and $S_h(E)$ are the normalized X-ray spectrum inclusively determined by the properties of the X-ray source and detector, and g_l and g_h are parameters that can be determined numerically if the X-ray source's spectra and the detector's spectral response are known, or via calibration in which materials at known thickness have to be employed.

It should be noted that the ρZ decomposition was proposed for post-reconstruction implementation and thus the reconstructed images in $\rho(x, y)$ and $Z(x, y)$ may suffer from the beam-hardening effect, since the initially obtained $\mu_l(x, y)$ and $\mu_h(x, y)$ may suffer from the beam-hardening effect. In practice, the beam-hardening effect can be reduced substantially, if not eliminated, by the techniques of beam-hardening correction that are default in state-of-the-art MDCT scanners. However, the accuracy of quantitative imaging may degrade, as those correction techniques are essentially empirical and hardly robust over clinical situations, especially if more than two kinds of materials, e.g., water, bone and iodine in blood compartments, are involved. Thus far, a few clinical applications have been reported in the literature, along with other image domain-based dual-energy CT techniques (Holms et al. 2008; Yu et al. 2009; McCollough 2015b).

7.1.3.3 Three-Material Decomposition Enabled by Mass Conservation

The approach of two-material decomposition can be utilized in a clinic for identifying the material of interest, such as bone, calcification or iodine, from other tissues in the human body. It is clinically common that decomposition of three or even more materials are of interest, e.g., in characterization of iodine/calcium in cardiovascular or iron/fat in hepatic cases. In principle, adding a third scan at another kVp makes three-material decomposition feasible, but such a straightforward way proportionally increases the radiation dose. Fortunately, resorting to the principle of mass conservation, one has (Liu et al. 2008, 2009)

$$f_{m1} + f_{m2} + f_{m3} = 1 \qquad (7.8.1)$$

$$\mu_m(x, y; E) = f_{m1}\mu_{m_1}(x, y; E) + f_{m2}\mu_{m_2}(x, y; E) + f_{m3}\mu_{m_3}(x, y; E)$$
$$= (\rho_1 f_{m1}\mu_{m_1}(x, y; E) + \rho_2 f_{m2}\mu_{m_2}(x, y; E) + \rho_3 f_{m3}\mu_{m_3}(x, y; E)) / \rho_{eff} \qquad (7.8.2)$$

where $m_1(\rho_1)$, $m_2(\rho_2)$ and $m_3(\rho_3)$ denote the mass fraction (density) of each constituent material, and ρ_{eff} is the effective mass density of the mixture. Then, the two-material decomposition can be extended for three-material decomposition via a two-step process specified next.

In the first step, the effective mass density and atomic number of the mixture is obtained using Equations 7.7.1–7.7.4 through an empirical lookup table. Subsequently, the mass fraction of materials 1 and 2 can be obtained by solving the following integral equations:

$$\mu_{eff,l} = C\rho_{eff} \int_0^{kVp_l} w_l(E)[f_{m1}\mu_{m_1}(x,y;E) + f_{m2}\mu_{m_2}(x,y;E) +$$

$$(1 - f_{m1} - f_{m2})\mu_{m_3}(x,y;E)]dE \tag{7.9.1}$$

$$\mu_{eff,h} = C\rho_{eff} \int_0^{kVp_h} w_h(E)[f_{m1}\mu_{m_1}(x,y;E) + f_{m2}\mu_{m_2}(x,y;E) +$$

$$(1 - f_{m1} - f_{m2})\mu_{m_3}(x,y;E)]dE \tag{7.9.2}$$

where $w_l(E)$ and $w_h(E)$ denote the normalized production of the source spectrum and detector response at low and high kVp, respectively, and C is a constant that can be determined via calibration. With f_{m1} and f_{m2} at hand, f_{m3} can be straightforwardly obtained using Equation 7.8.1. As indicated in the literature (Liu et al. 2009), the accuracy of the effective mass density ρ_{eff} may degrade if the effective atomic number Z_{eff} is larger than 30. Moreover, three-material decomposition may suffer from the beam-hardening effect as the operation specified earlier is carried out post-reconstruction. It also should be noted that, though the approach specified in Equations 7.7–7.9 is implemented in the image domain, its extension to the projection domain should be straightforward. Readers who are interested in three-material decomposition are referred to the literature (Liu et al. 2009)for details.

7.1.4 PHOTON-COUNTING SPECTRAL CT WITH SPECTRAL CHANNELIZATION

Suppose the photon-counting detector used in spectral CT with a polychromatic X-ray source is of energy resolution denoted by energy bin width ΔE_j, and $S_j(E)$ ($j = 1, 2, ..., J$) is the polychromatic spectrum associated with each bin. Given a detector element with its spectral response denoted by $D(E)$, Equation 3.10 needs to be modified to

$$N_j(E) = \int_{E_j - 0.5\Delta E_j}^{E_j + 0.5\Delta E_j} S_j(E) e^{-\int_L \mu(x,y;E)dl} D(E)dE \tag{7.10}$$

Then, the photon-counting detection of X-rays in spectral CT with a polychromatic X-ray source can be treated as a vector $N = [N_1, N_2, ..., N_J]^T$, with the total number of energy bins $J \geq 2$. Moreover, after taking the $-\log$ operation, Equation 3.1 can be extended into vector form (Ehn 2017; Tang and Ren 2021; Ren et al. 2021)

$$\mu\left(x, y; E\right) = \sum_{k=1}^{K} a_k\left(x, y\right) f_k\left(E\right) \tag{7.11}$$

where $f_k(E)$ $(k = 1, 2, ..., K)$ denotes the energy-dependent basis function and $a_k(x, y)$ the associated decomposition coefficients. Furthermore, by defining $A_k = \int_L a_k(x, y)dl$, one has

$$\int_L \mu(x, y; E)dl = \sum_{k=1}^{K} A_k(x, y) f_k(E) \tag{7.12}$$

where $A_k\left(x, y\right) = \int_L a_k\left(x, y\right)dl$. Hence, one can denote the projection data (attenuation) as a vector $A = [A_1, A_2, ..., A_k]^T$, with the dimensionality of functional space $K \geq 2$.

7.1.5 Multi-Material Decomposition (K-Edge Imaging) in Photon-Counting Spectral CT

The availability of multiple energy bins in a photon-counting detector provides the opportunity for decomposition of multiple materials, especially in clinical scenarios wherein contrast agent is administered. In general, since the materials for contrast agents in CT have a high atomic number with its K-edge within the diagnostic energy range, one has to extend Equation 7.5 by including a third material (usually the material generating the contrast)

$$\mu(x, y; E) = a_1(x, y)\mu_1\left(x, y; E\right) + a_2(x, y)\mu_2\left(x, y; E\right) + a_{CA}(x, y)\mu_{CA}(x, y; E) \tag{7.13}$$

where the subscript CA denotes the contrast agent, e.g., iodine or gadolinium that are commonly used in the clinic, or other high atomic number materials, e.g., gold, barium or bismuth that may be used in future contrast agents in the form of macromolecule or nanoparticles (see more detail in Chapter 9). In principle, Equation 7.13 can be expanded further to accommodate more materials, e.g., iodine and gadolinium, simultaneously, but caution needs to be exercised in dealing with the number of energy bins and dimensionality of functional space (see more detail in Chapter 8).

7.2 DATA ACQUISITION (SCAN) IN SPECTRAL CT

The earliest prototype of spectral CT was implemented in the image domain, in which two images at 80 kVp and 140 kVp were subtracted for better characterization of hemotoma (Marshall et al. 1981). Much spectral information in the interaction between X-rays and tissues is compromised in the simple and straightforward subtraction. Following the work by Alvarez and Macoviski, the vast majority of investigation in spectral CT, especially in the 1970s to mid-1980s, was carried out in the projection domain, aimed at exploring the advantages and potentials that can be offered by spectral CT. With the advent of DSDD CT in 2006, spectral CT resurged as a prevalent subject in CT technologies R&D and clinical applications, though the dominant goal behind the DSDD CT is mainly to improve (double) the temporal resolution of cardiovascular CT, especially CT coronary angiography. Since then, tremendous effort has been devoted by researchers to developing and optimizing the technologies for implementing spectral CT.

Historically, at least seven approaches have been proposed to implement spectral CT: slow kVp-switching, fast kVp-switching, spectral splitter, detector with spectral splitter, layered (sandwiched) detector, dual-source–dual-detector, and photon-counting detector, of which, except for the last one, are all energy-integration based. To date, the spectral splitter technique has not gained sufficient momentum in the industry, as the detector with a spectral splitter was proposed for the xenon gas detector that was almost phased out of the CT industry. Herein we focus on the four remaining technologies for implementing spectral CT (Figure 7.2), with their major properties listed in Table 7.1 and a brief discussion given next.

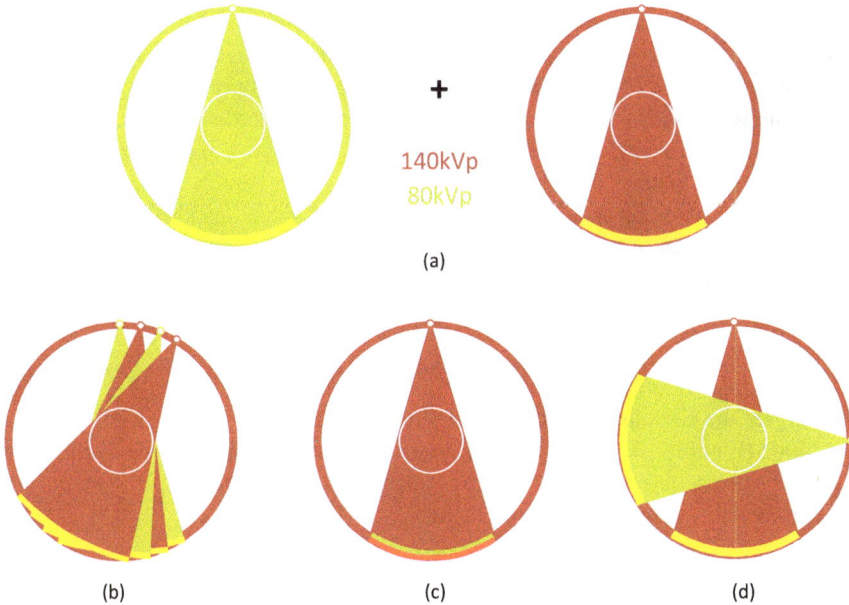

FIGURE 7.2   Schematics showing the four techniques to implement spectral CT: (a) slow kVp-switching, (b) fast kVp-switching, (c) dual layered detector and (d) dual-source–dual-detector.

TABLE 7.1

Primary Pros and Cons of Each Scan Mode and Associated Image Reconstruction Algorithms (FBP: filtered backprojection; IIR: iterative image reconstruction; T-resolution: temporal resolution; N-uniformity: noise uniformity.)

X-Ray Detection	Pros	Cons	Raw Data/Image	In Clinic
Slow kV	FBP/IIR	Balanced IQ	T-resolution	Y
Fast kV	FBP/IIR	T-resolution	Noise, N-uniformity	Y
Layered detector	FBP/IIR	T-resolution	Noise, N-uniformity	Y
Dual-source–dual-detector	FBP (IIR)	Accuracy	T-resolution, workflow	Y
Photon counting	FBP (IIR)	Accuracy	T-resolution, workflow	Y

7.2.1 Slow kVp-Switching in Energy-Integration Spectral CT

The slow kVp-switching technique (Figure 7.2a) is carried out by acquiring one set of projection data at one kVp and subsequently another set at the other kVp. If the angular positions of the second data set line up with those of the first set, the slow kVp-switching spectral CT can be implemented in the projection domain. Otherwise, it can only be implemented in the image domain, because of the angular mis-registration. Apparently, this is the easiest way to implement spectral CT with almost no impact on the CT architecture and hardware, and indeed was the first implementation of spectral CT by Hounsfield in the EMI CT (Hounsfield 1973). However, the slow kVp-switching is subject to time lag between the cascaded scans and prone to the inconsistency that may be induced by cardiovascular, respiratory and involuntary visceral motions. Moreover, though this way makes the partition of X-ray dose (see Section 7.4.5.1) at low and high kVps relatively easy, it is hard for the slow kVp-switching spectral CT to separate X-ray source spectra at low and high kVps, which, as elaborated in Chapter 8, Section 8.1.1, may compromise the system's performance considerably.

7.2.2 Fast kVp-Switching in Energy-Integration Spectral CT

To mitigate the risks associated with the inter-scan time lag, the fast kVp-switching technique (Figure 7.2b) is proposed, in which two sets of projection data at low and high kVps are acquired in an interleaved manner (Forghani 2017a, 2017b), but this mode may lead to the following situations:

- Given a total number of projection views per gantry rotation, the number of projection views in the scans at low and high kVps are cut in half. Consequently, unless the trigger frequency of data acquisition increases accordingly, the azimuthal resolution spectral CT can be degraded, which may impact some advanced clinical applications in which high spatial resolution is needed.

- Given a gantry rotation time and unless the tube current increases adequately, the noise in the images corresponding to low and high kVps increases by the square root of two, which may impact some advanced clinical applications where the noise property is of relevance.
- Care needs to be taken in partitioning the X-ray dose between the data acquisitions at low and high kVps, since, in general, the X-ray photons at lower kVp are less penetrating and may result in significantly higher noise in projection data, but the implementation of spectral CT needs the noise in low and high kVp scans to be comparable in intensity.
- Similar to the situation in slow kVp-switching, it is even harder, if not impossible, for fast kVp-switching spectral CT to separate X-ray source spectra, which may inevitably degrade the system's performance.

7.2.3 LAYERED DETECTION IN ENERGY-INTEGRATION SPECTRAL CT

Immediately after the invention of CT, the layered detector was proposed as a candidate technique for implementing spectral CT, in which, the X-ray photons at relatively lower energy are absorbed by the front layer with the rest at high energy by the rear layer (Sones and Barnes 1989). Layered detector technology was approached by a major CT vendor for implementation of spectral CT (Figure 7.3c), and it is currently offered in the marketplace (Duan et al. 2018). Since the two sets of projection data acquired at low and high kVps line up, this mode avoids the temporal and spatial mis-registration that occurs in both fast and slow kVp-switching. However, the separation of X-ray source spectra in this mode solely depends on the difference in absorption property between the front and rear layers. Moreover, the X-ray photons that have penetrated the human body and impinging at the detector cell may vary dramatically in its spectrum, due to the variation in the attenuation property over various routes. On the other hand, the spectral response of each detector element is energy dependent and its calibration may become more complicated than that in a single-layer detector, particularly if an interlayer filtration is embedded in between for spectral separation. This might be the underlying reason that it took relatively longer for the vendor to deliver its energy-integration spectral CT product to the marketplace.

7.2.4 DUAL-SOURCE AND DUAL-DETECTOR IN ENERGY-INTEGRATION SPECTRAL CT

The advent of DSDD CT marked the beginning of a renaissance in the R&D of spectral CT, though it is mainly aimed at doubling the temporal resolution in CT coronary angiography. Due to its architecture, DSDD CT (Figure 7.3d) has the desired flexibility in source spectral separation, dose partitioning between scans at low and high kVps, maintains the azimuthal resolution and uses established spectral calibration techniques that are proprietary to CT vendors. Notably, the approximately orthogonal layout of DSDD architecture leads to the fact that this mode can only be carried out in the image domain. Though image domain implementation is initially carried out in the slow kVp-switching mode, its functionality has been expanded substantially in DSDD CT with innovations in hardware and algorithms, making it quite successful in clinical practice and research, as evidenced by the numerous papers published so far. It should be noted that the roughly orthogonal DSDD layout does not render any time lag between the projection data (and thus the images) acquired at low and high kVps, which is the major advantage over the spectral CT implemented by slow kVp-switching.

7.2.5 PHOTON COUNTING WITH SPECTRAL CHANNELIZATION

The four techniques for data acquisition in spectral CT presented earlier are based on energy integration. Actually, in their milestone paper (Alvarez and Macovski 1976), the concept of dual-energy CT was proposed with X-ray detection in the manner of photon counting. Later on, the photon-counting detector was equipped with spectral resolution (binning in energy) (Shikhaliev 2005, 2006 and 2012; Roessl and Herrmann 2007; Ren et al. 2021), which possesses a few advantages over the energy-integration detector for implementation of spectral CT (see more details in Chapter 3, Sections 3.4.1–3.4.3).

7.2.6 PHOTON COUNTING AND ENERGY INTEGRATION: A JOINT APPROACH

The data acquisition modes introduced so far are dependent on either energy-integration or photon-counting detection, but in fact, a combination of them, which is termed *joint photon-counting and energy-integration detection* in this book, can also be an approach for data acquisition in spectral CT (Roessl et al. 2011), in which the noise in the data acquired by photon counting and energy integration, respectively, is correlated. A theoretical analysis and experimental evaluation (phantom study) carried out in the paper (Roessl et al. 2011) have shown that such a correlation in noise in fact may help the imaging performance of spectral CT, rather than degrade it as initially thought.

7.3 IMAGE FORMATION IN SPECTRAL CT

The formation of images in spectral CT implemented in the image domain undergoes a process similar to that of conventional single energy CT, in which sophisticated and proprietary spectral correction approaches are inherited. Correction of the beam-hardening effect carried out at low and high kVps can remove artifacts from the final spectral CT image, but it may undermine the physical basis upon which the spectral CT is grounded. Though tremendous effort has been devoted to making the image domain in spectral CT as effective as the projection domain solution, it should be kept in mind that, if pushed to the end of reaching the most achievable potential, the projection domain approach should outperform image domain implementation.

7.3.1 INTERACTION DECOMPOSITION: A MAPPING FROM PROJECTION SPACE TO INTERACTION SPACE

Starting from the maximum likelihood estimation in their milestone paper (Alvarez and Macovski 1976), Alvarez and Macovski approached Equations 7.1.1 and 7.1.2 and came up with a numerical (Newton–Raphson) solution to a pair of non-linear equations. Via algebra, the relationship between (I_{low}, I_{high}) and (A_α, A_β) can actually be obtained via polynomial data fitting, e.g., a third-order fitting with known materials at various thicknesses:

$$I_l \equiv \lambda_0 + \lambda_1 A_\alpha + \lambda_2 A_\beta + \lambda_3 A_\alpha^2 + \lambda_4 A_\alpha A_\beta + \lambda_5 A_\beta^2 + \lambda_6 A_\alpha^3 + \lambda_7 A_\beta^3 \quad (7.14.1)$$

$$I_h \equiv \chi_0 + \chi_1 A_\alpha + \chi_2 A_\beta + \chi_3 A_\alpha^2 + \chi_4 A_\alpha A_\beta + \chi_5 A_\beta^2 + \chi_6 A_\alpha^3 + \chi_7 A_\beta^3 \quad (7.14.2)$$

The coefficients λ_0, λ_1, λ_2, ..., λ_7 and χ_0, χ_1, χ_2, ..., χ_7 can be attained either analytically or experimentally, known as *calibration*, in which the linear least square with the Moore–Penrose pseudoinverse may be used (Buzug 2008). In principle, Equations 7.14.1 and 7.14.2 can be perceived as a mapping from the projection space (*P*-space) to the interaction space.

7.3.2 MATERIAL DECOMPOSITION: A MAPPING FROM PROJECTION SPACE TO *A*-SPACE

Starting from Equation 7.4 we can obtain the following equations in a way similar to attaining Equations 7.1.1 and 7.1.2:

$$I_l = \int_{E_l} S_l(E) \int_L a_1(x,y) dl\mu_1(x,y;E) dE + \int_{E_l} S_l(E) \int_L a_2(x,y) dl\mu_2(x,y;E) dE$$

$$\equiv \int_{E_l} S_l(E) A_1(x,y) \mu_1(x,y;E) dE + \int_{E_l} S_l(E) A_2(x,y) \mu_2(x,y;E) dE \quad (7.15.1)$$

$$I_h = \int_{E_h} S_h(E) \int_L a_1(x,y) dl\mu_1(x,y;E) dE + \int_{E_h} S_h(E) \int_L a_2(x,y) dl\mu_2(x,y;E) dE$$

$$\equiv \int_{E_h} S_h(E) A_1(x,y) \mu_1(x,y;E) dE + \int_{E_h} S_h(E) A_2(x,y) \mu_2(x,y;E) dE \quad (7.15.2)$$

Note that $S_l(E)$ and $S_h(E)$ are inclusively defined by the source spectrum, filtration and detector response.

7.3.2.1 Data Fitting

Analytically, we can turn Equations 7.15.1 and 7.15.2 into

$$A_1 \equiv \xi_0 + \xi_1 I_l + \xi_2 I_h + \xi_3 I_l^2 + \xi_4 I_l I_h + \xi_5 I_h^2 + \xi_6 I_l^3 + \xi_7 I_l^2 I_h + \xi_8 I_l I_h^2 + \xi_9 I_h^3 \qquad (7.16.1)$$

$$A_2 \equiv \zeta_0 + \zeta_1 I_l + \zeta_2 I_h + \zeta_3 I_l^2 + \zeta_4 I_l I_h + \zeta_5 I_h^2 + \zeta_6 I_l^3 + \zeta_7 I_l^2 I_h + \zeta_8 I_l I_h^2 + \zeta_9 I_h^3 \qquad (7.16.2)$$

which in principle can be perceived as a mapping from the P-space to the so-called A-space (Alvarez 2010, 2011 and 2013). Then, the task becomes to determine the coefficients $\xi_0, \xi_1, \xi_2, ..., \xi_9$ and $\zeta_0, \zeta_1, \zeta_2, ..., \zeta_9$, and at least two ways exist to get the solution. The first way is numerically for the scenario where $S_l(E)$ and $S_h(E)$ are exactly or quasi-exactly known. Given base materials, i.e., $[\mu_1, \mu_2]$ are known, a set of $[I_l, I_h]_{N \times 2}$ can be computed according to Equations 7.15.1 and 7.15.2 for a known material at the appropriately determined thickness $[A_1, A_2]_{N \times 2}$, where $N \times 2$ specifies the data dimension. The second way is experimental for the scenario where $S_l(E)$ and $S_h(E)$ are not exactly known. By placing a set of known materials at the appropriate thickness, i.e., given $[A_1, A_2]_{N \times 2}$, in the X-ray beam, one can attain the data set $[I_l, I_h]_{N \times 2}$ by measuring the X-ray intensity penetrating the materials. Then, the coefficients $\xi_0, \xi_1, \xi_2, ..., \xi_9$ and $\zeta_0, \zeta_1, \zeta_2, ..., \zeta_9$ may be obtained numerically from the data $[A_1, A_2]_{N \times 2}$ and $[I_l, I_h]_{N \times 2}$. Notably, the experimental method may provide a more robust solution because one may not be able to exactly modify the spectra $S_l(E)$ and $S_h(E)$ in practice.

7.3.2.2 Lookup Table

The approach specified in Equations 7.16.1 and 7.16.2 is termed the *direct approximation method*, and its accuracy, especially its accuracy at large object thickness, can be implemented via the sub-region direct approximation method and the iso-transmission line method (Chuang and Huang 1988). In fact, the direct approximation method can alternatively be implemented via lookup tables, in which known materials at appropriate thicknesses are used to attain a high sampling ratio in the functional space spanned by the base materials and interpolation can be carried out if inter-entry sampling in the material space is needed.

7.3.3 MATERIAL DECOMPOSITION IN IMAGE DOMAIN

As mentioned, the earliest practice in spectral CT was Hounsfield's attempt in the EMI scanner, which was just a subtraction of two CT images acquired at low and high kVps (Hounsfield 1973) – the simplest form of linear algebra. Right after the paper published by Alvarez and Macovski, Di Chiro investigated the feasibility of carrying out material decomposition in the image domain and indicated that it is equivalent to a linear combination of photoelectric absorption and Compton scattering in the projection domain (Di Chiro et al. 1979) . Notably, however, such a material decomposition in the image domain is in principle only an approximation of the material decomposition in the projection domain, since the cross-production terms in Equations 7.14.1, 7.14.2, 7.16.1 and 7.16.2 were actually absent from the image domain material decomposition, though the X-ray polychromatics-induced beam-hardening artifacts can be removed via system calibration carried out separately in forming the two images at low and high kVps. Via a joint calibration cross the two images, the performance of the image domain material decomposition can be improved moderately, as presented in the paper (Maass et al. 2009).

7.3.4 ITERATIVE MAXIMUM LIKELIHOOD ESTIMATION

The integral equations (Equations 7.2.1–7.2.2) and their polynomial approximations (Equations 7.16.1–7.16.2) are derived under the framework of maximum likelihood estimation (MLE) (Alvarez and Macovski 1976). However, given the X-ray dose, the number of photons recorded in each energy bin (and thus the signal-to-noise ratio (SNR) in data) is proportionally reduced with increasing number of energy bins, which imposes a significant challenge to image formation in photon-counting spectral CT, though there is no longer electronic noise and dark current-induced non-random noise. In general, statistical estimation carried out in an iterative manner can outperform analytical solutions in dealing with noise, and thus the iterative maximum likelihood estimation has been pursued to cope with the extremely low SNR that may occur in energy bins, especially at the low or high energy end.

The maximum likelihood estimation has been studied for data extraction in photon-counting spectral CT. Suppose $I_k(A_\alpha)$ ($k = 1, ..., K$), which observes the Poisson distribution, denotes the random variables corresponding to the number of photons recorded in energy bin B_k with mean value $\lambda(A_\alpha)$, where A_α denotes the set of line integrals. Given an object with its specific composition denoted by A_α, the likelihood of counting m_i photons in each bin B_i, i.e., $(I_1 = i_1, ..., I_K = i_K)$, can be written as

$$P(i_1,...,i_K \mid \lambda_1(A_\alpha),...\lambda_K(A_\alpha)) = \prod_{k=1}^{K} \frac{[\lambda_k(A_\alpha)]^{i_k}}{i_k!} e^{-\lambda_k(A_\alpha)} \tag{7.17}$$

For algebraic convenience, one may take the negative log-likelihood and get

$$L(i_1,...,i_K \mid A_\alpha) = -\ln(P(i_1,...,i_N \mid \lambda_1(A_\alpha),...\lambda_K(A_\alpha))$$

$$= \sum_{k=1}^{K} [\lambda_k(A_\alpha) + \ln(i_k!) - i_k \ln(\lambda_k(A_\alpha))] \tag{7.18}$$

$$\cong \sum_{k=1}^{K} [\lambda_k(A_\alpha) - i_k \ln(\lambda_k(A_\alpha))].$$

Notably, the constant term $ln(i_k!)$ is removed from the final result in Equation 7.18, and quite a few algorithms, e.g., those proposed in Reference (Roessl and Proksa 2007), can be readily utilized for solving Equation 7.18 numerically.

7.3.5 Alvarez's Method

As indicated in Reference (Alvarez 2011), in addition to being computationally inefficient, there is in theory no guarantee for the aforementioned iterative algorithm to converge. Alvarez proposed an algorithm consisting of two steps: (i) the logarithm of maximum likelihood estimation is linearized via Taylor expansion to get an initial solution using the Moore–Penrose pseudoinverse, and subsequently (ii) the initial solution is used in a lookup table to retrieve an entry to be added to the initial solution. As such, the accuracy of data extraction can be maintained with no concern about the convergence, while its computation time can be substantially shortened. For details about this two-pass algorithm, readers are referred to Reference (Alvarez 2011).

7.3.6 Multi-Channel Joint Material Decomposition and Image Reconstruction

Both the analytic and iterative (statistical or optimization-based) image reconstruction algorithms that have been used in conventional CT can be reused in spectral CT for image formation, no matter if the material decomposition is carried out in the projection or image domain. In general, however, a straightforward reuse of the analytic and iterative image reconstruction algorithms may not be an optimal solution in image formation, since it (i) usually requires inter-kVp spatial consistency and thus may impose constraints on the system architecture, and (ii) ignores the inter-kVp and/or inter-energy bin correlation in the spectral and/or noise properties, which can be used to make the image reconstruction better in noise property and/or robustness (Cai et al. 2013; Nakada et al. 2015; Zhao et al. 2015; Sukovle and Clinthorne 1999; Long and Fessler 2014; Zhang et al. 2014; Barber et al. 2016; Zhang et al. 2018). Hence, a joint scheme for material decomposition and image reconstruction, which has to be in the fashion of an iterative algorithm, is needed, as illustrated in the following sections.

7.3.7 Extended Algebraic Reconstruction Technique (E-ART)

Once the beam-hardening effect in projection data is corrected, the image reconstruction in conventional CT starts from Equations 3.7 and 3.9 and can be formulated as the solution to a system of linear equations that are hyper-planes, i.e., the intersection of those hyper-planes. The solution can be found via the algebraic reconstruction technique (ART), in which iterative orthogonal projection on the hyper-planes is carried out, as done by Hounsfield in the EMI scanner. The ART can certainly be reused to reconstruct an image in spectral CT once the material decomposition (and thus the beam-hardening correction) is carried out. Nevertheless, with joint material decomposition and image reconstruction, one has to start from Equations 3.10 and 3.11 in energy-integration spectral CT (or Equation 7.10 in photon-counting spectral CT). Consequently, the forward projection becomes non-linear and the joint material decomposition and image reconstruction is thus tantamount to finding the solution to a system of non-linear equations (hyper-surfaces), i.e., the intersection of those hyper-surfaces (Zhao et al. 2015).

In mathematics, it is difficult to carry out orthogonal projection onto hyper-surfaces. Using first-order Taylor expansion, Equations 3.10 and 3.11 (or equivalently Equation 7.10) can be approximated to a linear forward-projection. Then, with adequate modification, the formulation in ART can be reused for joint material decomposition and image reconstruction in spectral CT. Notably, the linearization using Taylor expansion has been a strategy that is frequently exercised in statistical (see next section) iterative image reconstruction. Impressive preliminary data of a phantom study was presented, and readers interested in the algorithmic derivation and more details of the result are referred to Reference (Zhao et al. 2015).

7.3.8 Statistical Approaches

The "joint-ness" in the E-ART is just a joint process of material decomposition and image reconstruction, in which there is no inter-kVp or inter-energy bin joint-ness at all. In fact, there exists inter-channel (low and high kVps in energy-integration spectral CT or energy bins in photon-counting spectral CT) correlation, which offers the opportunity for even better imaging performance and robustness if statistical modeling is combined with the iterative algorithms for joint material decomposition and image reconstruction (Nakada 2015).

7.3.8.1 Statistical Approaches with Quadratic Approximation of Objective Function

Under the framework of statistical image reconstruction, if one has no knowledge of the statistical property of the image to be reconstructed but assumes that the noise associated with projection data (observation) is random, least squares is the most fundamental approach to get the solution in an iterative manner (Buzug 2008). In fact, the projection data obeys the Poisson distribution, while the observation noise is in Gaussian distribution. Then, statistical approaches, such as maximum likelihood (ML) or maximum *a posteriori* probability (MAP) estimation, can be employed for material decomposition and image reconstruction in an iterative manner (Fessler 2009) ML and MAP are mathematically equivalent to the penalized weighted least squares (PWLS), and it is the penalty-based weighting that enables them to deliver images with better noise properties or robustness in dealing with challenging situations, e.g., data missing in a sonogram (Lange and Fessler 1999; Fessler 2009).

Usually, regularization is added to ML or replaces the prior in MAP for better properties in reconstruction, and the regularized ML and MAP can be expressed as

$$\hat{\mu} = \arg\max_{\mu \geq 0}(L(\mu) - \beta \cdot R(\mu)), \tag{7.19}$$

where $\hat{\mu}$ denotes the image to be reconstructed, $\mu \geq 0$ is the constraint on pixel value based on the fact that in reality no material is of a negative attenuation coefficient and β is a parameter to control the speed of convergence. Starting from Equations

3.7 and 3.9, the likelihood function $L(\mu)$ and regularization function $R(\mu)$ are in quadratic form and quite a few algorithms can be used to solve Equation 7.19 iteratively (Fessler 2009). Again, however, we can only start from Equations 3.10 and 3.11 in spectral CT and the X-ray source's polychromatics induces non-linearity, leading to the situation that the likelihood function $L(\mu)$ (and/or the regularization function $R(\mu)$ as well) is no longer quadratic (Long and Fessler 2014).

The earliest attempt under statistical framework for joint material decomposition and image reconstruction was reported in Reference (Sukovle and Clinthorne 1999), in which the Gaussian–Seidel algorithm was used to minimize the non-quadratic objective function. By adequately defining surrogate functions and applying optimization transfer principles, the non-quadratic likelihood (and/or regularization function) can be approximated into a quadratic form that is equivalent to the PWLS and thus quite a few algorithms can be used to find the solution (Long and Fessler 2014). By exercising a similar strategy, both the likelihood and edge-preserving regularization (objective function) in the joint material decomposition and image reconstruction can be approximated into voxel-wise separable surrogate functions that are quadratic, and thus existing algorithms can be reused.

It should be noted that the likelihood function $L(\mu)$ is formed jointly by taking all data channels (low and high kVps in energy integration or multi-energy bins in photon counting) into account simultaneously, leading to the fact that the image formed in this way has made use all the available information, i.e., not only jointly in material decomposition and image reconstruction but also jointly over the data channels. Another joint material decomposition and image reconstruction algorithm was proposed in Reference (Cai et al. 2013), in which, by applying the Bayesian rule and Gaussian observation modeling, the joint MAP estimation is converted into the minimization of a non-quadratic objective function with a modified conjugate gradient algorithm to find the solution. Impressive preliminary data from phantom study was presented in References (Cai et al. 2013) and readers interested in the algorithmic derivation are referred to them for more details.

7.3.8.2 Statistical Approaches with Quadratic Approximation of Objective Function and Material Constraint

The performance of statistical image reconstruction can be optimized by choosing the functional form and/or tweaking the associated parameters in regularization (or *a priori*). An algorithm called joint estimation maximum *a posteriori* (JE-MAP) was proposed in Reference (Nakada et al. 2015) for joint material decomposition and image reconstruction, in which, the regularization is modeled as a voxel-wise coupled Markov random field (MRF) by taking into account the correspondence between the voxel value and tissue types. In fact, the tissue type associated with each voxel is treated as a latent variable, as inspired by its successful applications in the field of image analysis. Using multivariate Gaussian distribution, both the likelihood and regularization terms can be approximated into quadratic forms and thus the iterated conditional modes (ICM) algorithm can be utilized to solve the problem. Impressive preliminary data from phantom study was presented in Reference

(Nakada et al. 2015) and readers interested in the algorithmic derivation are referred to it for more details.

7.3.9 POST-DECOMPOSITION STATISTICAL APPROACHES

As indicated in Reference (Zhang et al. 2014), if the statistical approaches start post-decomposition, the likelihood function $L(\mu)$ in Equation 7.19 becomes quadratic. By adopting an MRF as the *a priori*, a joint model-based iterative reconstruction (JDE-MBIR) was proposed for image formation in dual-energy spectral CT implemented via fast kVp-switching. Presented in Figure 7.3 are the preliminary results of a patient study obtained with water and iodine as the basis for material decomposition and monochromatic analysis (see Section 7.4.3), which shows that the JDE-MBIR algorithm outperforms its counterparts with independent analytic (FBP) or iterative (MBIR) image reconstruction in the images formed for material decomposition. Additionally, the proposed JDE-MBIR behaves well in convergence, and readers interested in the details are referred to Reference (Zhang et al. 2014).

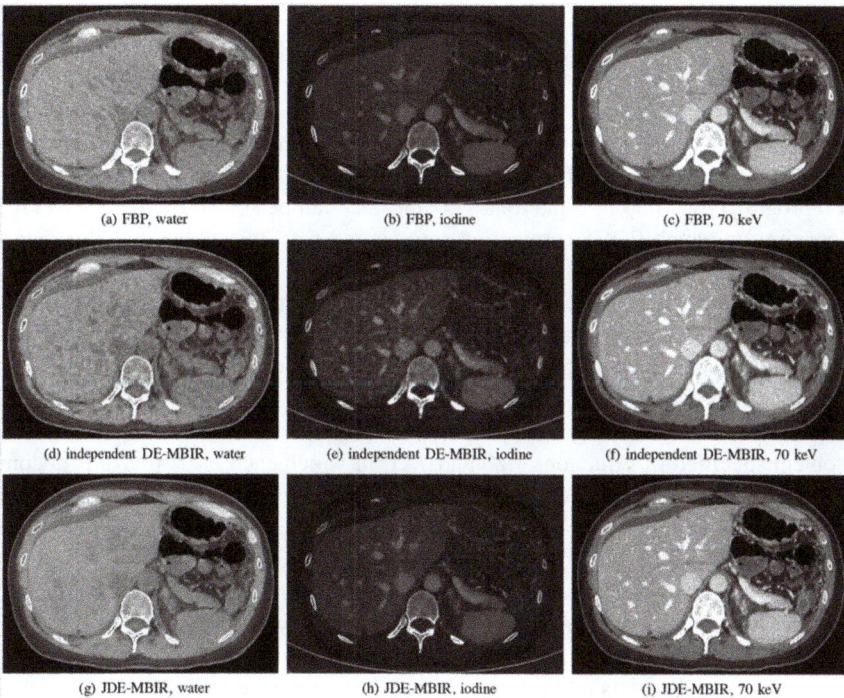

(a) FBP, water	(b) FBP, iodine	(c) FBP, 70 keV
(d) independent DE-MBIR, water	(e) independent DE-MBIR, iodine	(f) independent DE-MBIR, 70 keV
(g) JDE-MBIR, water	(h) JDE-MBIR, iodine	(i) JDE-MBIR, 70 keV

FIGURE 7.3 Illustration of the performance of joint estimation maximum *a posterior* (JE-MAP) algorithm in spectral imaging (material decomposition and virtual monochromatic imaging) and its advantage over independent estimation maximum *a posterior* (JE-MAP) algorithm and FBP algorithm, respectively. (Images are adopted with permission from Zhang et al. 2014.)

7.3.10 OPTIMIZATION-BASED APPROACHES

Statistical image reconstruction, which has played a dominant role in PET/SPECT and an increasingly important role in CT, is formulated as a problem of parameter estimation, in which the variables and noise are adequately modeled based on an insightful understanding of the observation process. Recently, optimization-based approaches, in which the image reconstruction is formulated as programming or optimization, is gaining momentum in CT image reconstruction, especially in situations wherein the projection data are acquired at low radiation dose or some of them are missing.

An optimization-based image reconstruction algorithm is proposed in Reference (Barber et al. 2016; Pan et al. 2018; Chen et al. 2018) and states

$$b^* = \arg\min_{b} \Psi(b) \qquad s.t. \qquad \Phi(b; g_M) \leq \varepsilon \qquad and \qquad b \succ 0 \qquad (7.20)$$

where b^* denotes the material-decomposed image to be reconstructed. $\Psi(b)$ is the objective function and is defined as

$$\Psi(b) = \sum_{k=1}^{K} b_{kTV}, \qquad (7.21)$$

and $\Phi(b; g_M)$ denotes the data divergence, where k indexes over all basis images given a pixel location. Ideally, if one starts from Equations 3.7 and 3.9, the optimization program specified in Equations 7.20 and 7.21 can be solved by the ASD-POCS algorithm, in which POCS (projection onto convex sets) lowers the data divergence and ASD (adaptive steepest descent) lowers the total variation objective function, respectively and alternatively. Unfortunately, however, the non-linearity induced by X-ray polychromatics in spectral CT (Equations 3.10 and 3.11) leads to data divergence, and consequently the optimization program specified in Equations 7.20 and 7.21 become non-convex.

The ASD-NC-POCS algorithm is proposed to solve the non-convex optimization problem specified in Equations 7.20 and 7.21, in which each basis image is decomposed into a "monochromatic component (linear term)" and "decomposition error (non-linear term)" (Pan et al. 2018; Chen et al. 2018). With respect to the monochromatic component, the formulation in the ASD-POCS algorithm can be directly reused, followed by updating with the decomposition error at each iteration, which is the key step to making the ASD-NC-POCS algorithm work. In principle, the ASD-NC-POCS algorithm is heuristic, though three necessary conditions for its convergence are given. Readers interested in its details are referred to Reference (Pan et al. 2018; Chen et al. 2018) for details.

Prior to concluding this section, I would like to point out that the multi-channel joint material decomposition and image reconstruction, regardless of their implementation with statistical or optimization-based approaches, may significantly increase the computational complexity. For example, in comparison to conventional CT with an $N×M$ system matrix, the dimension of the system matrix in the multi-channel joint material decomposition and image reconstruction increases to $O((S×N)×M)$. Additionally, a joint treatment may create difficulty in maintaining the system matrix's conditioning that is crucial to the convergence and robustness of image reconstruction over measurement noise (Fessler and Booth 1999; Barber et al. 2016; Mory 2018).

7.4 IMAGE PRESENTATION IN SPECTRAL CT

The spectral CT offered by leading CT vendors provides an assembly of functionalities, termed *image presentation* in this section, for clinical applications and preclinical research. Starting from the earliest concept of material decomposition in the projection domain, we go over those major functionalities.

7.4.1 ANALYSIS IN MATERIAL SPACE

7.4.1.1 Contrast Enhancement

A close inspection of Equation 7.5 tell us that, by adjusting energy E, the slope of the linear combination varies, which is equivalent to changing the angle of projection, as illustrated in Figure 7.4a. It is interesting to note that, given any material, there exists a characteristic angle in the functional space spanned by the base materials, and the characteristic angle is determined by (Lehmann et al. 1981)

$$\varphi = \arctan\left[\frac{a_2(x,y)}{a_1(x,y)} \right]. \tag{7.22}$$

Using bone and water as the base materials, Figure 7.4b may be more helpful for us to understand the concept of projection in the functional space, in which the clustered dots classify the distribution of calcium, iodine, fat and water. The azimuthal

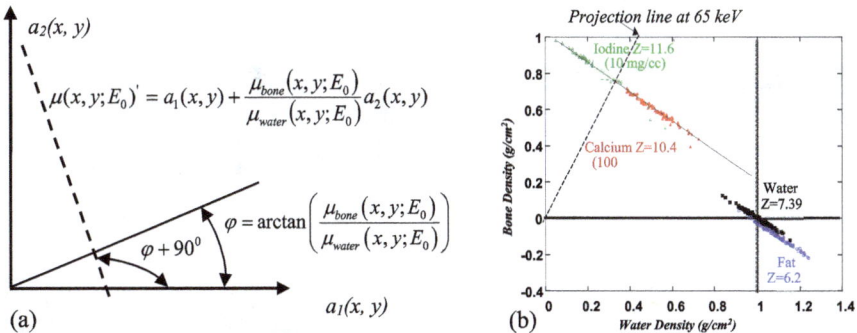

FIGURE 7.4   (a) Schematic showing the projection in a functional space spanned by two base materials, with the projection angle φ determined by the base materials at energy E_0, and (b) an example of clustered distribution of material in the functional space spanned by bone and water.

angle corresponds to the material's atomic number and the intra-cluster spreading out in each material is due to quantum, electronic or other noise in data acquisition (Lehmann 1981; Alvarez 2010).

Shown in Figure 7.5 is the result of a phantom study of contrast enhancement that is of clinical relevance in cardiovascular imaging. The phantom is configured of multiple targets with calcium and iodine at various concentrations. The image in Figure 7.5a is a conventional CT image acquired at 120 kVp, in which the calcium–iodine targets at concentration ratio over 10:1 is not discernible. Nevertheless, all those targets become readily differentiable in the dual-kVp spectral CT image (Figure 7.5b), which, in fact, corresponds to a projection onto the solid line in the functional space spanned by water and bone (Figure 7.4b).

7.4.1.2 Contrast Cancellation

A revisit of Figure 7.4 tells us that, rather than the one onto the solid line, the projection can also be carried out onto the dashed line in the material space. As such, the contrast between calcium and iodine decreases substantially or may even disappear. The functionality of contrast cancellation in spectral CT is of relevance in quite a few clinical applications, e.g., virtual non-contrast in neurovascular CT to differentiate between hemorrhagic and calcification (Wiggins et al. 2019).

7.4.2 MATERIAL ANALYSIS IN IMAGE DOMAIN

Material analysis was initially carried out in image domain, though it was just a subtraction of images acquired at low and high kVps (Hounsfield 1973), respectively. With the advent of spectral CT implemented with a dual source and dual detector, the material analysis carried out in the image domain with functionality similar to that in the projection domain has been developed to fulfill the requirements imposed by clinical applications. Overall, the image domain material analysis, which is carried out in the CT-value space spanned by the CT numbers of a pixel generated in the CT images corresponding to low and high kVps, respectively,

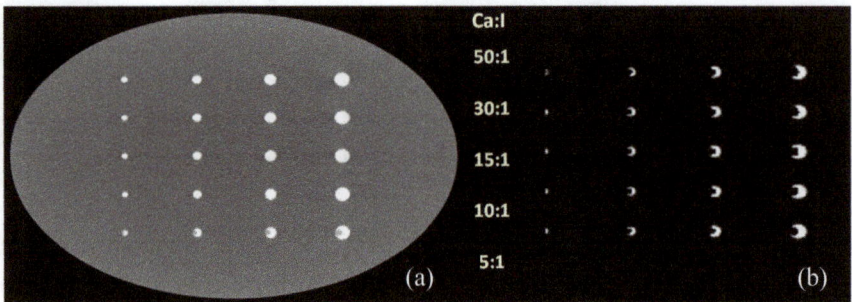

FIGURE 7.5 Illustration of material enhancement via projection in the functional space spanned by base materials: (a) almost no contrast between calcium (Ca) and iodine (I) before projection; (b) strong contrast between them after projection.

falls into two categories: (i) material projection and (ii) material classification (Jin 2011).

7.4.2.1 Material Projection

As illustrated in Figure 7.6a, except for the replacement of abscissa and coordinate axes, the image domain material projection is carried out in a manner that is similar to the material projection in the A-space (see Figure 7.4). The CT number of soft tissues, including adipose, water and blood, should roughly be on the line at slope k_{st}, in the CT-number space, while any of the soft tissue (denoted by (x, y) in the CT-number diagram) mixed with iodine, the most commonly used CT contrast in the clinic, moves to the spot (x_0, y_0) along the line with slope k_{iod}. Then, as illustrated in Figure 7.6a, virtual non-contrast CT can be carried out specifically as (Jin 2011)

$$ x = \frac{k_{iod}x_0 - y_0}{k_{iod} - k_{st}}, \qquad y = k_{st}x. \qquad (7.23) $$

Usually, the noise in the low and high kVps CT images are comparable, i.e., $\sigma_{x0} = \sigma_{y0} = \sigma_0$, leading to the noise in projected image as

$$ \sigma = \sqrt{\frac{\sigma_x^2 + \sigma_y^2}{2}} = \sqrt{\frac{1 + k_{st}^2}{2}} \cdot \frac{\sqrt{1 + k_{iod}^2}}{|k_{st} - k_{iod}|} \cdot \sigma_0. \qquad (7.24) $$

Notably, depending on the slopes k_{st} and k_{iod}, the noise in the projected image may be significantly larger than that in the original images acquired at either low or high kVps.

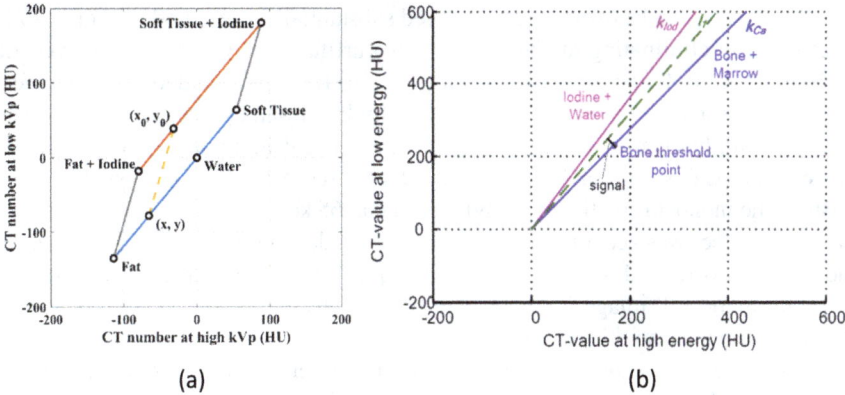

FIGURE 7.6 Diagrams showing the schematic of material analysis and classification in the image domain.

7.4.2.2 Material Classification

It is clinically relevant in practice to differentiate the iodine-based contrast from bony tissues, but such a task is difficult to accomplish in conventional CT, as the contrast agent at varying concentrations may mix with blood and coexist in bone marrow. However, in the material space spanned by the CT number acquired at low and high kVps, these two materials can be classified if a bisector is drawn between their trajectories over concentration, as illustrated in Figure 7.6b. Notably, the functionality of material classification not only enhance CT's capability as a quantitative imaging modality in general, but also facilitate the removal of material, such as virtual non-contrast, replacement of bone and removal of calcification, as well as other clinically relevant applications (Sodickson et al. 2021; Wiggins et al. 2019; McCollough et al. 2015b; Danad 2015).

7.4.3 VIRTUAL MONOCHROMATIC IMAGING AND ANALYSIS

Again, recalling from Equation 7.16, in the functional space spanned by two base materials, one has

$$\mu(x, y; E) = a_1(x, y)\mu_1(x, y; E) + a_2(x, y)\mu_2(x, y; E) \qquad (7.25)$$

at (monochromatic) energy E. It is straightforward to imagine that, once $a_1(x, y)$ and $a_2(x, y)$ are acquired with the approaches presented in Sections 7.3.1–7.3.10, the attenuation of a material at any other energy E can be synthesized using Equation 7.25 (Alvarez and Macovski 1976; Alvarez and Seppi 1979). This means that though only a polychromatic X-ray source is available for diagnostic imaging in reality, virtually we can obtain a monochromatic CT image at any energy level in spectral CT implemented via dual-kVp scan. The significance of this virtual monochromatics can never be overestimated, since quite a few issues in clinical practice, such as beam-hardening artifacts and quantification inaccuracy in calcium scoring or bone marrow density, can be overcome or reduced substantially. Presented in Figure 7.7 is an example of eliminating the beam-hardening artifacts via virtual monochromatic analysis. Three rods corresponding to fat, calcium (100 mg/cc) and iodine (10 mg/cc) dissolved in water are embedded in a 25 cm cylindrical water phantom. It is observed that the beam-hardening artifacts exist between the calcium and iodine rods in the conventional CT images at 140 kVp and 80 kVp, respectively, but no such artifact exists in the monochromatic image synthesized at 65 keV, since the nonlinear beam-hardening effect was accounted for in the material decomposition (see Equation 7.5 and the context related to it). Moreover, it should be noted that the noise level of a monochromatic CT image is lower than either polychromatic image employed to obtain the monochromatic image.

As indicated and shown in Reference (Lehmann et al. 1981), the synthesis of a virtual monochromatic image using Equation 7.25 is actually equivalent to carrying out the projection in the functional space spanned by the basis materials. Both the

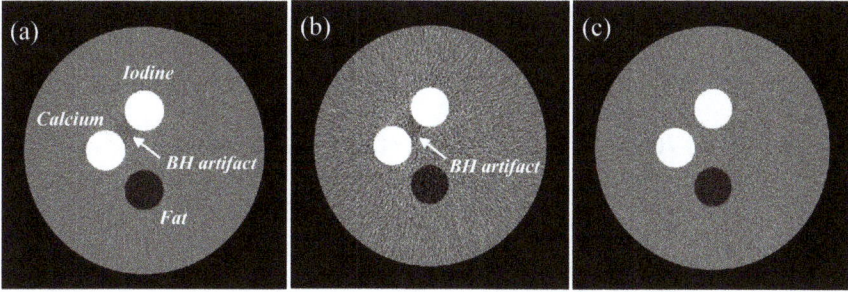

FIGURE 7.7 Illustration of eliminating beam-hardening artifacts in spectral CT via dual-kVp scan: the image acquired at (a) 140 kVp and (b) 80 kVp, and (c) the virtual monochromatic image at 65 keV (display: w/l = 200/1000 HU; iodine: 10 mg/cc; calcium: 100 mg/cc).

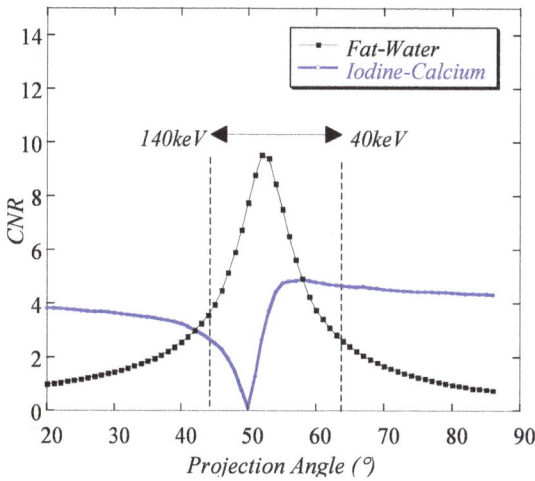

FIGURE 7.8 Schematic showing the variation of CNR as a function over the monochromatic energy E_0 that corresponds to the projection angle (Lehmann et al. 1981).

contrast and noise in the projected images vary with the angle of projection, resulting in fluctuation in the contrast-to-noise ratio (CNR), as illustrated in Figure 7.8. Note that the CNR between the materials reach the maximum that can be achieved in the polychromatic scan at the dose that is the sum of dual-kVp scans (Alvarez and Seppi 1979). Moreover, it is observed that the calcium–iodine and fat–tissue targets reach their maximum CNR at different energies, implying that the performance of spectral CT is task dependent and thus its assessment should be task specific too, as to be illustrated later in Section 8.3.3.

In addition to being implemented in the projection domain, the virtual monochromatic analysis can be carried out in the image domain via linear weighted combination (Yu et al. 2009)

$$I(x, y; E) = w(E)I_{low}(x, y) + (1 - w(E))I_{high}(x, y), \tag{7.26.1}$$

$$w(E) = \frac{\mu_1(E)\mu_2^{high} - \mu_2(E)\mu_1^{high}}{\mu_1^{low}\mu_2^{high} - \mu_1^{high}\mu_2^{low}} \cdot \frac{\mu_2^{low}}{\mu_2(E)}, \tag{7.26.2}$$

The virtual monochromatic image can reach the minimum noise at energy E that is determined by solving

$$\frac{\mu_1(E)}{\mu_2(E)} = \frac{\left(\dfrac{\mu_1^{low}}{\mu_2^{low}} + \dfrac{\mu_1^{high}}{\mu_2^{high}}\right) \cdot \dfrac{\sigma_{low}^2}{\sigma_{high}^2}}{1 + \dfrac{\sigma_{low}^2}{\sigma_{high}^2}} \tag{7.27.1}$$

while reaching the maximum CNR between iodine and water at energy E by solving

$$\frac{\mu_1(E)}{\mu_2(E)} = \frac{\left(\dfrac{\mu_1^{low}}{\mu_2^{low}} + \dfrac{\mu_1^{high}}{\mu_2^{high}}\right) \cdot \dfrac{C_{high}}{C_{low}} \cdot \dfrac{\sigma_{low}^2}{\sigma_{high}^2}}{1 + \dfrac{C_{high}}{C_{low}} \cdot \dfrac{\sigma_{low}^2}{\sigma_{high}^2}} \tag{7.27.2}$$

In Equations 7.27.1 and 7.27.2, the noise levels in the image acquired at low (σ_{low}) and high kVps (σ_{low}), which is dependent on patient size and dose partitioning between the two scans, play an important role in determining the noise levels in the two cases (Yu et al. 2009). Meanwhile, notably, in the criterion toward maximum CNR (Equation 7.27.2), the contrast of the targeted signal against a background at low (C_{low}) and high (C_{high}) kVps, also plays an important role, reinforcing that the imaging performance of spectral CT is task dependent and thus its assessment should be task driven.

7.4.4 M-ANALYSIS IN SPECTRAL CT: A UNIFIED PERSPECTIVE

As elaborated earlier, both material analysis (projection and classification) and monochromatic analysis, regardless of whether implemented in the projection or image domain, or by the one-step approach (see Sections 7.3.6–7.3.10), have their roots in the interaction space spanned by photoelectric absorption and Compton scattering (namely, interaction space), as originally proposed by Alvarez and Macovski in their milestone paper (Alvarez and Macovski 1976). We should have a unified perspective of both of them (namely, M-analysis henceforth) in the interaction space, as pictorially illustrated in Figure 7.9, in which each of them is a form of M-analysis (Forghani et al. 2017c; Noguchi et al. 2017).

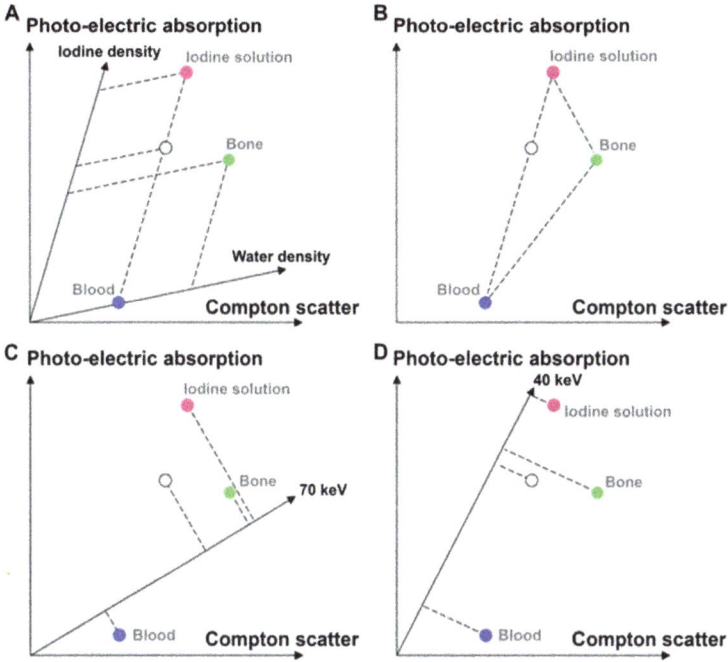

FIGURE 7.9 Pictorial view of *M*-analysis in the interaction space: (a) mapping from the interaction space to material space, (b) material analysis, and (c and d) monochromatic analysis at 70 keV and 40 keV. (Adopted from Forghani et al. 2017c with permission.)

7.4.5 SYNTHESIS OF CONVENTIONAL CT IMAGE IN SPECTRAL CT

7.4.5.1 Synthesis via Linear Weighting

With the two polychromatic CT images acquired at high and low kVps, the spectral CT images in the sense of material decomposition can be obtained using the approaches depicted earlier. In fact, the two polychromatic CT images themselves may be of clinical relevance to provide supplemental information to support diagnostic decision-making. However, a direct presentation of them may be not a good choice since they may be either inferior in noise (low kVp image) or contrast (high kVp image), necessitating a joint presentation of them as a linear weighted combination. As such, more information can be provided in a way similar to the routine polychromatic CT images acquired at 100 kVp or 120 kVp in the clinic. As investigated in Reference (Yu et al. 2009) in depth, there are two criteria for linear weighted combination. The first criteria is toward the goal that the rendered image is of minimum noise:

$$I^{\sigma}(x,y) = w_{low}^{\sigma}(x,y)I_{low}(x,y) + w_{high}^{\sigma}(x,y)I_{high}(x,y) \qquad (7.28.1)$$

$$\sigma_{min}(x,y) = \frac{\sigma_{low,b}(x,y)\sigma_{high,b}(x,y)}{\sqrt{\sigma_{high,b}^2(x,y) + \sigma_{low,b}^2(x,y)}} \qquad (7.28.2)$$

$$w_{low}^{\sigma}(x,y) = \frac{\sigma_{high,b}^2(x,y)}{\sigma_{high,b}^2(x,y) + \sigma_{low,b}^2(x,y)} \qquad (7.28.3)$$

$$w_{low}^{\sigma}(x,y) + w_{high}^{\sigma}(x,y) = 1 \qquad (7.28.4)$$

where the subscripts b and s denote "background" and targeted "signal" in the CT images acquired at high and low kVps. The second criteria is toward the goal that the rendered image is of maximum CNR

$$I^{CNR}(x,y) = w_{low}^{CNR}(x,y)I_{low}(x,y) + w_{high}^{CNR}(x,y)I_{high}(x,y) \qquad (7.29.1)$$

$$CNR_{max}(x,y) = \sqrt{\frac{2C_{low}^2}{(\sigma_{low,b}^2 + \sigma_{low,b}^2)} + \frac{2C_{high}^2}{(\sigma_{high,b}^2 + \sigma_{high,b}^2)}} \qquad (7.29.2)$$

$$w_{low}^{CNR}(x,y) = \frac{C_{low}(\sigma_{high,b}^2(x,y) + \sigma_{high,s}^2(x,y))}{C_{low}(\sigma_{high,b}^2(x,y) + \sigma_{high,s}^2(x,y)) + C_{high}(\sigma_{low,b}^2(x,y) + \sigma_{low,s}^2(x,y))} \qquad (7.29.3)$$

$$w_{low}^{CNR}(x,y) + w_{high}^{CNR}(x,y) = 1 \qquad (7.29.4)$$

The phantom study in Reference (Yu et al. 2009) shows that the CNR in the linear weighted combination toward maximum CNR is between the polychromatic images at 80 kVp and 140 kVp, and comparable or slightly better than that at 120 kVp, which is the most frequently utilized kVp in the clinic. Equations 7.28.1–7.28.4 and 7.29.1–7.29.4 show that the noise level at each kVp image ($\sigma_{low,b}$, $\sigma_{low,s}$, $\sigma_{high,b}$ and $\sigma_{high,s}$), which depends on patient size and dose partitioning between the two scans at different kVps, plays an important role in both criteria (Yu et al. 2009). Notably, in the criterion toward maximum CNR (Equations 7.29.1–7.29.4), the contrast of the targeted signal at low and high kVps also plays an important role, stating that the imaging performance of spectral CT is task dependent and thus its assessment should be task driven. Moreover, the linear weighted combination is approximately equivalent to a projection in the functional space spanned by the basis material.

7.4.5.2 Synthesis via Non-Linear Weighting

In principle, the linear weighted combination is a global approach. Intuitively, it may be a better strategy if blending of the two polychromatic CT images at high and low kVps is carried out in a local and non-linear way. The modal (modified sigmoid) blending function – a local and non-linear blending approach – has been investigated via phantom and patient studies in hepatic imaging (Holms et al. 2008; Kim et al. 2010). Using the CNR^2 normalized by X-ray exposure as the figure of merit (FOM), an observer study (Wilcoxon signed-rank test) was conducted in Reference (Holms et al. 2008) and the preliminary data show that the non-linear image fusion can only slightly outperform the linear blending at weighting factor 0.5 (i.e., 50%–50% blending between low and high kVps) at the scenarios wherein the lesions are of hyper-attenuation (>70 HU), and comparable while the contrast is relatively low (<65 HU).

7.4.6 Principal Component Analysis in Spectral CT

With an increasing number of energy bins, the signal detection in each bin, especially the signal detected in high-energy bins, may suffer from photon starvation, especially while the object to be imaged is relatively large in size. Moreover, there is no doubt that redundancy exists in the data acquired over multiple energy bins, and the inter-bin redundancy can be used to make spectral CT more effective and efficient in material decomposition and/or noise reduction. Principal component analysis (PCA) has established itself as one of the most popular and potent multivariate statistical analysis for extracting redundant information from multi-channel data and has found application in almost all scientific fields. Following is a customization of PCA for its application in spectral CT.

Suppose there are p energy bins in a spectral CT, and X_i ($i = 1, ..., K{\times}M{\times}N$) denote the mean-deviated multi-spectral data at the ith detector cell, where $M{\times}N$ is the detector dimension and K is the number of total projection views in the data acquisition. Then, let $X_{p{\times}(K{\times}M{\times}N)}$ denote the measured spectral data sorted and arranged as $[X_1, X_2, ..., X_{K{\times}M{\times}N}]$, and $\Sigma_{X,p{\times}p}$ denote the covariance matrix associated with $X_{p{\times}(K{\times}M{\times}N)}$. Via singular value decomposition (SVD), the eigenvalues $\lambda_1, \lambda_2, ...$ λ_p and the associated unit eigenvectors $\mathbf{u}_1, \mathbf{u}_2, ... \mathbf{u}_p$ can be obtained. Applying an orthogonal transformation $P_{p{\times}p}$ composed of the eigenvectors on the data as $X_{p{\times}(K{\times}M{\times}N)}$ $= P_{p{\times}p}Y_{p{\times}p{\times}(K{\times}M{\times}N)}$, i.e., at each data index i, one has

$$\begin{bmatrix} x_1 & x_2 & ... & x_p \end{bmatrix}^T = \begin{bmatrix} \mathbf{u}_1 & \mathbf{u}_2 & ... & \mathbf{u}_p \end{bmatrix}\begin{bmatrix} y_1 & y_2 & ... & y_p \end{bmatrix}^T \quad (7.30)$$

or, equivalently, since $P_{p{\times}p}$ is an orthogonal matrix, one has $Y_{p{\times}(K{\times}M{\times}N)} = P^T_{p{\times}p}$ $X_{p{\times}(K{\times}M{\times}N)}$, i.e.,

$$\begin{bmatrix} y_1 & y_2 & ... & y_p \end{bmatrix}^T = \begin{bmatrix} \mathbf{u}_1 & \mathbf{u}_2 & ... & \mathbf{u}_p \end{bmatrix}^T\begin{bmatrix} x_1 & x_2 & ... & x_p \end{bmatrix}^T \quad (7.31)$$

and the covariance matrix $\Sigma_{Y,p{\times}p}$ associated with $Y_{p{\times}(K{\times}M{\times}N)}$ becomes diagonal.

The PCA in spectral CT can be carried out in either the projection or image domain (Xie et al. 2021). If FBP is adopted for image formation, the implementation of PCA in the projection domain may offer better performance than that in the image domain, since noise, especially the noise in high-energy bins, may lead to difficulty in image reconstruction. However, the computation complexity of implementation in the projection domain $O_{(p \times (K \times M \times N))}$ is much higher than that in the image domain. Notably, in material decomposition, the image corresponding to each material is meaningful in physics, but with PCA, each composite image may no longer be meaningful, and thus its interpretation in clinical applications and preclinical research may not be as straightforward any more.

7.5 DISCUSSION

With the landscape of technological and clinical advancements in spectral CT sketched in this chapter, it is fair for us to state that photon-counting spectral CT is gaining momentum in its research and development, while energy-integration spectral CT has been well accepted in the clinic. With the technological advancements made in photon-counting spectral CT and the success made by energy-integration CT in the clinic (see more in Chapter 8) it is encouraging to optimistically anticipate that, with the potential technological solutions to improve its imaging performance and its synergy with novel contrast agents, spectral CT, especially the one that works in photon-counting mode, would be able to eventually advance CT's clinical utility in a manner that can be more significant than incremental, if not breakthrough.

8 Spectral MDCT (Part 2)
Optimization of Image Quality for Clinical Applications

With the fundamentals of physics and existing data acquisition and image formation schemes presented in Chapter 7, we are ready to investigate the approaches that can optimize the image quality (imaging performance) of spectral computed tomography (CT). In principle, as indicated in the previous chapter, material-specific imaging, including two-material and three-material decomposition based, and the virtual monochromatic CT, can be treated as a mapping from the projection space (*P*-space) (Tang and Ren 2021; Ren et al. 2021) to the so-called *A*-space (Alvarez 2010, 2011, 2013). Aimed at optimizing image quality for clinical applications, the properties of material decomposition, specifically the properties in signal detection, noise propagation, the dimensionality of *P*-space and material space, the matching of dimensionality between these two spaces, the conditioning of material space and the conditioning of spectral channelization, are thoroughly analyzed in this chapter.

8.1 OPTIMIZATION OF IMAGE QUALITY IN ENERGY-INTEGRATION SPECTRAL CT

In currently available spectral CT, the energy-integration detector works in indirect mode (Bushberg et al. 2012; Huda 2016), wherein X-ray photons interact with a scintillator of high atomic number and convert into visible light photons that reach the photodiode and generate electrons (current) to be captured by the data acquisition system (DAS). The imaging performance of energy-integration spectral CT is similar to that of the conventional CT in many aspects, but here we are concerned about those that are specific to spectral CT.

8.1.1 ARTIFACTS AND THEIR SUPPRESSION

As mentioned, the implementation of spectral CT requires that the noise levels in low and high peak kilovoltage (kVp) scans are roughly the same or comparable, which necessitates an uneven dose partitioning between the two scans. It has been reported in the literature that, via adequate dose partitioning, the total dose associated with state-of-the-art energy-integration spectral CT is slightly larger or comparable with that of conventional single-energy CT (Flohr et al. 2008; Yu et al. 2009).

DOI: 10.1201/9780429028465-8

One of the major advantages of energy-integration spectral CT over conventional CT is its potential of eliminating beam-hardening artifacts caused by intensive attenuating materials, such as bone and iodinated contrast media. Theoretically speaking, the beam-hardening artifacts should disappear in spectral CT. However, due to imperfections in the imaging chain, residual artifacts due to the beam-hardening effect may still exist in spectral CT, as shown by the phantom study presented in Figure 8.1, in which a cardiac phantom consisting of chambers filled with iodinated contrast agent is used for illustration. Compton scattering impinging on the energy-integration detector may contaminate the projection data and adversely affect the material-specific imaging and virtual monochromatic imaging/analysis in spectral CT, since, in Equation 3.1 and Equation 7.5, it is assumed that no Compton scattering is detected in the signal. However, in practice, though the anti-scatter grid (ASG) in state-of-the-art multi-detector CT (MDCT) can do a good job, there may still be a small amount of Compton scattering detected in the signal, even in the scenario in which 2D ASG is used, that undermines the physical foundation of material decomposition (Equation 3.1) and virtual monochromatic imaging/analysis (Equation 7.5).

Additionally, the energy-integration spectral CT may suffer from all the artifacts encountered in conventional CT, e.g., ring artifacts caused by the inter-detector channel variation in the gain and spectral response, but an in-depth coverage on those artifacts is beyond the scope of this chapter, and readers interested in details are referred to the literature (Cody et al. 2005; Hsieh 2009).

8.1.2 De-Noising in Spectral Domain

In general, the images acquired at low and high kVps in the energy-integration spectral CT implemented with a dual source and dual detector are closely correlated in structure (anatomy), while there is almost no correlation in their noise, providing the opportunity of de-noising in the spectral domain. For example, by (i)

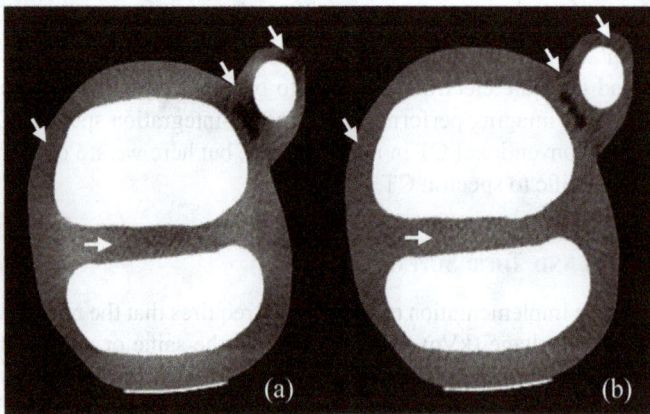

FIGURE 8.1 Suppression of beam-hardening artifacts in a cardiac chamber phantom study: (a) polychromatic CT at 120 kVp and (b) virtual monochromatic image at 70 keV.

forming a composite image as the average of the images at low and high kVps and (ii) scaling the composite image into ones corresponding to the low and high kVp images, respectively, the original images at low and high kVps can be effectively de-noised. Though the scaling factor at each image pixel is obtained from the ratio of low-pass filtered composite images over the images at low and high kVps that have undergone the same low-pass filtering, the spatial resolution assessed by the modulation transfer function remains almost identical, i.e., the anatomic details can be preserved. Impressive performance in de-noising has been demonstrated and readers interested in the details are referred to References (Leng et al. 2011, 2015). Moreover, note that such spectral domain de-noising can also be implemented in the projection domain, especially in data acquisition with a dual-layer detector.

8.1.3 SEPARATION OF X-RAY SOURCE SPECTRA

It has been known from the very beginning that the separation of the X-ray source's spectra at high and low kVps are of paramount relevance in spectral CT's imaging (interaction decomposition) performance. Initially, attention was mainly paid to characterizing the noise in spectral CT images and the relationship of noise between the images acquired at low and high kVps, as originally done by Alvarez and Macovski in their milestone paper (Alvarez and Macovski 1976):

$$\sigma_{A_1} = \frac{(\frac{m_{low,2}^2}{I_2} + \frac{m_{high,2}^2}{I_1})^{1/2}}{(m_{low,1}m_{high,2} - m_{low,2}m_{high,1})} = \frac{(\frac{m_{low,2}^2}{I_2} + \frac{m_{high,2}^2}{I_1})^{1/2}}{m_{low,1}m_{high,2}(1 - \frac{m_{low,2}}{m_{high,2}} \cdot \frac{m_{high,1}}{m_{low,1}})} \tag{8.1}$$

$$\sigma_{A_2} = \frac{(\frac{m_{low,1}^2}{I_2} + \frac{m_{high,1}^2}{I_1})^{1/2}}{(m_{low,1}m_{high,2} - m_{low,2}m_{high,1})} \tag{8.2}$$

where

$$m_{low,1} = \frac{\partial \ln I_1}{\partial A_1}, \qquad m_{low,2} = \frac{\partial \ln I_1}{\partial A_2} \tag{8.3}$$

$$m_{high,2} = \frac{\partial \ln I_2}{\partial A_1}, \qquad m_{high,2} = \frac{\partial \ln I_2}{\partial A_2} \tag{8.4}$$

Apparently, the denominator in Equations 8.1 and 8.2 plays a critical role in determining the noise in the A-space and thus in the image domain, since it vanishes as the two spectra approach each other. In fact, the denominator is the Jacobian of Equations 7.1.1 and 7.1.2, which was also defined as the spectral quality factor (SQF) in Reference (Alvarez et al. 2004). It should be noted that, as indicated by Alvarez, a spectral separation refers to no spectral overlapping, other than just a large difference between the effective energies of the spectra corresponding to the two kVps (Alvarez 2010, 2011, 2013).

Similar analysis in optimizing the X-ray source spectra was made in material decomposition and it was found that $(R_1 - R_2)$, where R_1 and R_2 are the ratio of the mass attenuation coefficients of materials 1 and 2 at low and high kVps, respectively, plays a critical role (Kelcz et al. 1979). By defining DE_{ratio}, the slope of the material's linear attenuation coefficient (LAC) as a function over the density at low and high kVps, the assessment of spectral quality can also be carried out in the image domain by evaluating $(DE_{ratio1} - DE_{ratio2})$, where the subscripts 1 and 2 indicate the two materials to be differentiated. As indicated in Reference (Primak et al. 2009), the difference in DE_{ratio} determines the contrast between two materials in spectral CT, in analogue to the linear attenuation coefficient that determines the contrast between two materials in conventional CT. Hence, by separating the source spectra, differentiating iodine (I) or gadolinium (Gd) that is of relatively high atomic number from other materials of low atomic number, e.g., soft tissues, can be improved substantially, but, notably, this would not be the case in the differentiation of soft tissue, since $(DE_{ratio1} - DE_{ratio2})$ corresponding to them are quite small. Notably, this again shows that the optimization of imaging performance is task dependent.

It has also been found that tin is an adequate material for X-ray source spectral optimization in spectral CT with an iodinated contrast agent. For a large body, the thickness of tin should roughly be 0.5 mm, while it may go up to 0.8 mm for a small body or head scan. The underlying reason may be that tin's K-edge is close to that of iodine and gadolinium, making $(DE_{ratio1} - DE_{ratio2})$ relatively large. Presented in Figure 8.2 is an example showing how tin can be used to separate the source spectra in an energy-integration spectral CT (Primak et al. 2009).

8.1.4 Radiation Dose in Energy-Integration Spectral CT

It has been reported in the early implementation of spectral dual-energy CT (DECT) that the radiation dose associated with DECT is roughly 25% larger than that of a single-energy conventional CT at 120 kVp. With improvement in implementation technologies, it was later reported that the dose of DECT is comparable to or slightly higher than that of conventional CT (Flohr et al. 2008; Yu et al. 2009).

8.2 PROPERTIES OF PHOTON-COUNTING X-RAY DETECTION FOR SPECTRAL MDCT

As indicated in Chapter 3, Sections 3.4.2 and 3.4.3, photon counting has been the approach for radiation detection since its discovery and the method of choice for data acquisition in nuclear medicine. In theory, photon-counting detection may be a best fit to spectral CT, as it facilitates spectral manipulation – either energy binning or spectral weighting, or both. Recently, with steady progress in refining detector pitch (1.0×1.0 mm^2 to 0.1×0.1 mm^2) (Ehn 2017; Danielsson et al. 2021) and dynamic beam-forming techniques (Hsieh and Pelc 2013; Szczykutowicz and Mistretta 2013a, 2013b), the risk of pulse pile-up in spectral CT is being mitigated to a level that

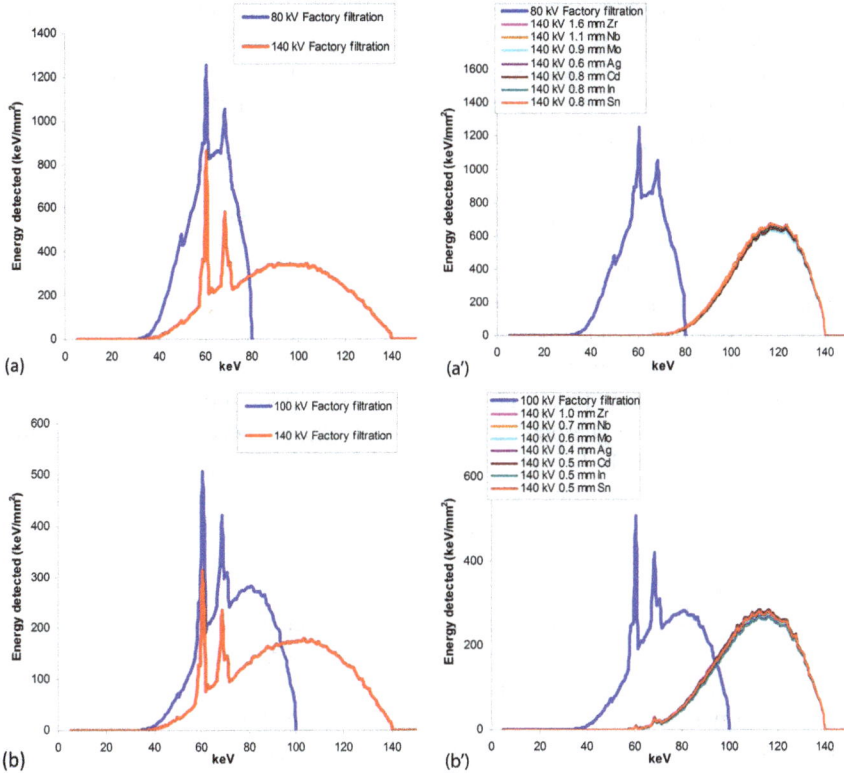

FIGURE 8.2 Examples showing the separation of X-ray source spectra in a clinical CT using metal tin: (a) default spectra, and (b) shaped by different metals at various thickness (Adopted from Primak et al. 2009 with permission).

is acceptable in practice. Following is coverage of X-ray photon-counting spectral CT, including its working mechanism, performance, issues to be addressed and potential.

8.2.1 IDEAL PHOTON-COUNTING X-RAY DETECTION FOR SPECTRAL CT

As noted earlier, separation of X-ray source spectra at low and high kVps is crucial to the image quality of energy-integration spectral CT. In fact, due to spectral overlapping and no chance for spectral matching or weighting, all four approaches presented in Chapter 7 (Sections 7.2.1–7.2.4) to implement energy-integration spectral CT are suboptimal. If X-rays are detected by counting each photon with its energy accurately labeled (infinite spectral resolution), there would be no spectral overlapping at all. More important, the counted photons can be manipulated to reduce the spectral mismatching between signal generation and detection, or to improve the detection efficiency by spectral binning and weighting (Tapiovaara and Wagner 1985) (see more in Section 8.5). The photon-counting detector in reality can only be of finite energy resolution, and the vast majority of photon-counting detectors are of two to eight energy bins at energy resolution that can be as good as 5 keV. As elaborated later in this chapter, even with spectral modulation at very coarse resolution, the image quality of photon-counting spectral CT can still be substantially improved, in comparison to energy-integration spectral CT.

8.2.2 Realistic Photon-Counting X-Ray Detection for Spectral CT

8.2.2.1 Pulse Pile-Up

We have briefly talked about pulse pile-up in Chapter 3, Sections 3.4.2 and 3.4.3 (Figure 3.7c), and a zoomed view of it is given in Figure 8.3 (left), which shows that, with an increasing number of incident X-ray photons roughly up to $0.5 \times 10^9/(mm^2 \cdot s)$, the detector's response is linear, i.e., almost no pulse pile-up occurs. Once exceeding the threshold, pulse pile-up happens, at the severity depending on the detector's working modes. Though the risk of pulse pile-up can be substantially reduced via detector cell refinement and/or dynamic bowtie, other system modeling-based algorithmic solutions may also help (Taguchi et al. 2010, 2022).

8.2.2.2 Charge Sharing

Charge sharing is an immediate consequence of detector cell refinement, as shown on the right of Figure 8.3. A cloud of electron–hole pairs spread cross neighboring detector cells and in turn lead to mis-registration (distortion) in both photon counting and energy labeling, which may degrade each energy bin's spectral property and result in extended tail or humping at the end, as indicated by the arrows in Figure 8.4 (left). Fortunately, with increasing complexity in ASIC, on-chip logics can detect the occurrence of charge sharing over neighboring cells and recover the accuracy in pulse counting and energy labeling, by detecting the coincidence and distributing all

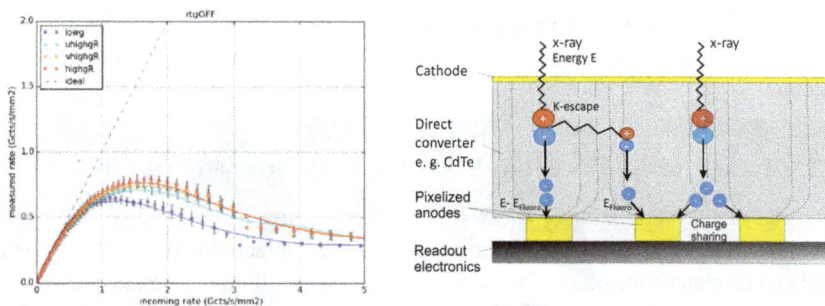

FIGURE 8.3   (Left) Schematic illustration of pulse pile-up in photon-counting detection of X-rays and (right) a microscopic view of charge sharing, fluorescence and K-escaping. (With permission, the plot on the left is adopted from Dectris AG, Switzerland (https://www.dectris .com/detectors/x-ray-detectors/), while the drawing on the right is from Flohr et al. 2020.)

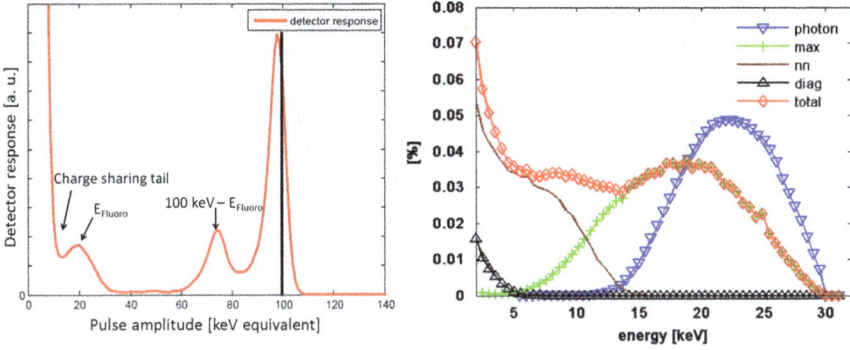

FIGURE 8.4 Schematic showing an example of the spectral response of an energy bin in a photon-counting detector in spectral CT: (left) distortion in spectral response and (right) its recovery via on-chip logics. (Adopted from Flohr et al. 2020 (left) and Tlustos 2010 (right) with permissions)

the detected energy to the cell at the highest energy (Figure 8.4, right) (Tlustos 2010), in addition to other algorithmic approaches (Taguchi 2020; Taguchi et al. 2022).

8.2.2.3 Scattering

Both Rayleigh (coherent) and Compton (incoherent) scattering inevitably occur when X-ray photons interact with the sensor materials (CdTe/CZT) in the photon-counting detector, exactly in the same way as X-ray photons propagate in other materials. Similar the charge sharing illustrated in Figure 8.3 (right), the scattered photons may create a cloud of electron–hole pairs at neighboring cells and result in mis-registration (distortion) in photon counting and energy labeling that contribute to the tailing effect. Though their root causes differ, the eventual effect on the spectral response property of the photon-counting detector is identical, since the time lag of scattering is extremely short. Hence, the on-chip logics used in anti-charge sharing can be readily adopted to suppress the effect of scattering in the photon-counting detector (Tlustos 2010).

8.2.2.4 Fluorescence Escaping

It is likely that, rather than creating a cloud of charges, the incident X-ray photon may knock out a K-shell electron in the sensor material (CdTe/CZT), and the resultant vacancy is then filled by an electron from outer shells, leading to a fluorescent event that may distort the registration in energy or trigger another cascade of scattering or fluorescent events. As shown on the left of Figure 8.4, as the difference in energy is constant, the peak of fluorescence occurs at a fixed difference in energy. Again, though the root cause differs, the eventual effect of fluorescence escaping on the spectral response is exactly the same as that of scattering. Hence, the strategy of on-chip logics mentioned earlier can be adopted to suppress the effect of fluorescence escaping on the mis-registration in pulse counting and energy labeling (Tlustos 2010).

8.2.2.5 Charge Trapping

In general, impurities and lattice defects may inevitably exist in the sensor materials of the photon-counting detector, which may form the centers that can trap charges in the detection process. In turn, the trapped charges may affect the biased electrical field and degrade the spectral response (charge collection efficiency) manifested as a lowered pulse counts, with more energy labeling toward the lower end and thus extended tailing. In general, charge trapping is a short-term event and can be reset if the charges escape the traps and return to the conduction or valence band because of thermal effect (Tlustos 2010).

8.2.2.6 Sensor Polarization

In contrast to charge trapping, the polarization of sensor materials in the photon-counting detector is a deep trapping and thus in general a long-term effect (reliability issue) associated with intensified X-ray radiation. The deeply trapped charges in the sensor material can diminish the efficiency of charge collection and result in a lowered pulse count. The mechanism of deep trapping formation is complicated, but CZT is notably less susceptible to it than CdZe. Moreover, a rigorous controlling of the fabrication process, e.g., material selection, surface preparation, contact deposition and surface passivation, is assumed to be helpful in improving the long-term reliability of sensor materials by reducing the likelihood of sensor polarization (Tlustos 2010; Ehn 2017; Danielsson et al. 2021; Flohr et al. 2020).

8.3 MULTI-MATERIAL DECOMPOSITION IN PHOTON-COUNTING SPECTRAL MDCT

Iodine, with its K-edge (33.2 keV) at the lower end of the energy range of diagnostic imaging, is utilized as an iodinated contrast agent in the vast majority (85%) of body CT scans for diagnostic imaging in clinics (ACR 2021; Lusic and Grinstaff 2013). Using singular value decomposition (SVD) analysis, Lehmann and Alvarez et al. studied how the dimensionality of material space changes if iodine is present in the materials to be imaged (Alvarez 1976; Roth 1984; Lehmann and Alvarez 1986). They found that the dimensionality of linear space for material decomposition becomes three and thus three basis materials, of which iodine is necessary, have to be used to span the space for material decomposition (Roth 1984; Sukovle and Clinthorne 1999). By extending Equation 7.5 into

$$\mu(x;E) = a_{m1}(x) \cdot \mu_{m1}(E) + a_{m2}(x) \cdot \mu_{m2}(E) + a_I(x) \cdot \mu_I(x) \qquad (8.5)$$

the three-material decomposition (3-MD) scheme is adopted for spectral imaging in photon-counting spectral CT (Roessl and Proksa 2007; Schlomka et al. 2008; Roessl et al. 2011; Zhao et al. 2018). Later on, 3-MD is extended to four-material decomposition (4-MD)–based spectral imaging of multi-contrast agents (e.g., iodine and gadolinium) by extending Equation 8.5 into

$$\mu(x;E) = a_{m1}(x) \cdot \mu_{m1}(E) + a_{m2}(x) \cdot \mu_{m2}(E) + a_I(x) \cdot \mu_I(E) + a_{Gd}(x) \cdot \mu_{Gd}(E) \quad (8.6)$$

which means that the dimensionality of the material space enclosing biological tissues and materials of two distinct K-edges equals to four, and the K-edge materials have to be in the basis materials.

Notably, the first two terms on the right side of Equations 8.5 and 8.6 are assumed to be associated with two basis materials. Initially, however, these two terms actually correspond to the photoelectric absorption and Compton scattering (Roessl and Proksa 2007; Schlomka et al. 2008; Roessl et al. 2011), which may serve as an experimental verification that the basis function can be either a function of energy that characterizes X-ray interaction with material or the material's attenuation coefficient. In other words, in the presence of material with its K-edge falling into the diagnostic energy range (*K-edge material* henceforth), one may choose the interaction function or material's attenuation function in a mixed manner as the basis function, as long as the dimensionality of basis function matches (equal to or larger than) that of the material space enclosing the materials to be imaged. Hence, it is not essential for us to distinguish between interaction and attenuation in the basis functions, despite the fact that such a hybrid decomposition may make the calibration process complicated in practice. Nevertheless, it is essential to include the K-edge material in the basis materials, otherwise the attenuation behavior of K-edge material can't be adequately characterized.

8.3.1 DIMENSIONALITY OF MATERIAL SPACE AND ITS DETERMINATION

Depending on the specific imaging task, many material pairs, e.g., PMMA/Teflon (Ehn 2017), PMMA/aluminum (Kalender 1986) and soft tissue/cortical bone (Alvarez 2010), have been selected as the basis materials for two-material decomposition (2-MD) of biological tissues ($1 \leq Z \leq 20$). Via principal component analysis, it has been found that the material decomposition carried out with the first and second principal components as the (virtual) basis materials performs the best in differentiation of soft tissues in the human body (Weaver and Huddleston 1985). It has been reported in a series of papers (Williamson et al. 2006; Han et al. 2016, 2017) that a dual basis vector model (polystyrene/H_2O for low-Z materials or H_2O/ C_aCl_2 (23%) for high-Z materials) outperforms the two-parametric model in characterization of biological tissues. To date, all of these basis materials and numerical solutions behave very well in 2-MD, mainly due to the fact that the dimensionality of the linear space for material decomposition of biological tissues equals to two, as investigated and verified by Lehmann and Alvarez through singular value decomposition (SVD) analysis (Alvarez 1976; Roth 1984; Lehmann and Alvarez 1986). On the other hand, it is interesting to note that as many as 12 interactions may occur while X-ray photons are propagating in biological tissues (Roth 1984), though the occurrence likelihood of most of them are very low and thus can be omitted. The dimensionality of the material space associated with the XCOM library has been further studied using a hypothesis-based approach and found to likely be up to four (Bornefalk 2012). Despite of existence of possible interactions in addition to the photoelectric absorption and Compton scattering, it has so far been a common practice to assume that the dimensionality of linear space for material decomposition of biological tissues is two.

In analogue to what has been done by Lehmann and Alvarez, the SVD analysis can be adopted to determine the dimensionality of material space for spectral imaging in photon-counting CT (Tang and Ren 2021). Suppose a total of M materials are to be imaged in an application in the energy range [18, 150] keV. Given the ith material, let $\{\mu_{ij}\}$ denote the sampling of its mass attenuation coefficient at an adequate interval, e.g., 1 keV, where $1 \leq j \leq N$ and N is the number of samplings in the energy range. A data matrix can be formed by sorting all of the sampled data row-wise into matrix $A_{M \times N} = \{\mu_{ij}\}$. Applying SVD, $A_{M \times N}$ can be decomposed into (Alvarez 2010, 2019)

$$A_{M \times N} = U_{M \times M} \, \Sigma_{M \times N} \, V_{N \times N}^{T}, \tag{8.7}$$

where $U_{M \times M}$ and $V_{N \times N}$ are orthogonal unity matrices and $\Sigma_{M \times N}$ a rectangular diagonal matrix with the eigenvalues $\{\sigma_i : 1 \leq i \leq M\}$ of $A_{M \times N}$ in descending order as its diagonal elements, i.e., $\{\Sigma_{ii} = \sigma_i\}$. By definition, the dimensionality of $A_{M \times N}$ (i.e., the dimensionality of material space) is the number of non-zero eigenvalues.

Listed in the first row of Table 8.1 are singular values of typical biological tissues in the human body. Through SVD, the dimensionality of the material space spanned by typical biological tissues is determined as two, consistent with what has been published in the literature (Alvarez 1976, 2013; Roth 1984). Presented in the second row are the singular values corresponding to a set of biological tissues, with its dimensionality being still two as all of them are just a subset of the tissues in human body (row 1). The third row shows that, with inclusion of gadolinium (5 mg/ml), the dimensionality of material space increases from two to three, which is again consistent with what has been published in the literature (Alvarez 1976, 2013; Roth 1984). The singular values displayed in the fifth row show that, with both iodine (5 mg/ml) and gadolinium (5 mg/ml) included, the dimensionality of materials becomes four.

8.3.2 CONDITIONING OF MATERIAL SPACE BASIS AND ITS IMPACT ON IMAGE QUALITY

Once the dimensionality of material space is determined, the next task in implementing photon-counting spectral CT is the selection of basis materials. As reported in the literature (Alvarez and Macovski 1976; Alvarez 1976, 2010, 2013, 2019; Kelcz et al. 1979; Kalender et al. 1986; Tang and Ren 2021), the performance of material decomposition, especially the noise property, is quite stable over the selection of basis materials in 2-MD supported by two spectral channels. However, in the investigation of 3-MD and 4-MD, it has been observed that its noise property is strongly dependent on the selection of basis materials (Tang et al. 2020; Ren et al. 2020; Tang and Ren 2021). Moreover, it has been noted that the material decomposition and virtual monochromatic imaging/analysis behave quite differently over basis material selection. Thus, to further understand the fundamentals of photon-counting spectral CTs and the guidelines on its analysis, design and implementation, a systematic study of the effective dimensionality of material space and the conditioning of basis materials and their impact on image quality of material-specific imaging and virtual

TABLE 8.1

Dimensionality of Typical Biological Tissues in the Human Body and the Tissues and Materials That Configure the Phantoms Used in the Study

Materials to Be Imaged	SV_1	SV_2	SV_3	SV_4	SV_5	Dim.
Common biological tissues in human body	8.8583e+00 (1.0)	2.4994e−01 (2.8215e−02)	2.6310e−02 (2.9701e−03)	1.7657e−02 (1.9932e−03)	1.5322e−02 (1.7297e−03)	2
Adipose, white matter, gray matter, cortical bone	4.8678e+01 (1.0)	5.3443e+00 (1.0979e−01)	2.0031e−02 (4.1149e−04)	2.2550e−05 (4.6324e−07)	—	2
Adipose, white matter, gray matter, cortical bone, I (10 mg/ml)	4.9393e+01 (1.0)	6.5469e+00 (1.3255e−01)	1.1973e+00 (2.4240e−02)	1.8286e−02 (3.7022e−04)	2.2551e−05 (4.5656e−07)	3
Adipose, white matter, gray matter, cortical bone, Gd (10 mg/ml)	4.9526e+01 (1.0)	6.3207e+00 (1.2762e−01)	6.7173e−01 (1.3563e−02)	1.9990e−02 (4.0363e−04)	2.2543e−05 (4.5517e−07)	3
Adipose, white matter, gray matter, cortical bone, I (10 mg/ml), Gd (10 mg/ml)	5.0237e+01 (1.0)	7.2997e+00 (1.4531e−01)	1.2820e+00 (2.5519e−02)	6.6460e−01 (1.3229e−02)	1.8204e−02 (3.6236e−04)	4

Source: Tang and Ren 2021.
Notes: Energy range: [18, 150] keV. SV: singular value.

monochromatic imaging/analysis performance in photon-counting CT is necessary. Notably, by "conditioning", we refer to (i) sufficiency in dimensionality, (ii) well-posedness in the condition number of basis functions and (iii) matching of K-edge materials (Tang and Ren 2021).

Given a set of basis materials, its dimensionality can be determined via SVD in exactly the same way as that in determining the dimensionality of material space, except for the difference in forming the data matrix $A_{M \times N}$. Letting $\{\mu'_{ij}\}$ denote sampling of the mass attenuation coefficient of the basis materials at an adequate interval, $A_{M \times N}$ can be formed by row-wise sorting all of the sampled data, i.e., $A'_{M \times N} = \{\mu'_{ij}\}$ (see the context related to Equation 8.7). Again, by definition, the dimensionality of matrix $A_{M \times N}$ (the dimensionality of basis materials) is the number of eigenvalues of matrix $A_{M \times N}$ that is larger than zero. In addition, the condition number (well-posedness) of matrix $A_{M \times N}$ (the condition number of basis materials) is defined as the square root of the ratio of the largest eigenvalue over the smallest non-zero eigenvalue $\sigma_{max} / \sigma_{min}$. In linear algebra, the condition number of a linear equation system is an indicator of the system's robustness over the measurement error and/or noise (Strang 2006; Leon 2006). It can also be considered as a quantity to assess the uniformity in the norm of the basis vectors that span a linear space (Strang 2006; Tang and Ren 2021). Intuitively, the condition number is a quantity to characterize the extent to which the vectors that span the linear space are uncorrelated. In general, the larger the condition number, the worse the situation. Potentially, the minimum condition number can go down to unity, in which the involved vectors are not only uncorrelated but also orthogonal.

In a simulation study of 3-MD–based photon-counting spectral CT (Tang and Ren 2021), six sets of basis materials (Table 8.2) have been designated: BM-0 (adipose, PMMA and Teflon), BM-1 (soft tissue, Gd (10 mg/ml) and cortical bone), BM-2 (soft tissue, Gd (20 mg/ml) and cortical bone), BM-3 (adipose, Gd (20 mg/ml) and PMMA), BM-4 (soft tissue, I (20 mg/ml), Gd (20 mg/ml) and cortical bone) and BM-5 (adipose, I (20 mg/ml), Gd (20 mg/ml) and Teflon). In the first case of 3-MD (first row of Table 8.2), the condition number corresponding to the basis materials adipose, PMMA and Teflon (BM-0) is larger than 3×10^4. Such a large condition number implies that the material decomposition carried out under this set of basis materials may be ill-posed. As shown in more cases of 3-MD (rows 2–4 of Table 8.2), the condition number of basis materials becomes approximately three orders smaller if Teflon, PMMA and adipose are in turn replaced by cortical bone, Gd (10–30 mg/ml) and soft tissue. The fifth row in Table 8.2 designates a special case in which adipose and PMMA are used as the basis materials to boost the contrast between soft tissues (see Figure 8.5 and related context for more detail). Moreover, as shown in rows 6–8 of Table 8.2, a similar phenomenon occurs when iodine (10–30 mg/ml) replaces gadolinium (10–30 mg/ml). With an increasing concentration of Gd (rows 2–4 in Table 8.2), the condition number of the basis materials declines and does so in the cases wherein iodine is one of the basis materials (rows 6–8 in Table 8.2). In the case of 4-MD using cortical bone, Gd (20 mg/ml), I (20 mg/ml) and soft tissue as the basis materials (row 9 in Table 8.2), it is observed that, given Gd and I

TABLE 8.2

Condition Numbers of the Basis Materials Employed in the Study

	Basis Materials	SV_1	SV_2	SV_3	SV_4	Condition
1	Adipose, PMMA and Teflon (BM-0)	1.8515e+01 (1.0)	1.9881e+00 (1.0738e−01)	5.8465e−04 (3.1577e−05)	—	3.1668e+04
2	Soft tissue, Gd (10 mg/ml) and cortical bone (BM-1)	4.8878e+01 (1.0)	4.7498e+00 (9.7178e−02)	5.3173e−01 (1.0879e−02)	—	9.1922e+01
3	Soft tissue, Gd (20 mg/ml) and cortical bone (BM-2)	4.9518e+01 (1.0)	5.1824e+00 (1.0466e−01)	9.7901e−01 (1.9771e−02)	—	5.0579e+01
4	Soft tissue, Gd (30 mg/m) and cortical bone	5.0337e+01 (1.0)	5.7120e+00 (1.1348e−01)	1.3222e+00 (2.6267e−02)	—	3.8070e+01
5	Adipose, PMMA and Gd (20 mg/ml) (BM-3)	1.5342e+01 (1.0)	2.1152e+00 (1.3788e−01)	2.6951e−02 (1.7567e−03)	—	5.6925e+02
6	Soft tissue, I (10 mg/ml) and cortical bone	4.8743e+01 (1.0)	5.0891e+00 (1.0441e−01)	9.1948e−01 (1.8864e−02)	—	5.3011e+01
7	Soft tissue, I (20 mg/m) and cortical bone	4.9164e+01 (1.0)	6.1021e+00 (1.2412e−01)	1.5460e+00 (3.1446e−02)	—	3.1800e+01
8	Soft tissue, I (30 mg/m) and cortical bone	4.9691e+01 (1.0)	7.3744e+00 (1.4840e−01)	1.9146e+00 (3.8529e−02)	—	2.5954e+01
9	Soft tissue, I (20 mg/ml), Gd (20 mg/ml) and cortical bone (BM-4)	5.0639e+01 (1.0)	7.0196e+00 (1.3862e−01)	2.3250e+00 (4.5913e−02)	9.2075e−01 (1.8183e−02)	5.4997e+01
10	Adipose, I (20 mg/ml), Gd (20 mg/ml) and Teflon (BM-5)	2.4833e+01 (1.0)	2.8444e+00 (1.1454e−01)	1.3544e+00 (5.4539e−02)	7.1303e−01 (2.8713e−02)	5.9015e+01

Source: Tang and Ren 2021.

Notes: Energy range: 18–150 keV. SV: singular value. Rows 1–8: 3-MD; rows 9–10: 4-MD. Normalized singular value is in bracket.

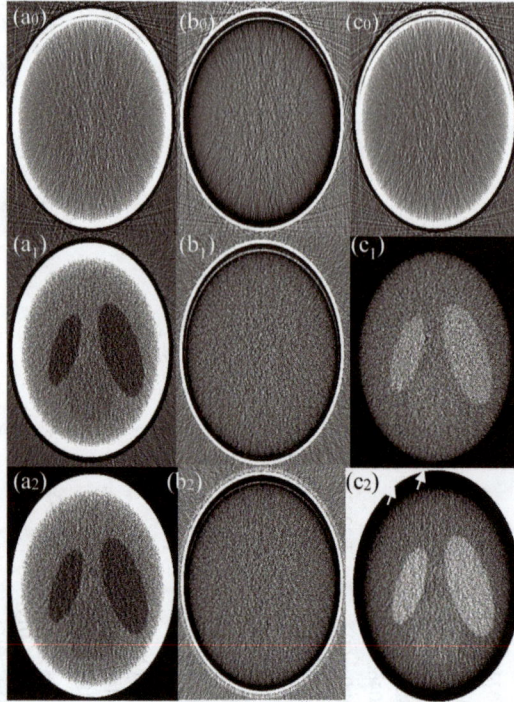

FIGURE 8.5 Material-specific images of Phan-0 corresponding to (a_0-c_0) Teflon, PMMA and adipose; (a_1-c_1) bone, Gd (20 mg/ml) and tissue; (a_2-c_2) Gd (20mg/ml), PMMA and adipose.

in the basis materials, the condition number of basis materials is reasonably small even though soft tissue and cortical bone are replaced by adipose and Teflon (row 10 in Table 8.2).

The humanoid head phantom images corresponding to various basis materials under realistic detector spectral response are shown in Figure 8.5 (WL: the level of brain parenchyma; WW: 8 times the noise of parenchyma). The images in the top row (a_0-c_0) correspond to the basis materials Teflon, PMMA, and adipose, in which, as predicted by the condition number in row 1 of Table 8.3, the noise is so severe that no internal structure of the head phantom is discernible. Using cortical bone, gadolinium (20 mg/ml) and soft tissue as the basis materials, the generated material-specific images are in the second row (a_1-c_1), in which the phantom's internal structure becomes discernible as the noise is substantially reduced. Moreover, if gadolinium (20 mg/ml) is kept but the other two basis materials are substituted with adipose and PMMA, the internal structure of Phan-0 becomes even more discernible (a_2-c_2), particularly in the basis image corresponding to adipose (Figure 8.5c_2). However, since PMMA and adipose behave very similarly in their attenuation as a function of energy, artifacts due to inaccurate material decomposition may appear, e.g., the bright peripheral areas indicated by the white arrowheads in Figure 8.5c_2.

TABLE 8.3

Noise (σ_1, σ_2, σ_3, σ_4) in the Image Corresponding to Each Basis Material and the Resultant Total Noise

Basis Materials	σ_1	σ_2	σ_3	σ_4	σ_t
1	Adipose, PMMA and Teflon (BM-0)	(1.8135e+01)	(1.5508e+01)	(3.5406e−01)	—	(2.3864e+1)
		1.2416e+01	1.2416e+01	2.8747e−01		1.7561e+01
2	Soft tissue, Gd (10 mg/ml) and cortical bone (BM-1)	(7.6896e−03)	(5.8727e−03)	(1.3848e−03)	—	(9.7743e−03)
		1.1554e−02	1.1821e−02	1.1821e−02		2.0322e−02
3	Soft tissue, Gd (20 mg/ml) and cortical bone (BM-2)	(5.3147e−03)	(2.8853e−03)	(1.3898e−03)	—	(6.2050e−03)
		7.1473e−03	5.8074e−03	3.0997e−03		9.7169e−03
4	Soft tissue, Gd (30 mg/ml) and cortical bone	(4.6839e−03)	(1.9066e−03)	(1.3908e−03)	—	(5.2448e−03)
		6.2662e−03	3.8383e−03	3.1057e−03		7.9777e−03
5	Adipose, PMMA and Gd (20 mg/ml) (BM-3)	(4.6309e−01)	(3.8133e−01)	(2.9078e−03)	—	(5.9989e−01)
		1.0835e+00	8.9526e−01	5.9209e−03		1.4055e+00
6	Soft tissue, I (10 mg/m) and cortical bone	(3.8834e−02)	(6.8703e−02)	(1.7887e−02)	—	(8.0920e−02)
		7.0074e−02	1.3031e−01	3.5281e−02		1.5210e−01
7	Soft tissue, I (20 mg/m) and cortical bone	(5.9368e−03)	(3.3968e−02)	(1.8196e−02)	—	(3.8989e−02)
		7.9022e−03	6.3897e−02	3.5593e−02		7.3567e−02
8	Soft tissue, I (30 mg/m) and cortical bone	(7.5598e−03)	(2.2457e−02)	(1.8237e−02)	—	(2.9901e−02)
		1.6910e−02	4.2251e−02	3.5677e−02		5.7827e−02
9	Soft tissue, cortical bone, I (20 mg/ml), Gd (20 mg/ml) (BM-4)	(5.8311e−03)	(3.2781e−02)	(6.6436e−02)	(1.1289e−02)	(7.5165e−02)
		7.5705e−03	2.3918e−01	4.4882e−01	4.1242e−02	5.1030e−01
10	Adipose, Teflon, I (20 mg/ml) and Gd (20 mg/ml) (BM-5)	(3.1791e−01)	(1.7872e−01)	(5.5780e−02)	(1.0411e−02)	(3.6907e−01)
		1.6238e+00	9.1713e−01	2.6367e−01	2.7597e−02	1.8837e+00

Source: Tang and Ren 2021.

Notes: Total noise: $\sigma_t = \sqrt{\sigma_1^2 + \sigma_2^2}$ in 2-MD; $\sigma_t = \sqrt{\sigma_1^2 + \sigma_2^2 + \sigma_3^2}$ in 3-MD; $\sigma_t = \sqrt{\sigma_1^2 + \sigma_2^2 + \sigma_3^2 + \sigma_4^2}$ in 4-MD. The measurement of noise corresponding to the ideal spectral response is presented in brackets.

The variation in noise and resultant discernibility of internal structures in the head phantom align well with variation in the condition number of the basis materials itemized in Table 8.2, and the noise gauged in Figure 8.5 is listed in Table 8.3.

The virtual monochromatic images at 18, 25, 35, 50, 65, and 80 keV obtained from the basis images in Figure 8.5 are shown in Figure 8.6 (WL: level of brain parenchyma; WW: 8 times parenchymatic noise). The best-case scenario in the contrast-to-noise ratio (CNR) occurs around 50 keV where gadolinium's K-edge is located. It is interesting and important to note that, despite the noise in the material-specific images varies dramatically due to the difference in the basis materials' conditioning, the noise in the virtual monochromatic images does not, owing to the intrinsic property in the noise correlation of the material-specific images (Kalender 1988; Roessl et al. 2007; Tang et al. 2023).

8.3.3 CONDITIONING OF SPECTRAL CHANNELIZATION AND ITS IMPACT ON IMAGE QUALITY

In principle, the number of spectral channels can be conceived as the dimensionality of P-space. As material decomposition is a linear mapping from the P-space to A-space, the number of spectral channels in photon-counting spectral CT should be larger than or at least equal to that of the material space, depending on the specific task in which the interested tissues are to be decomposed into a linear combination

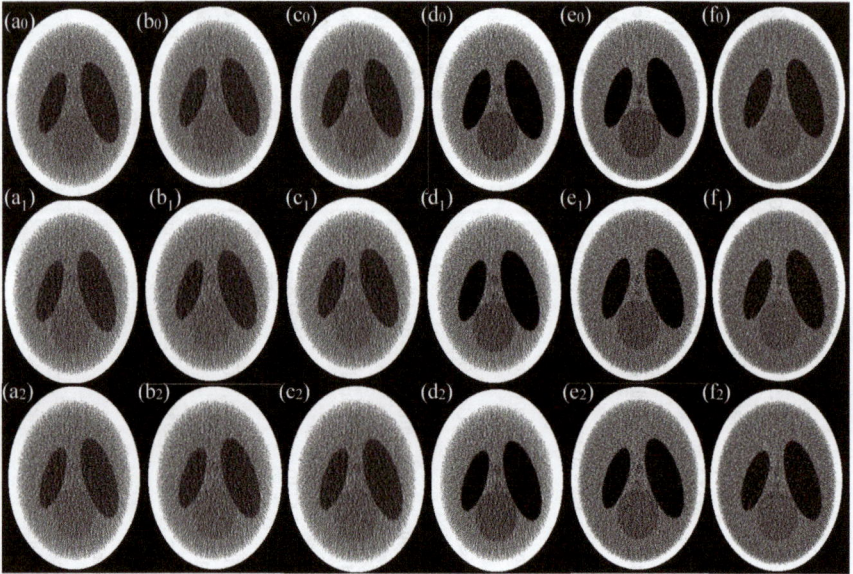

FIGURE 8.6 Virtual monochromatic images at 18, 25, 35, 50, 65 and 80 keV of Phan-0 obtained from 3-MD with basis materials: Teflon, PMMA and adipose; bone, Gd (20 mg/ml), and tissue; Gd (20 mg/ml), PMMA and adipose.

of the number of basis materials (Tang and Ren 2021; Ren et al. 2021). More research has recently been carried out to address this fundamental question via various approaches. For example, based on signal detection theory, Alvarez studied the dimensionality of material space and the influence of the number of spectral channels on image quality (mainly signal-to-noise ratio (SNR)) (Alvarez 2010, 2011, 2013, 2019). In practice, given a radiation dose, the number of X-ray photons falling into each spectral channel declines with the increasing number of channels, which may lead to degraded SNR in the basis image. Especially in the channel of lowest energy, a reduction in the number of X-ray photons may induce photon starvation that may offset the benefit offered by photon-counting spectral CT over the conventional CT. Hence, given a specific task, the number of spectral channels (dimensionality of projection space) in photon-counting spectral CT should be as few as possible as long as it is sufficient (equal to or larger than) to accommodate the dimensionality of the basis materials.

The detection of signals by the photon-counting detector in a spectral channel implemented via energy thresholding can be modeled as (Alvarez and Macovski 1976; Tang and Ren 2021; Ren et al. 2021)

$$I_k(L) = \int_{E_{min}^k}^{E_{max}^k} D_k(E) N_0(E) \exp\left(-\int_L \mu(x;E)dl\right)dE \qquad (8.8)$$

where L denotes the path of the X-ray beam. The subscript k indexes the spectral channel in data acquisition, while $[E_{min}^k, E_{max}^k]$ defines the kth spectral channel's energy range. $N_0(E)$ is the normalized X-ray source spectrum expressed in X-ray photon counts and the spectrum corresponding to a typical X-ray tube employed in CT, e.g., the one that is schematically presented in Figure 3.4b. Note that the X-ray photons at energy lower than 20 keV are removed by source filtration and the peak voltage can go up to 140–150 keV.

$D_k(E)$ denotes the inclusive effects of the detector's efficiency $\eta(E)$ and response $S_k(E)$ in the kth spectral channel:

$$D_k(E) = S_k(E)\eta(E) \qquad (8.9)$$

In practice, the spectral channelization in 2-MD– and 3-MD–based spectral imaging in photon-counting CT can be carried out by setting the detector's efficiency $\eta(E)$. Analytically, the spectral response of the kth channel is defined as

$$S_k(E) = \int_{E_{min}^k}^{E_{max}^k} R(E,E)dE \qquad (8.10)$$

where E denotes the incident energy. In the case of ideal detector spectral response, $R(E, E')$ is defined as a pulse function. However, in reality wherein the distortion induced by scattering, charge sharing and fluorescent escaping exists, $R(E, E')$ is modeled as a summation of Gaussian functions (Ehn 2017; Tang and Ren 2021; Ren et al. 2021). Illustrated in Figure 8.7 are examples of spectral channels in

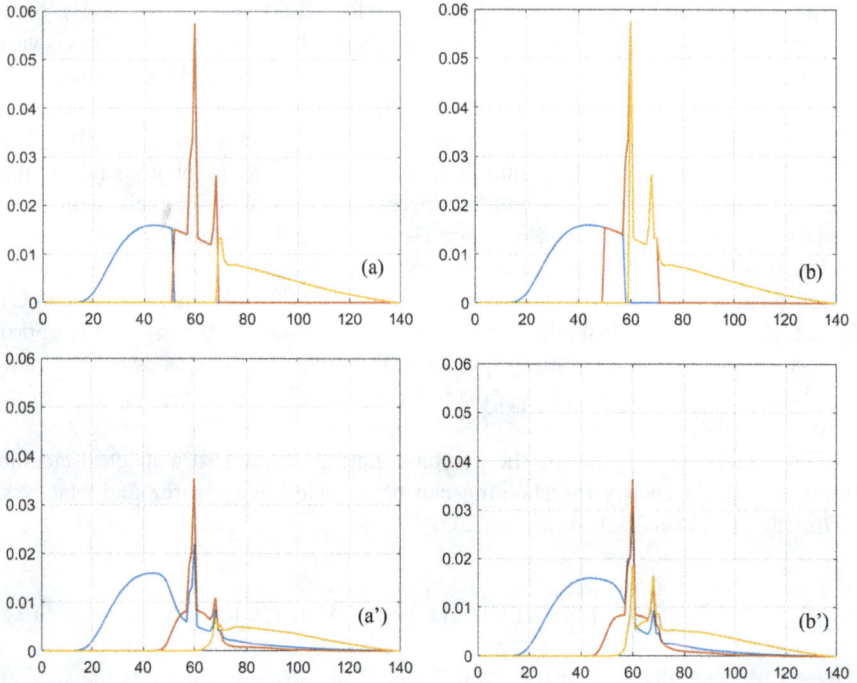

FIGURE 8.7   Spectral channels in 3-MD at 0% (column 1: a and a′) and 25% (column 2: b and b′) spectral overlapping, under ideal (row 1: a and b) and realistic (row 2: a′ and b′) detector response.

photon-counting spectral CT for 3-MD–based spectral imaging with (right column) and without (left column) spectral overlapping, and under ideal (top row) and realistic (bottom row) detector spectral response.

In addition to being used to determine the dimensionality of material space and the conditioning of basis materials as presented earlier, the SVD approach can also be employed to study the conditioning of spectral channelization for spectral imaging in photon-counting CT. Suppose a total of M spectral channels in the energy range [18, 150] keV are to be utilized for spectral imaging in photon-counting CT. Given the kth spectral channel, let $\{q_{kj}\}$ denote the sampling of its intensity profile $(D_k(E) \cdot N_0(E)$ in Equations 8.8–8.10 over the entire energy range [18, 150] keV at 1 keV interval, where $1 \leq j \leq N$ and N is the number of samplings in the energy range. A data matrix can be formed by sorting all of the sampled data row-wise into a matrix $Q_{M \times N} = \{q_{kj}\}$, which, via SVD, can be decomposed into the product of three matrices

$$Q_{M \times N} = U_{M \times M} \, \Sigma_{M \times N} \, V_{N \times N}^T \tag{8.11}$$

where $U_{M \times M}$ and $V_{N \times N}$ are orthogonal matrices and $\Sigma_{M \times N}$ is a rectangular diagonal matrix with the singular values $\{\lambda_i : 1 \leq i \leq M\}$ of $Q_{M \times N}$ in descending order as its diagonal elements, i.e., $\{\Sigma_{ii} = \lambda_i\}$. Again, the condition number (well-posedness) of $Q_{M \times N}$ (conditioning of spectral channelization) is defined as the square root of the ratio of the largest singular value over the smallest non-zero singular value $\lambda_{max} / \lambda_{min}$ (Strang 2006; Leon 2006).

Given soft tissue, gadolinium (20 mg/ml) and cortical bone as the basis materials, the condition number and associated noise under both ideal and realistic detector spectral response and their variation over the cases of spectral overlap are graphically charted in Figure 8.8. Regarding the condition number, it is noted that (i) under ideal detector spectra response, the condition number corresponding to the case of no overlap reaches the minimum, while that corresponding to other cases grows along with increasing spectral overlap (Figure 8.8b); (ii) under realistic detector spectral response, the condition number over all cases increases considerably, due to the distortion in the detector's spectral response; (iii) the distortion in the detector's spectral response degrades the conditioning of spectral channelization more in the cases wherein no or small spectral overlapping occurs than the cases wherein relatively large spectral overlapping exists. Regarding noise, the distortion in the detector's spectral response degrades the noise property of material-specific imaging considerably, while the variation in the property of noise is consistent with that in the conditioning of spectral channelization.

Under both ideal and realistic detector spectral response, the noise gauged at the targeted region of interest (ROI) and CNR against the background are plotted in Figure 8.9a and b, respectively, in which the cases corresponding to up to 50% overlapping in detector spectral channels at 5% steps are enclosed. Again, the profiles plotted in Figure 8.9 quantitatively confirm that the overlapping in spectral channels indeed degrades the noise in virtual monochromatic images across the entire energy range, though almost no effect at the sweet spot (~70 keV) wherein the highest CNR is reached. Nevertheless, it is interesting and important to note that there exists a sweet spot in CNR around 50 keV, i.e., the K-edge of gadolinium. Notably, the overlapping in spectral channels improves the CNR at the sweet spots, but degrades once it leaves.

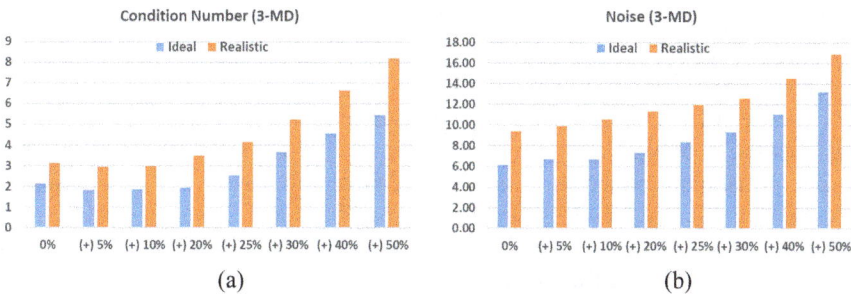

FIGURE 8.8   (a) The condition number and (b) the corresponding noise in 3-MD under both ideal and realistic detector spectral response ("+" indicates overlap).

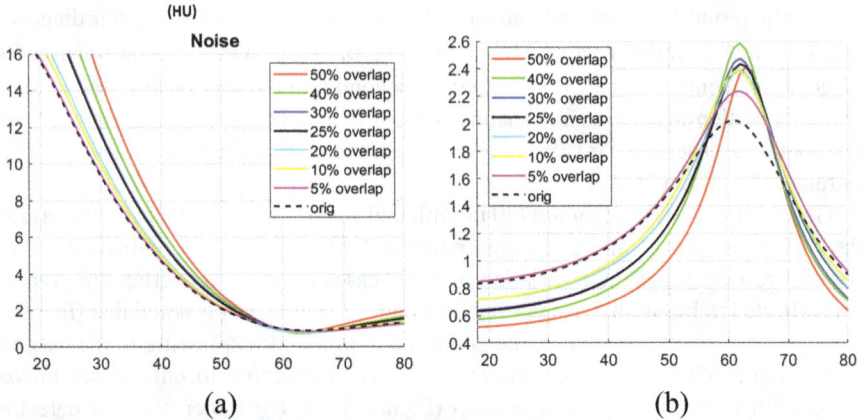

FIGURE 8.9   Variation of (a) noise and (b) CNR in virtual monochromatic analysis over energy, corresponding to the cases in spectral overlap, under realistic detector response (unit of all abscissa: keV).

8.4 NOISE CORRELATION OF MULTI-MATERIAL DECOMPOSITION IN PHOTON-COUNTING SPECTRAL MDCT

It has been known from the beginning that the noise in projection data acquired at two distinct peak voltages are of relevance in determining the image quality of spectral CT (Alvarez and Macovski 1976; Alvarez 1976). Using maximum likelihood estimation, Alvarez and Macovski showed that the Jacobian of transform from the P-space to A-space determines the noise property that is governed by the Cramér–Rao lower bound (CRLB) (Alvarez and Macovski 1976; Alvarez 1976, 2013). Alternatively, Kelcz et al. studied the same issue by taking noise as the uncertainty in estimation of the basis material mass density (Kelcz et al. 1979). Using the first-order Taylor expansion, Kelcz et al found that the so-called R-quantity, which is the ratio of mass attenuation coefficients associated with the two interested materials at the two distinct peak voltages, plays a key role that is almost identical to the Jacobian of the transform from P-space to A-space (Primak et al. 2009).

Initially, Alvarez and Macovski assumed no correlation in noise between projection data acquired at the two peak voltages (*correlation vanishing* henceforth), as this is indeed the case in data acquisition via photon-counting under ideal spectral response or voltage switching (fast kV-switching). They showed that though the noise correlation in projection data vanishes, there still exists a negative noise correlation in the image corresponding to each basis material (Alvarez and Macovski 1976; Alvarez 1976; Alvarez and Seppi 1979; Kalender et al. 1988) (*material-specific image* henceforth). Notably, the assumption of correlation vanishing seems invalid in the case of data acquisition via a layered (sandwiched) detector, but, through an in-depth statistical analysis, it turns out that the noise correlation in the data acquired by the first and second layers is in fact negligibly small and thus can be treated as another case of correlation vanishing (Sones and Barnes 1989). Nevertheless, the correlation-vanishing assumption is actually not valid in photon-counting data acquisition if the realistic detector response is taken in account, as the spectral distortion inevitably induces overlapping in adjacent spectral channels (Ren et al. 2020, 2021; Tang and Ren 2021).

In 2-MD–based spectral imaging, an investigation to reveal the effect of noise correlation in the projection data on noise and noise correlation in the material-specific images has been reported (Roessl et al. 2007). It was shown that the correlation of noise in the two material-specific images is negative, and, if the correlation in the projection data vanishes, the analytics degenerates to the case initially derived by Alvarez and Macovski (Alvarez 1976; Alvarez and Macovski 1976; Alvarez and Seppi 1979). Notably, the work in Reference (Roessl et al. 2007) was focused on the counting-integration mode in data acquisition and only analytic plots were given, though the conclusion is in fact general and applicable to other cases of 2-MD–based spectral imaging via different data acquisition schemes.

With increasing multi-spectral channels and multi-basis materials, the dimension of Jacobian increases, which complicates the way in which the noise correlation in projection data acquired in each spectral channel impacts the noise and noise correlation in the material-specific images. Specifically, the sign of the off-diagonal elements in the inverse of an $M \times M$ ($M > 2$) matrix may vary, implying that the correlation in the noise corresponding to each material-specific image in the m-MD–based spectral imaging may not always be negative, as has been the case in 2-MD–based spectral imaging (Kalender et al. 1988). By treating $I_k(L)$ ($k = 1, \ldots, K$) and $A_p(L)$ ($p = 1, \ldots, P$) as random variables in the P-space and A-space, respectively, the mapping from the former to the latter can be written as (Tang et al. 2023)

$$I_k\left(L\right) = f_k\left(A_1\left(L\right),\ldots,A_p\left(L\right)\right)\left(k = 1,\ldots,K\right) \tag{8.12}$$

Then, we have the covariance matrix of A as (Roessl et al. 2007; Cowan 1998)

$$V\left[A\right] = \left(F^{-1}\right) \cdot V\left[I\right] \cdot \left(F^{-1}\right)^{T} \tag{8.13}$$

where each entry of the mapping matrix F is defined as $F_{kp} = \partial I_k / \partial A_p$. In analogue to the way in Reference (Roessl et al. 2007), we define the effective attenuation coefficient, SNR, and correlation coefficient in the P-space and A-space, respectively, as In analogue to the way in Reference (Roessl et al. 2007), we define the effective attenuation coefficient, SNR, and correlation coefficient in the P-space and A-space, respectively, as

$$\mu_{kp} = -\frac{1}{I_k}\frac{\partial I_k}{\partial A_p}, SNR_k = \frac{I_k}{\sigma_{I_k}} \tag{8.14}$$

$$\rho_{I_{k1}I_{k2}} = \frac{\sigma_{I_{k1}I_{k2}}}{\sigma_{I_{k1}}\sigma_{I_{k2}}}, \quad \rho_{A_{p1}A_{p2}} = \frac{\sigma_{A_{p1}A_{p2}}}{\sigma_{A_{p1}}\sigma_{A_{p2}}} \tag{8.15}$$

Once the material-specific images are generated, the Pearson correlation coefficient (R-coefficient), as defined next, can be adopted to quantitatively assess the correlation of noise in those images:

$$R = \frac{\sum_{i=1}^{N}(x_i - \bar{x})(y_i - \bar{y})}{\sqrt{\sum_{i=1}^{N}(x_i - \bar{x})^2}\sqrt{\sum_{i=1}^{N}(y_i - \bar{y})^2}} \tag{8.16}$$

where x_i and y_i denote the pixels at the identical location in each of the two material-specific images. $\bar{x}$ and $\bar{y}$ are the averaged intensity of all the pixels in each of the two images, and N is the total number of pixels in each of the images engaged in the measurement.

8.4.1 NOISE CORRELATION OF TWO-MATERIAL DECOMPOSITION IN PHOTON-COUNTING SPECTRAL MDCT

In 2-MD, we have the Jacobian

$$\Delta_{2\times2} = \mu_{11}\mu_{22} - \mu_{21}\mu_{12} \underset{A_1 A_2}{\underline{\Delta}} \frac{1}{A_1 A_2} \det(F) \tag{8.17}$$

According to Equation 8.13, the covariance matrix $V[A]$ becomes

$$V_{2\times2}[A] = \begin{bmatrix} \sigma_{A_1}^2 & \sigma_{A_1 A_2} \\ \sigma_{A_2 A_1} & \sigma_{A_2}^2 \end{bmatrix} \tag{8.18}$$

where the entries are

$$\sigma_{A_1}^2 = \frac{1}{\Delta_{2\times2}^2}\left(\frac{\mu_{22}^2}{SNR_1^2} + \frac{\mu_{12}^2}{SNR_2^2} - 2\rho_{I_{12}}\frac{\mu_{22}}{SNR_1}\frac{\mu_{12}}{SNR_2} \right) \tag{8.19}$$

$$\sigma_{A_2}^2 = \frac{1}{\Delta_{2\times2}^2}\left(\frac{\mu_{21}^2}{SNR_1^2} + \frac{\mu_{11}^2}{SNR_2^2} - 2\rho_{I_{12}}\frac{\mu_{11}}{SNR_2}\frac{\mu_{21}}{SNR_1} \right) \tag{8.20}$$

$$\sigma_{A_1 A_2} = \sigma_{A_2 A_1} = -\frac{1}{\Delta_{2\times2}^2}\left(\frac{\mu_{21}\mu_{22}}{SNR_1^2} + \frac{\mu_{12}\mu_{11}}{SNR_2^2} - \rho_{I_{12}}\left(\frac{\mu_{11}}{SNR_2}\frac{\mu_{22}}{SNR_1} + \frac{\mu_{12}}{SNR_2}\frac{\mu_{21}}{SNR_1} \right) \right) \tag{8.21}$$

Furthermore, we have the cross-correlation

$$\rho_{A_1 A_2} = \rho_{A_2 A_1}$$

$$= \frac{-\left(\dfrac{\mu_{21}\mu_{22}}{SNR_1^2} + \dfrac{\mu_{12}\mu_{11}}{SNR_2^2} - \rho_{I_{12}}\left(\dfrac{\mu_{11}}{SNR_2}\dfrac{\mu_{22}}{SNR_1} + \dfrac{\mu_{12}}{SNR_2}\dfrac{\mu_{21}}{SNR_1}\right)\right)}{\left(\dfrac{\mu_{22}^2}{SNR_1^2} + \dfrac{\mu_{12}^2}{SNR_2^2} - 2\rho_{I_{12}}\dfrac{\mu_{22}}{SNR_1}\dfrac{\mu_{12}}{SNR_2}\right)^{\!1/2}\left(\dfrac{\mu_{21}^2}{SNR_1^2} + \dfrac{\mu_{11}^2}{SNR_2^2} - 2\rho_{I_{12}}\dfrac{\mu_{11}}{SNR_2}\dfrac{\mu_{21}}{SNR_1}\right)^{\!1/2}}$$

$$(8.22)$$

If there is no correlation between the projection data acquired at the two peak voltages, Equations 8.19–8.22 degenerate into

$$\sigma_{A_1}^2 = \frac{1}{\Delta_{2\times 2}^2}\left(\frac{\mu_{22}^2}{SNR_1^2} + \frac{\mu_{12}^2}{SNR_2^2}\right) \tag{8.19'}$$

$$\sigma_{A_2}^2 = \frac{1}{\Delta_{2\times 2}^2}\left(\frac{\mu_{21}^2}{SNR_1^2} + \frac{\mu_{11}^2}{SNR_2^2}\right) \tag{8.20'}$$

$$\sigma_{A_1 A_2} = -\frac{1}{\Delta_{2\times 2}^2}\left(\frac{\mu_{21}\mu_{22}}{SNR_1^2} + \frac{\mu_{12}\mu_{11}}{SNR_2^2}\right) \tag{8.21'}$$

$$\rho_{A_1 A_2} = \frac{-\left(\dfrac{\mu_{21}\mu_{22}}{SNR_1^2} + \dfrac{\mu_{12}\mu_{11}}{SNR_2^2}\right)}{\left(\dfrac{\mu_{22}^2}{SNR_1^2} + \dfrac{\mu_{12}^2}{SNR_2^2}\right)^{\!1/2}\left(\dfrac{\mu_{21}^2}{SNR_1^2} + \dfrac{\mu_{11}^2}{SNR_2^2}\right)^{\!1/2}} \tag{8.22'}$$

which is exactly the same as that originally given by Alvarez and Macovski (Alvarez 1976; Alvarez and Macovski 1976). In general, an inter-channel spectral overlapping under realistic detector spectral response induces positive correlation between the data acquired in each channel, i.e., $\rho_{I_{12}} 0$, which decreases the magnitude of nominators in Equations 8.19–8.22. Meanwhile, however, the inter-channel overlapping may decrease the magnitude of $\Delta_{2\times 2}^2$ in the denominator to a larger extent. Together, these changes may increase the magnitude of noise and noise correlation in the data denoted by A_1 and A_2 that are obtained via material decomposition.

The noise correlation in the material-specific images corresponding to basis materials soft tissue and cortical bone obtained via 2-MD under ideal and realistic detector spectral response are presented in the scatterplots in Figure 8.10a and Figure 8.10b, respectively. The noise in the material-specific images under 2-MD is in negative correlation, which is consistent to what has been reported in the literature (Alvarez and Seppi 1979; Kalender et al. 1988; Roessl et al. 2007). Moreover, it is observed that, the inter-channel overlapping in the detector's spectral response

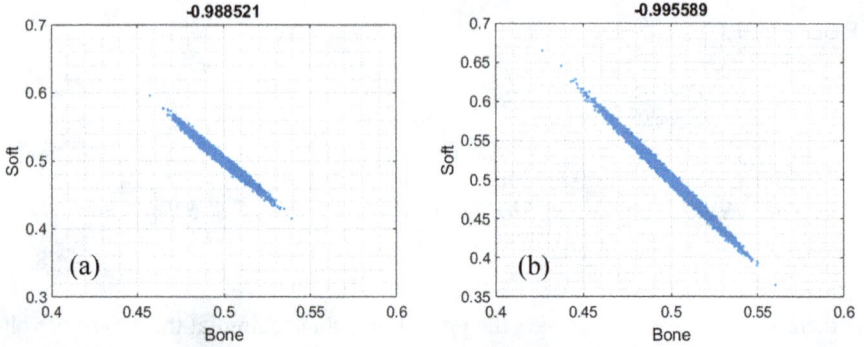

FIGURE 8.10 Correlation of noise between material-specific images acquired via 2-MD under (a) ideal and (b) realistic detector spectral response.

modestly increases the magnitude of noise correlation coefficient, as the magnitude of noise in each material-specific image markedly increases.

8.4.2 NOISE CORRELATION OF THREE-MATERIAL DECOMPOSITION IN PHOTON-COUNTING SPECTRAL MDCT

In 3-MD, we have the Jacobian

$$\Delta_{3\times3} = \mu_{11}\mu_{22}\mu_{33} + \mu_{12}\mu_{23}\mu_{31} + \mu_{21}\mu_{32}\mu_{13} - \mu_{31}\mu_{22}\mu_{13} - \mu_{32}\mu_{23}\mu_{11} - \mu_{11}\mu_{21}\mu_{33}$$

$$\Delta \stackrel{}{=} \frac{1}{A_1 A_2 A_3} \det(F) \tag{8.23}$$

Again starting from Equation 8.13, the covariance matrix $V[A]$ becomes

$$V_{3\times3}[A] = \begin{bmatrix} \sigma_{A_1}^2 & \sigma_{A_1 A_2} & \sigma_{A_1 A_3} \\ \sigma_{A_2 A_1} & \sigma_{A_2}^2 & \sigma_{A_2 A_3} \\ \sigma_{A_3 A_1} & \sigma_{A_3 A_2} & \sigma_{A_3}^2 \end{bmatrix} \tag{8.24}$$

With algebra, we can specifically and deliberately arrive at the results presented next, though the results may be analytically expressed in a more compact form.

$$\sigma^2_{A_1A_1} = \left(\mu_{23}\mu_{32} - \mu_{33}\mu_{22}\right)^2 / SNR^2_1 + \left(\mu_{13}\mu_{32} - \mu_{33}\mu_{12}\right)^2 / SNR^2_2 + \left(\mu_{13}\mu_{22} - \right.$$

$$\mu_{12}\mu_{23}\big)^2 / SNR^2_3 - 2\rho_{I12}\left(\mu_{13}\mu_{23}\mu^2_{32} + \mu^2_{33}\mu_{12}\mu_{22} - \mu_{33}\mu_{12}\mu_{23}\mu_{32} - \mu_{33}\mu_{13}\mu_{22}\mu_{32}\right)$$

$$/SNR_1 SNR_2 - 2\rho_{I23}(\mu^2_{13}\mu_{22}\mu_{32} + \mu_{33}\mu^2_{12}\mu_{23} - \mu_{12}\mu_{13}\mu_{23}\mu_{32} - \mu_{33}\mu_{12}\mu_{13}\mu_{22}) /$$

$$SNR_2 SNR_3 - 2\rho_{I13}(\mu_{12}\mu^2_{23}\mu_{32} + \mu_{33}\mu_{13}\mu^2_{22} - \mu_{13}\mu_{22}\mu_{23}\mu_{32} - \mu_{33}\mu_{12}\mu_{22}\mu_{23}) /$$

$$SNR_1 SNR_3) / \Delta^2_{3\times3}$$

$$(8.25)$$

$$\sigma^2_{A_2A_2} = ((\mu_{23}\mu_{31} - \mu_{33}\mu_{21})^2 / SNR^2_1 + \left(\mu_{13}\mu_{31} - \mu_{33}\mu_{11}\right)^2 / SNR^2_2 + \left(\mu_{11}\mu_{23} - \mu_{13}\mu_{21}\right)^2 /$$

$$SNR^2_3 - 2\rho_{I12}\left(\mu_{13}\mu_{23}\mu^2_{31} + \mu^2_{33}\mu_{11}\mu_{21} - \mu_{33}\mu_{11}\mu_{23}\mu_{31} - \mu_{33}\mu_{13}\mu_{21}\mu_{31}\right) / SNR_1 SNR_2$$

$$- 2\rho_{I23}(\mu^2_{13}\mu_{21}\mu_{31} + \mu_{33}\mu^2_{11}\mu_{23} - \mu_{11}\mu_{13}\mu_{23}\mu_{31} - \mu_{33}\mu_{11}\mu_{13}\mu_{21}) / SNR_2 SNR_3$$

$$- 2\rho_{I13}(\mu_{11}\mu^2_{23}\mu_{31} + \mu_{33}\mu_{13}\mu^2_{21} - \mu_{13}\mu_{21}\mu_{23}\mu_{31} - \mu_{33}\mu_{11}\mu_{21}\mu_{23}) / SNR_1 SNR_3) / \Delta^2_{3\times3}$$

$$(8.26)$$

$$\sigma^2_{A_3A_3} = ((\mu_{11}\mu_{32} - \mu_{12}\mu_{31})^2 / SNR^2_2 + \left(\mu_{21}\mu_{32} - \mu_{22}\mu_{31}\right)^2 / SNR^2_1 + \left(\mu_{11}\mu_{22} - \mu_{12}\mu_{21}\right)^2 /$$

$$SNR^2_3 - 2\rho_{I12}\left(\mu_{11}\mu_{21}\mu^2_{32} + \mu_{12}\mu_{22}\mu^2_{31} - \mu_{11}\mu_{22}\mu_{31}\mu_{32} - \mu_{12}\mu_{21}\mu_{31}\mu_{32}\right) / SNR_1 SNR_2 -$$

$$2\rho_{I23}(\mu^2_{12}\mu_{21}\mu_{31} + \mu^2_{11}\mu_{22}\mu_{32} - \mu_{11}\mu_{12}\mu_{21}\mu_{32} - \mu_{11}\mu_{12}\mu_{22}\mu_{31}) / SNR_2 SNR_3 -$$

$$2\rho_{I13}(\mu_{12}\mu^2_{21}\mu_{32} + \mu_{11}\mu^2_{22}\mu_{31} - \mu_{11}\mu_{21}\mu_{22}\mu_{32} - \mu_{12}\mu_{21}\mu_{22}\mu_{31}) / SNR_1 SNR_3) / \Delta^2_{3\times3}$$

$$(8.27)$$

$$\sigma_{A_1A_2} = \sigma_{A_2A_1} = -((\mu^2_{23}\mu_{31}\mu_{32} + \mu^2_{33}\mu_{21}\mu_{22} - \mu_{33}\mu_{21}\mu_{23}\mu_{32} - \mu_{33}\mu_{22}\mu_{23}\mu_{31}) / SNR^2_1 +$$

$$(\mu^2_{33}\mu_{11}\mu_{12} + \mu^2_{13}\mu_{31}\mu_{32} - \mu_{33}\mu_{11}\mu_{13}\mu_{32} - \mu_{33}\mu_{12}\mu_{13}\mu_{31}) / SNR^2_2 + (\mu_{11}\mu_{12}\mu^2_{23} + \mu^2_{13}\mu_{21}\mu_{22}$$

$$-\mu_{11}\mu_{13}\mu_{22}\mu_{23} - \mu_{12}\mu_{13}\mu_{21}\mu_{23}) / SNR^2_3 - \rho_{I12}(\mu^2_{33}\mu_{11}\mu_{22} + \mu^2_{33}\mu_{12}\mu_{21} + 2\mu_{13}\mu_{23}\mu_{31}\mu_{32} -$$

$$\mu_{33}\mu_{11}\mu_{23}\mu_{32} - \mu_{33}\mu_{13}\mu_{21}\mu_{32} - \mu_{33}\mu_{12}\mu_{23}\mu_{31} - \mu_{33}\mu_{13}\mu_{22}\mu_{31}) / SNR_1 SNR_2 - \rho_{I23}(\mu^2_{13}\mu_{21}\mu_{32}$$

$$+2\mu_{33}\mu_{11}\mu_{12}\mu_{23} + \mu^2_{13}\mu_{22}\mu_{31} - \mu_{11}\mu_{13}\mu_{23}\mu_{32} - \mu_{12}\mu_{13}\mu_{23}\mu_{31} - \mu_{33}\mu_{11}\mu_{13}\mu_{22} -$$

$$\mu_{33}\mu_{12}\mu_{13}\mu_{21}) / SNR_2 SNR_3 - \rho_{I13}(\mu_{12}\mu^2_{23}\mu_{31} + 2\mu_{33}\mu_{13}\mu_{21}\mu_{22} + \mu_{11}\mu^2_{23}\mu_{32} -$$

$$\mu_{13}\mu_{21}\mu_{23}\mu_{32} - \mu_{13}\mu_{22}\mu_{23}\mu_{31} - \mu_{33}\mu_{11}\mu_{22}\mu_{23} - \mu_{33}\mu_{12}\mu_{21}\mu_{23}) / SNR_1 SNR_3) / \Delta^2_{3\times3}$$

$$(8.28)$$

$$\sigma_{A_1A_3} = \sigma_{A_3A_1} = -\Big(\big(\mu_{21}\mu_{23}\mu^2{}_{32} + \mu_{33}\mu^2{}_{22}\mu_{31} - \mu_{22}\mu_{23}\mu_{31}\mu_{32} - \mu_{33}\mu_{21}\mu_{22}\mu_{32}\big)\big/ SNR^2{}_1 +$$

$$\big(\mu_{11}\mu_{13}\mu^2{}_{32} + \mu_{33}\mu^2{}_{12}\mu_{31} - \mu_{12}\mu_{13}\mu_{31}\mu_{32} - \mu_{33}\mu_{11}\mu_{12}\mu_{32}\big)\big/ SNR^2{}_2 + \big(\mu^2{}_{12}\mu_{21}\mu_{23} +$$

$$\mu_{11}\mu_{13}\mu^2{}_{22} - \mu_{12}\mu_{13}\mu_{21}\mu_{22} - \mu_{11}\mu_{12}\mu_{22}\mu_{23}\big)\big/ SNR^2{}_3 - \rho_{I12}(\mu_{11}\mu_{23}\mu^2{}_{32} + 2\mu_{33}\mu_{12}\mu_{22}\mu_{31} +$$

$$\mu_{13}\mu_{21}\mu^2{}_{32} - \mu_{12}\mu_{23}\mu_{31}\mu_{32} - \mu_{13}\mu_{22}\mu_{31}\mu_{32} - \mu_{33}\mu_{11}\mu_{22}\mu_{32} - \mu_{33}\mu_{12}\mu_{21}\mu_{32})\big/ SNR_1SNR_2 -$$

$$\rho_{I23}(\mu^2{}_{12}\mu_{23}\mu_{31} + 2\mu_{11}\mu_{13}\mu_{22}\mu_{32} + \mu_{33}\mu^2{}_{12}\mu_{21} - \mu_{11}\mu_{12}\mu_{23}\mu_{32} - \mu_{12}\mu_{13}\mu_{21}\mu_{32} -$$

$$\mu_{12}\mu_{13}\mu_{22}\mu_{31} - \mu_{33}\mu_{11}\mu_{12}\mu_{22})\big/ SNR_2SNR_3 - \rho_{I13}(\mu_{13}\mu^2{}_{22}\mu_{31} + 2\mu_{12}\mu_{21}\mu_{23}\mu_{32} +$$

$$\mu_{33}\mu_{11}\mu^2{}_{22} - \mu_{11}\mu_{22}\mu_{23}\mu_{32} - \mu_{13}\mu_{21}\mu_{22}\mu_{32} - \mu_{12}\mu_{22}\mu_{23}\mu_{31} - \mu_{33}\mu_{12}\mu_{21}\mu_{22})\big/$$

$$SNR_1SNR_3\big)\big/ \Delta^2{}_{3\times3}$$

$$(8.29)$$

$$\sigma_{A_2A_3} = \sigma_{A_3A_2} = -\Big(\big(\mu_{33}\mu^2{}_{21}\mu_{32} + \mu_{22}\mu_{23}\mu^2{}_{31} - \mu_{21}\mu_{23}\mu_{31}\mu_{32} - \mu_{33}\mu_{21}\mu_{22}\mu_{31}\big)\big/ SNR^2{}_1 +$$

$$\big(\mu_{33}\mu^2{}_{11}\mu_{32} + \mu_{12}\mu_{13}\mu^2{}_{31} - \mu_{11}\mu_{13}\mu_{31}\mu_{32} - \mu_{33}\mu_{11}\mu_{12}\mu_{31}\big)\big/ SNR^2{}_2 +$$

$$\big(\mu^2{}_{11}\mu_{22}\mu_{23} + \mu_{12}\mu_{13}\mu^2{}_{21} - \mu_{11}\mu_{12}\mu_{21}\mu_{23} - \mu_{11}\mu_{13}\mu_{21}\mu_{22}\big)\big/ SNR^2{}_3 -$$

$$\rho_{I12}(\mu_{12}\mu_{23}\mu^2{}_{31} + 2\mu_{33}\mu_{11}\mu_{21}\mu_{32} + \mu_{13}\mu_{22}\mu^2{}_{31} - \mu_{11}\mu_{23}\mu_{31}\mu_{32} - \mu_{13}\mu_{21}\mu_{31}\mu_{32} -$$

$$\mu_{33}\mu_{11}\mu_{22}\mu_{31} - \mu_{33}\mu_{12}\mu_{21}\mu_{31})\big/ SNR_1SNR_2 - \rho_{I23}(\mu^2{}_{11}\mu_{23}\mu_{32} + 2\mu_{12}\mu_{13}\mu_{21}\mu_{31} +$$

$$\mu_{33}\mu^2{}_{11}\mu_{22} - \mu_{11}\mu_{13}\mu_{21}\mu_{32} - \mu_{11}\mu_{12}\mu_{23}\mu_{31} - \mu_{11}\mu_{13}\mu_{22}\mu_{31} - \mu_{33}\mu_{11}\mu_{12}\mu_{21})\big/$$

$$SNR_2SNR_3 - \rho_{I13}(\mu_{13}\mu^2{}_{21}\mu_{32} + 2\mu_{11}\mu_{22}\mu_{23}\mu_{31} + \mu_{33}\mu_{12}\mu^2{}_{21} - \mu_{11}\mu_{21}\mu_{23}\mu_{32} -$$

$$\mu_{12}\mu_{21}\mu_{23}\mu_{31} - \mu_{13}\mu_{21}\mu_{22}\mu_{31} - \mu_{33}\mu_{11}\mu_{21}\mu_{22})\big/ SNR_1SNR_3\big)\big/ \Delta^2{}_{3\times3}$$

$$(8.30)$$

where $\Delta_{3\times3} = \mu_{11}\mu_{23}\mu_{32} - \mu_{13}\mu_{21}\mu_{32} - \mu_{12}\mu_{23}\mu_{31} + \mu_{13}\mu_{22}\mu_{31} - \mu_{33}\mu_{11}\mu_{22} + \mu_{33}\mu_{12}\mu_{21}$ (8.31)

If no correlation exists in projection data, ($\rho_{I_{ij}} = 0, i = 1,2,3; j = 1,2,3$), Equations 8.25–8.30 break down into

$$\sigma^2_{A_1A_1} = \Big(\big(\mu_{23}\mu_{32} - \mu_{33}\mu_{22}\big)^2 \big/ SNR^2{}_1 + \big(\mu_{13}\mu_{32} - \mu_{33}\mu_{12}\big)^2 \big/ SNR^2{}_2 +$$

$$\big(\mu_{13}\mu_{22} - \mu_{12}\mu_{23}\big)^2 \big/ SNR^2{}_3\Big)\big/ \Delta^2{}_{3\times3}$$

$$(8.25')$$

$$\sigma^2_{A_2A_2} = \left(\left(\mu_{23}\mu_{31} - \mu_{33}\mu_{21}\right)^2 / SNR^2_1 + \left(\mu_{13}\mu_{31} - \mu_{33}\mu_{11}\right)^2 / SNR^2_2 +\right.$$

$$\left.\left(\mu_{11}\mu_{23} - \mu_{13}\mu_{21}\right)^2 / SNR^2_3\right) / \Delta^2_{3\times3} \tag{8.26'}$$

$$\sigma^2_{A_3A_3} = \left(\left(\mu_{11}\mu_{32} - \mu_{12}\mu_{31}\right)^2 / SNR^2_2 + \left(\mu_{21}\mu_{32} - \mu_{22}\mu_{31}\right)^2 / SNR^2_1 +\right.$$

$$\left.\left(\mu_{11}\mu_{22} - \mu_{12}\mu_{21}\right)^2 / SNR^2_3\right) / \Delta^2_{3\times3} \tag{8.27'}$$

$$\sigma_{A_1A_2} = \sigma_{A_2A_1} = -\left(\left(\mu^2_{23}\mu_{31}\mu_{32} + \mu^2_{33}\mu_{21}\mu_{22} - \mu_{33}\mu_{21}\mu_{23}\mu_{32} - \mu_{33}\mu_{22}\mu_{23}\mu_{31}\right) / SNR^2_1 +\right.$$

$$(\mu^2_{33}\mu_{11}\mu_{12} + \mu^2_{13}\mu_{31}\mu_{32} - \mu_{33}\mu_{11}\mu_{13}\mu_{32} - \mu_{33}\mu_{12}\mu_{13}\mu_{31}) / SNR^2_2 + (\mu_{11}\mu_{12}\mu^2_{23} +$$

$$\mu^2_{13}\mu_{21}\mu_{22} - \mu_{11}\mu_{13}\mu_{22}\mu_{23} - \mu_{12}\mu_{13}\mu_{21}\mu_{23}) / SNR^2_3) / \Delta^2_{3\times3}$$

$$\tag{8.28'}$$

$$\sigma_{A_1A_3} = \sigma_{A_3A_1} = -\left(\left(\mu_{21}\mu_{23}\mu^2_{32} + \mu_{33}\mu^2_{22}\mu_{31} - \mu_{22}\mu_{23}\mu_{31}\mu_{32} - \mu_{33}\mu_{21}\mu_{22}\mu_{32}\right) / SNR^2_1 +\right.$$

$$(\mu_{11}\mu_{13}\mu^2_{32} + \mu_{33}\mu^2_{12}\mu_{31} - \mu_{12}\mu_{13}\mu_{31}\mu_{32} - \mu_{33}\mu_{11}\mu_{12}\mu_{32}) / SNR^2_2 + (\mu^2_{12}\mu_{21}\mu_{23} +$$

$$\mu_{11}\mu_{13}\mu^2_{22} - \mu_{12}\mu_{13}\mu_{21}\mu_{22} - \mu_{11}\mu_{12}\mu_{22}\mu_{23}) / SNR^2_3) / \Delta^2_{3\times3}$$

$$\tag{8.29'}$$

$$\sigma_{A_2A_3} = \sigma_{A_3A_2} = -\left(\left(\mu_{33}\mu^2_{21}\mu_{32} + \mu_{22}\mu_{23}\mu^2_{31} - \mu_{21}\mu_{23}\mu_{31}\mu_{32} - \mu_{33}\mu_{21}\mu_{22}\mu_{31}\right) / SNR^2_1 +\right.$$

$$(\mu_{33}\mu^2_{11}\mu_{32} + \mu_{12}\mu_{13}\mu^2_{31} - \mu_{11}\mu_{13}\mu_{31}\mu_{32} - \mu_{33}\mu_{11}\mu_{12}\mu_{31}) / SNR^2_2 + (\mu^2_{11}\mu_{22}\mu_{23} +$$

$$\mu_{12}\mu_{13}\mu^2_{21} - \mu_{11}\mu_{12}\mu_{21}\mu_{23} - \mu_{11}\mu_{13}\mu_{21}\mu_{22}) / SNR^2_3) / \Delta^2_{3\times3}$$

$$\tag{8.30'}$$

Similarly, the inter-channel spectral overlap induces positive correlation between the data acquired in different channels, i.e., $\rho_{I_{12}} > 0$, $\rho_{I_{23}} > 0$, and $\rho_{I_{13}} > 0$, which in general decreases the magnitude of nominators in Equations 8.25–8.30. Also, the inter-channel overlap may decrease the magnitude of $\Delta^2_{3\times3}$ in the denominator to a larger extent. Jointly, these changes may increase the magnitude of noise and noise correlation in the data denoted by A_1, A_2 and A_3 after material decomposition. As shown earlier, the analytic expression of each entry of matrix $V_{3\times3}[A]$ becomes exhaustively complicated in 3-MD, though their derivation can be carried out according to Equation 8.13. Hence, an analysis of the noise and noise correlation via simulation

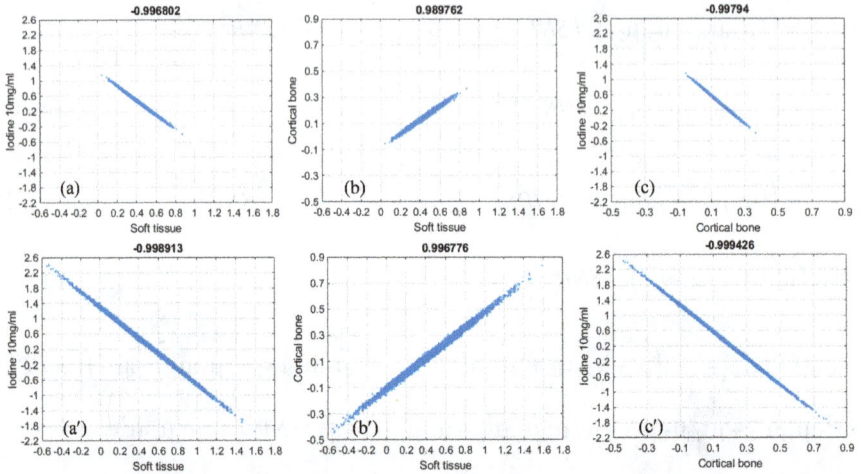

FIGURE 8.11 Correlation of noise between the material specific images acquired via 3-MD under both (a–c) ideal and (a′–c′) realistic detector response.

study makes more sense in terms of feasibility in the case of 4-MD–based (and beyond) spectral imaging in photon-counting CT.

The correlation of noise in the material-specific images corresponding to the basis materials soft tissue, 10 mg/ml iodine and cortical bone under ideal detector spectral response are presented in the scatterplots in Figure 8.11a–c. The polarity of noise correlation over the material-specific images in 3-MD–based spectral imaging alternates between +1 and −1. The inter-channel overlap induced by the spectral distortion in a realistic detector's spectral response modestly increases the magnitude of noise correlation, which is again expected according to Equations 8.25′–8.28′.

8.5 OPTIMIZATION OF IMAGE QUALITY IN PHOTON-COUNTING SPECTRAL CT VIA SPECTRAL WEIGHTING

Once the dimensionality (number of energy bins) of P-space is determined, the deployment of energy bins (termed *binning*) and spectral weighting are the determinants for photon-counting spectral CT to reach optimal imaging performance. This section, prior to diving into the optimization of weighting schemes and energy binning, indicate that, in general, the de-noising approach in the spectral domain for the energy-integration spectral CT (Section 8.1.2) can also be reused for de-noising in spectral domain in photon-counting spectral CT. Meanwhile, it should be noted that, with an increasing number of energy bins, the data acquired in the energy bins toward the high (fewer X-ray photons) and low (softer X-ray photons) energy ends may suffer from photon starvation. Hence, intuitively, the data acquired in the energy bins toward the low energy end or the composite data obtained by averaging data over all the energy bins may be more trustful in providing the guide map in de-noising.

8.5.1 SPECTRAL MATCHING: GENERAL

As illustrated in Figure 3.7c (see Chapter 3), the response in an energy-integration detector is proportional to the energy carried by the detected X-ray photons, while that in a photon-counting detector is merely proportional to the number of X-ray photons. On the other hand, as stated in Equations 3.1–3.3, the photoelectric absorption behaves as a function of $1/E^3$, which mismatches the spectral property of the energy-integration detector substantially ($1/E^3$ vs. E^1) and that of photon-counting detector to a slightly less severity ($1/E^3$ vs. E^0). As indicated by T-W in Reference (Tapiovaara and Wagner 1985), the signal formed in radiography bears information in both spatial (actually temporal–spatial in fluoroscopy) and spectral domains. Hence, in addition to matching the signal's spatial or temporal–spatial property, the spectral response of an optimal detector should also match that of the signal to be detected. A photon-counting detector offers the opportunity for spectral matching and/or weighting, though the matching/weighting in practice may be relatively coarse because of the finite width of energy bins. Notably, however, the data acquisition in CT is usually carried out at higher energy, e.g., 100 kVp or 120 kVp, than that in radiography and thus the Compton scattering plays a more important role. So one has to be cautious that, since the Compton scattering varies little over energy, the effectiveness of spectral matching/weighting may intrinsically declines in CT, including spectral CT, in comparison to that in radiography.

8.5.2 TASK-DEPENDENT SPECTRAL WEIGHTING

By removing electronic noise and dark current via thresholding in pulse height, a photon-counting spectral CT can outperform energy-integration spectral CT in situations wherein the radiation is extremely low, as exemplified in the example presented in Figure 3.7c. Moreover, as indicated earlier, the much bigger benefit offered by the photon-counting detector with multiple energy bins is the opportunity for spectral weighting, which, in theory, can substantially improve the imaging performance of CT in general and spectral CT in specific, as elucidated later.

Under the framework of statistical signal detection and using the detective quantum efficiency (DQE) as the figure of merit, T-W treated the imaging task in radiography as a two-alternative forced-choice event and pointed out that the image quality is task dependent (Tapiovaara and Wagner 1985). By assuming the detected X-ray photons are in Poisson distribution, the image quality (squared SNR) was formulated as

$$SNR^2 = A \frac{\left[\int_0^{kVp} \left(\overline{N_1(E)} - \overline{N_2(E)} \right) D(E) w(E) dE \right]^2}{\int_0^{kVp} \left(\overline{N_1(E)} + \overline{N_2(E)} \right) D(E) w^2(E) dE} \tag{8.32}$$

where A denotes the area corresponding to the signal, and $\overline{N_1(E)}$ and $\overline{N_2(E)}$ are the averaged intensity in the signal and background areas defined in the event. $D(E)$ denotes the fraction of absorbed X-ray photons and $w(E)$ is a weighting function. To fully extract the information conveyed in the spectral domain, i.e., to make the detector's SNR^2 reach that of an ideal detector from the spectral point of view

$$SNR^2_{ideal} = A \int_0^{kVp} \frac{\left(\overline{N_1(E)} - \overline{N_2(E)}\right)^2}{N_1(E) + N_2(E)} dE \qquad (8.33)$$

the weighting function $w(E)$ has to take the form

$$w(E) = \frac{\overline{N_1(E)} - \overline{N_2(E)}}{N_1(E) + N_2(E)} \qquad (8.34)$$

Moreover, if the imaging task is to identify an object at low contrast against the background, which is the case that is most likely encountered in practice, it turned out the weighting function should be

$$w(E) \cong \mu_1(E) - \mu_2(E) \qquad (8.35)$$

where $\mu_1(E)$ and $\mu_2(E)$ are the LACs of the materials in the signal and background areas, respectively. Notably, this is again consistent with the statement that the imaging performance of an optimal detector is task dependent. The weighting scheme specified in Equation 8.35 was evaluated in Reference (Cahn et al. 1999; Giersch et al. 2004), with the presence of glandular–adipose and other soft tissues as the targeted material to be identified, and the Monte Carlo–based investigation showed that the LAC–based weighting strategy indeed works in both radiography and CT.

Using sufficient statistics as the criterion, the optimization of spectral weighting in spectral imaging was investigated in Reference (Wang and Pelc 2011). It turns out that, once the basis materials spanning the A-space for material decomposition is determined, the optimal spectral weighting functions are actually the basis materials' LACs (termed as μ-weights henceforth). Notably, sufficient statistics means that the imaging performance – material decomposition in the case herein – is quantum limited, i.e., its noise reaches the Cramér–Rao lower bound. Moreover, the μ-weights are dependent on the X-ray source spectrum, but not on the properties, e.g., constituent materials and geometric dimension, of the object to be imaged.

With the availability of multiple energy bins, one can carry out the spectral weighting as depicted earlier to optimize the detection efficiency. However, it should be noted that, given the radiation dose that has been established in existing clinical practice, with an increasing number of energy bins, there are a decreasing number of X-ray photons allotted to each energy bin, leading to a situation that photon starvation may occur in some of the bins at the high-energy end, which may offset the benefit that can be offered by multiple energy bins (Tang and Ren 2021). This means, given a task of detecting a specific material, the number of energy bins should be optimized in a systematic manner, other than presumably making assumptions, based on quite a few criteria under the framework of signal detection and estimation.

8.5.3 TASK-DEPENDENT SPECTRAL CHANNELIZATION

In order to suppress noise (induced by scatter and fluorescence), the lower end of the first energy bin is usually set at 10–15 keV, while the setting of the upper end of the last bin is dependent on applications, e.g., 60 keV for preclinical imaging of small animals, 90–100 keV for clinical imaging of a human head and 120–130 keV for clinical imaging of other anatomy. Using the CRLB, which is actually the diagonal element of the inverse Fisher information matrix as criterion (Roessl and Herrmann 2009), the optimization of binning in multi-material decomposition has been investigated and found that, given a basis material with its K-edge being in the interested energy range, e.g., gadolinium or iodine used in the contrast agent for MRI and CT, the SNR in the corresponding basis image reaches its highest while the central thresholding of a paired energy bin is being set close to the K-edge. It was also found that, with a 5%–10% energy resolution that is readily available in existing photon-counting detectors, the SNR varies modestly (Roessl and Proksa 2007; Schlomka et al. 2008; Roessl et al. 2011).

In practice, the determination or computation of the Fisher information matrix and resultant CRLB is not trivial. Alternatively, by still treating the material decomposition as a problem of statistical estimation, a surrogate measure, which is the area (or volume) circumscribing the confidence region (namely, the confidence region map), was proposed in References (Nik et al. 2011) as the criterion for optimization of energy binning. In addition to similar findings with respect to binning's influence on differentiating the targeted material (iodine this time) with its K-edge within the interested energy range, it was found that the energy binning actually does almost no favor to material decomposition for differentiating soft tissues, such as water and adipose, perhaps mainly because their K-edge is far outside the interested energy range.

Using CRLB as the criterion again, the optimization of energy binning is further investigated in Reference (Wang and Pelc 2011), showing that the performance of material decomposition can be improved by adding more energy bins or even with notch filtration (though its implementation is questionable in reality), but the optimal solution is dependent on the habitus of the object to be imaged and the X-ray source spectrum. In other words, there is no solution in energy binning that can fit all applications, which is another manifestation that the imaging performance of photon-counting spectral CT is task dependent.

8.6 SURVEY OF IMAGE QUALITY IN SPECTRAL CT OVER DATA ACQUISITION SCHEMES

Under the framework of statistical signal detection, the generalized SNR d^2 (deflection coefficient) was adopted by Alvarez to analyze the imaging performance of spectral CT with data acquisition by conventional energy integration, photon counting, joint photon counting and energy-integration, and ideal detection (photon counting with infinite spectral resolution) (Alvarez 2010, 2011).

8.6.1 DATA ACQUISITION SCHEMES

The imaging task is again formulated as a two-alternative forced-choice test, in which cortical bone and soft tissue are chosen as the basis materials and a whitening (orthogonal) transformation is carried out in the A-space to facilitate the analysis. Presented at descending order next are the analytic results in d^2 corresponding to the four types of data acquisition, wherein $\langle \cdot \rangle_N$ and $\langle \cdot \rangle_Q$ denote the average over photons and energy, respectively; λ is the average of all detected photons; t_f is the thickness of target; and $F = \langle E^2 \rangle / \langle E \rangle^2$ is the ratio of the second moment of energy over the squared first moment of energy (Alvarez 2010, 2011):

$$d_{ideal}^2 = \frac{\lambda t_f^2}{2} \cdot \left\langle \left[\mu_t(E) - \mu_b(E) \right]^2 \right\rangle_N \tag{8.36}$$

$$d_{N2Q}^2 = \frac{\lambda t_f^2}{2} \cdot \left\langle \left[\mu_t(E) - \mu_b(E) \right]^2 \right\rangle_N \tag{8.37}$$

$$d_{NQ}^2 = d_{conv}^2 + \frac{\lambda t_f^2}{2} \cdot \frac{\left(\left\langle \mu_t(E) - \mu_b(E) \right\rangle_N - \left\langle \mu_t(E) - \mu_b(E) \right\rangle_Q \right)^2}{F - 1} \tag{8.38}$$

$$d_K^2 = \frac{\lambda t_f^2}{2} \cdot \sum_{k=1}^{K} \lambda_k \left\langle \mu_t(E) - \mu_b(E) \right\rangle_k^2 \tag{8.39}$$

$$d_{convN}^2 = \frac{\lambda t_f^2}{2} \cdot \left\langle \mu_t(E) - \mu_b(E) \right\rangle_N^2 \tag{8.40}$$

$$d_{convQ}^2 = \frac{t_f^2}{2F} \cdot \left\langle \mu_t(E) - \mu_b(E) \right\rangle_Q^2 \quad d_{convQ}^2 = \frac{\lambda t_f^2}{2F} \cdot \left\langle \mu_t(E) - \mu_b(E) \right\rangle_Q^2 \tag{8.41}$$

A simulation study was carried out in Reference (Alvarez 2011) to investigate the imaging performance of the three most fundamental modes of spectral CT: (i) N2Q (photon-counting detection with two energy bins), (ii) NQ (joint photon counting and energy integration), and (iii) N2 (energy-integration detection at low and high kVps), in which the spectral CT with ideal signal detection and conventional energy integration are taking as the references. Presented in Figure 8.12a and Figure 8.12b are their d^2 normalized by that of ideal spectral CT as the functions over kVps and object thickness, respectively. It is observed that the spectral CT implemented with N2Q, NQ or N2 data acquisition outperforms the conventional

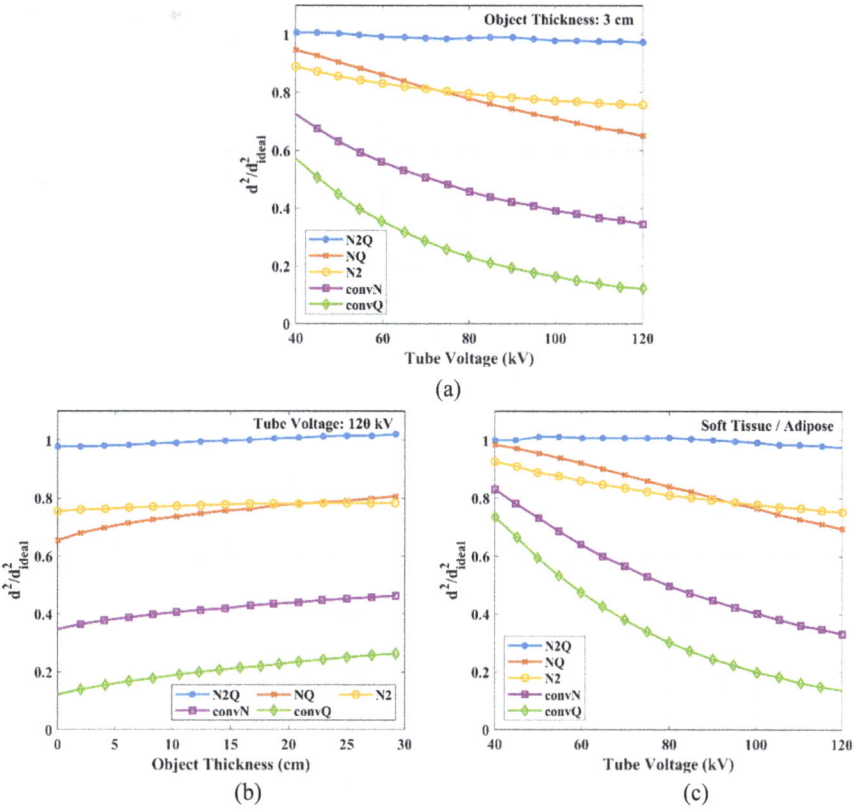

FIGURE 8.12 Variation of generalized signal-to-noise ratio d^2 (a) of a 3 cm object as a function over tube voltage, (b) at 120 kVp as a function over object thickness, (c) of soft tissue/adipose over tube voltage. (Adopted from Alvarez 2010 with permission.)

CT (energy-integration and photon-counting data acquisition) substantially, as the N2Q spectral CT approaches the imaging performance of spectral CT with ideal signal detection. The gain in the imaging performance (as assessed by d^2) of the N2Q spectral CT over other modes of spectral CT and the conventional energy-integration CT improves with increasing tube peak voltage and decreasing object thickness. It is important to note that, at 120 kVp and 5 cm object thickness that are clinically relevant for CT imaging of the human body, the N2Q's gain in imaging performance over other modes reaches its highest.

8.6.2 Potential of Photon-Counting Spectral CT in Soft-Tissue Differentiation

Compared to MRI and PET/SPECT, the capability of CT in soft-tissue differentiation, which is of paramount relevance in clinical applications, is limited. Hence, the clinical prominence of spectral CT against conventional CT is largely hinged on whether spectral CT can offer much better soft-tissue differentiation. With soft tissue

(10 cm thickness) and adipose as the target and background materials, a simulation study is carried out in Reference (Alvarez 2011) to investigate the normalized imaging performance of different implementations of spectral CT (d^2/d^2_{ideal}), and presented in Figure 8.12 is their variation as functions over tube peak voltage. Notably, the imaging performance (generalized SNR) of N2Q spectral CT in differentiating soft tissue and adipose is quite stable with increasing tube peak voltage, while that of conventional CT, either implemented with energy integration or photon counting, drops significantly. Particularly, at tube peak voltage 80–120 keV that is clinically relevant, the imaging performance of N2Q spectral CT is potentially three to seven times better than that of the conventional CT that is routinely employed in clinical practice. Alongside other preliminary data presented in Reference (Malusek et al. 2013), this observation should encourage the technological community to invest more effort in the research and development of spectral CT, especially in light of the increasing availability of photon-counting detectors for implementing spectral CT.

8.7 CLINICAL APPLICATIONS OF SPECTRAL CT

Since its advent in the marketplace in 2005, spectral CT has played an increasing relevant role in clinical applications of diagnostic imaging, ranging from characterization of monosodium urate deposits in the synovial fluid of joints and soft tissues (gouty arthritis), analysis of composition in renal stones (uric or non-uric), depiction of mass and metastasis, and assessment of therapeutical efficacy in oncology, to visualization of the vasculature and micro-vascular environment under urgent settings in neurology and cardiology. With the functionalities of two-material decomposition (or three-material decomposition under mass/volume conservation) and analysis supported by virtual monochromatic imaging/analysis, the common clinical uses of spectral CT include (i) material-specific mapping and virtual monochromatic imaging/analysis at adequate energy for better detection and characterization of lesions; (ii) virtual monochromatic imaging/analysis at adequate energy for better

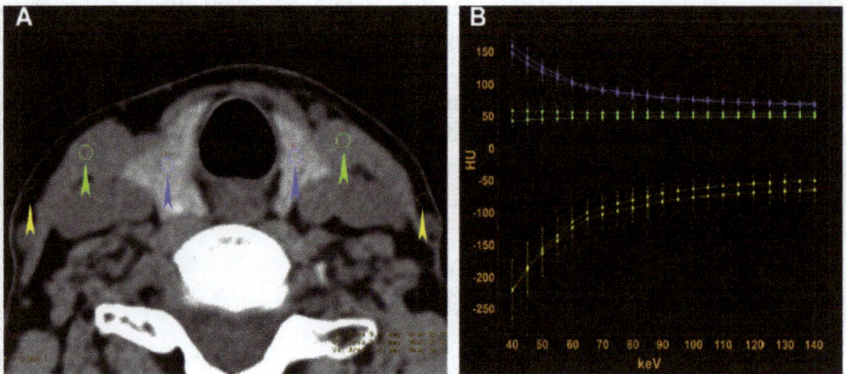

FIGURE 8.13   (A) Selection of ROIs in a head and neck scan and (B) the profiles of virtual monochromatic analysis corresponding to the ROIs. (Adopted from Forghani 2017c with permission.)

conspicuity of iodinated contrast agents to lower the risk of nephropathy in patients with pre-existing conditions, such as renal functional vulnerability, hypertension, hyperlipidemia and diabetes; (iii) virtual monochromatic imaging/analysis at adequate energy to suppress the beam-hardening artifacts induced by metallic implants or stents/clips; and (iv) spectral analysis endorsed by virtual monochromatic imaging/analysis as a function over energy level (see Figure 8.13). Aimed at inspiring more research and development activities to advance its ability to address more clinical challenges, the following is a brief survey of spectral CT applications and potentials in a number of clinically relevant sub-specialties.

8.7.1 Oncologic Applications

Currently, spectral CT is making significant contributions to the diagnosis, staging, treatment planning and assessment in oncology via:

- Material-specific iodine mapping to facilitate the characterization of lesions, such as hepatocellular carcinoma, and their underlying micro-vascular environment with iodine uptake as a surrogate biomarker (see Figure 8.14).

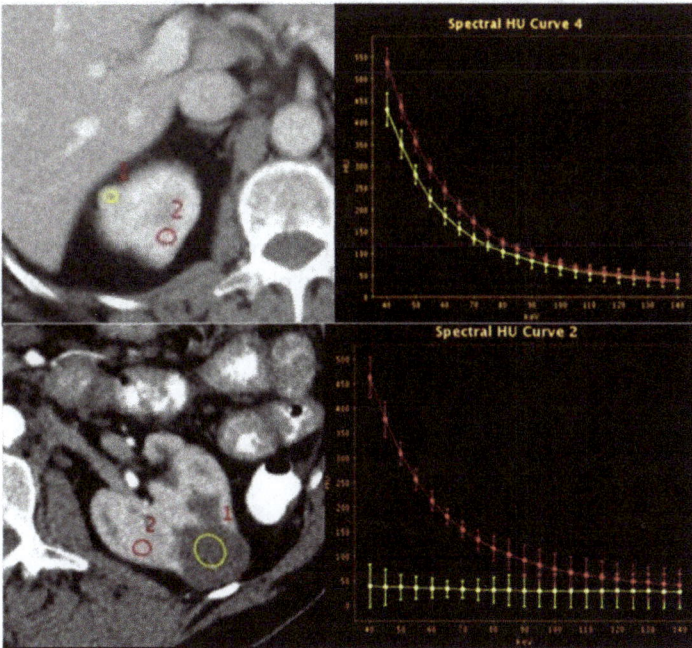

FIGURE 8.14 (Left) Selection of ROIs in an abdominal scan and (right) the profiles of virtual monochromatic analysis corresponding to the ROIs. (Adopted from Agrawal et al. 2014 with permission.)

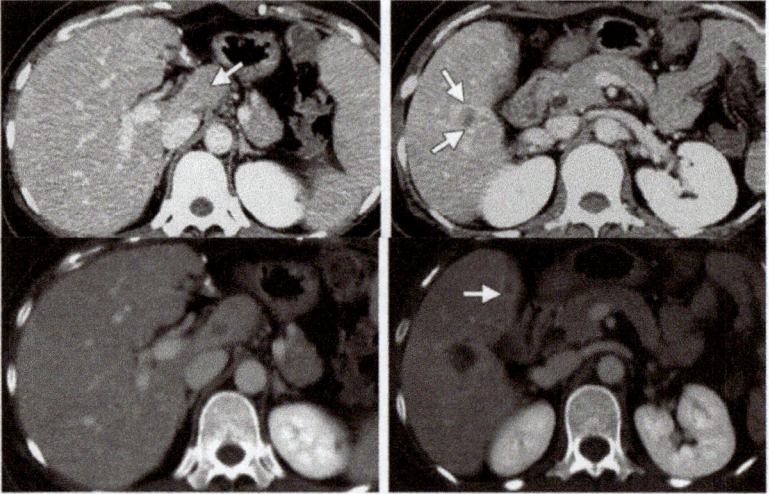

FIGURE 8.15 (Top) contrast-enhanced CT images of colon carcinoma metastases to the liver and (bottom) corresponding iodine-specific images. (Adopted from Agrawal et al. 2014 with permission.)

- Virtual non-contrast imaging to facilitate the characterization of lesions, e.g., colon carcinoma metastases in the liver, by providing complementary information on co-existing features, such as calcification, fat and hemorrhage (see Figure 8.15).
- Spectral analysis endorsed by virtual monochromatic imaging to facilitate differentiation of malignant lesion, for example, renal carcinoma, from benign pathologies (e.g., renal cysts).

Potentially, with quantitative material-specific mapping and virtual monochromatic imaging/analysis, spectral CT would be able to play a more significant role in tumor staging, treatment planning and assessment, by providing functional (e.g., angiogenesis, micro-vascular environment and tumor viability) rather than only morphological (e.g., variation in tumor size in response to therapy) information for initial and continued decision-making in oncology.

8.7.2 CARDIOVASCULAR APPLICATIONS

Spectral CT is making significant contributions to clinical excellence in cardiovascular imaging via:

- Virtual non-contrast imaging to generate images from one single data acquisition for calcium scoring and angiography simultaneously.

- Virtual monochromatic imaging/analysis at high voltage (>80 keV) to remove the blooming artifacts induced by metallic parts (stents, bypass clips, sterna wire), calcification and/or bulky iodinated contrast agents to improve the assessment of lumen patency.
- Virtual monochromatic imaging/analysis at low voltage (<60 keV) to reduce the dose of contrast agents up to ~50% and thus lower the risk of contrast-induced nephrology.

Increasing data in cardiovascular pathophysiology suggest that plaque burden, inflammatory infiltration, fibroatheroma, intra-plaque hemorrhage, micro-calcification and lipid-rich necrotic core may jointly play critical roles in plaque's vulnerability. Potentially, with further improved capability of differentiating soft tissues, spectral CT would play a significant role in atherosclerotic plaque analysis to prevent rupture-induced acute cerebral/coronary syndromes. Moreover, as a non-invasive imaging modality at high sensitivity, CT angiography has been a breakthrough in the management of coronary arterial diseases. Integrated with myocardium assessment, spectral CT-based angiography and perfusion together may provide a robust solution for diagnosis and management of acute coronary syndromes.

8.7.3 NEUROVASCULAR APPLICATIONS

Spectral CT is regaining its ground in neurology, especially under emergency settings or in patients with MRI contraindication, for imaging acute intracranial hemorrhage and other life-threatening neurotraumas:

- Virtual non-calcium imaging to generate images with bone removal for improved visualization of vascular malformation, e.g., stenosis, aneurysms and spot sign in head and neck CT angiography.
- Virtual non-contrast imaging to differentiate hemorrhage from iodine for risk assessment of systemic hemorrhage post intra-arterial revascularization via thrombolysis and/or thrombectomy.
- Virtual monochromatic imaging/analysis at adequate energy for better delineation of gray and white matter, and detection of tumors in the brain.
- Virtual monochromatic imaging/analysis at adequate energy to reduce beam-hardening artifacts for better visualization of the pathophysiology in the posterior fossa (75 keV) or transpedicular screw fixation (110 keV) in the spine.

Potentially, spectral CT may gain more ground in the paradigm of neurovascular imaging, such as ischemic or hemorrhagic stroke and other intracranial hemorrhage, or even imaging of intracranial tumors, with its increasing capability of differentiating soft tissues and providing surrogate functional information complementary to the anatomic (morphological) information.

8.8 DISCUSSION

With the landscape of technological and clinical advancements in spectral CT sketched herein, it is fair to state that photon-counting spectral CT is gaining momentum in its research and development, while energy-integration spectral CT is ramping up for acceptance in the clinic. The technological advancements made in photon-counting spectral CT and the preliminary success made by energy-integration CT in the clinic are encouraging the community to optimistically anticipate that, with the potential technological solutions to improve its imaging performance and its synergy with novel contrast agents, spectral CT, especially one that works in photon-counting mode, would be able to eventually advance CT's clinical utility in a manner that can be more significant than incremental, if not breakthrough.

9 Contrast Agents for MDCT

Fundamentals, State of the Art and Outlook

Among all the major factors that have enabled clinical success of computed tomography (CT), of special note is the iodinated contrast agent and its prominent efficacy in all diagnostic imaging applications. The utility of iodine as an agent for contrast enhancement in X-ray imaging was found as early as 1901 when Guerbet developed an oil-based iodine contrast medium called lipiodol (Bonnemain and Guerbet 1995; Shahid et al. 2020) soon after Roentgen's discovery of the X-ray in 1895. In the 1920s, Osborne et al. found that the urine of patients who were treated with iodine-containing compound was radiopaque, leading to an angiogram in which an iodine salt such as sodium iodine was utilized (Osborne et al. 1923; Brooks 1924). In the early days, the clinical utility of iodinated contrast agents was mainly for radiological imaging of the gastrointestinal track and other tubular organs or cavities in the human body. The advent of CT in the early 1970s fueled the practice of intravenous administration of iodinated contrast agents. By taking advantage of the mechanism of body compartments, the conspicuity of either a vascular or parenchymal lesion, or both, can be boosted substantially owing to iodine's much stronger X-ray attenuation compared to soft tissues. Since then, the clinical utility of iodinated contrast agents for diagnostic imaging has been continuously extending and advancing (Schöckel et al. 2020; Lusic and Grinstaff 2013).

In concert with pathophysiology, pharmacokinetics and CT physics, the iodinated contrast agent plays an indispensable role for physicians to make diagnostic decisions in detection and characterization of vascular anomalies (aortic dissection, aneurism, stenosis, thrombosis and/or embolism) and neoplasm (benign and malignant) in the head and neck, thorax, abdomen, pelvis, extremities and other parts of the human body. Approximately, 40% of the 300 million CT scans that are conducted each year worldwide are carried out under administration of iodinated contrast agents, while the percentage goes up substantially to 80% if only the thoracic and abdominal cases are surveyed (Shahid et al. 2020; Schöckel et al. 2020). More than 3500 tons of iodine are used annually by healthcare providers worldwide, sustaining the iodinated contrast agents industry that currently consists of only four vendors (GE Healthcare, Bayer, Guerbet and Bracco), with an annual market volume that is projected well above $1 billion (Shahid et al. 2020; Schöckel et al. 2020; Lusic and Grinstaff 2013).

DOI: 10.1201/9780429028465-9

Except for calcium that is of relatively large atomic number and abundance in the bone, hydrogen, oxygen, carbon and nitrogen, which are the four major compositions of soft tissues that interface with blood and other body fluids, are all of relatively small atomic number and virtually exist at iso-density. In physics, the subject contrast in CT is generated by attenuation of X-ray photons (radiopacity) at the atomic level and accordingly the subject contrasts between soft tissues in CT are relatively low, limiting CT's sensitivity in detection and characterization of pathophysiological lesions against normal surroundings in comparison to other imaging modalities, such as MRI, nuclear medicine, and optical and ultrasonic imaging. This perhaps is the most striking reason that contrast agents have been accompanying X-ray–related imaging modalities from the very beginning, and thus far iodine has been the material of choice for intravascular administration.

As a metalloid element, iodine possesses an atomic number of 53 and K-edge of 33.2 keV that is close to the effective energy of X-ray photons for radiography and CT, leading to much stronger attenuation in comparison to soft tissues, body fluids and even bone. With its strong radiopacity, a straightforward application of iodinated contrast agent is in angiogram and/or angiography for assessment of lumen patency and detection of other cardiovascular pathophysiologic lesions. In physiology, multiple compartments have been identified in the human microcirculation system. For example, there are four compartments in the liver: blood, interstitial fluid, hepatocyte and reticuloendothelial (RE) cellular compartments (Bae 2003; Bae 2010; Mattrey and Aguirre 2003). In comparison to normal hepatic parenchyma, a hepatic lesion may differ in its volume and particularly mean transit time of each compartment. Angiogenesis is in general associated with malignance and forms immature capillaries in the lesion's microenvironment. Hence, hyper- or hypo-attenuation can in principle be generated corresponding to hepatic lesions in CT if hemokinetics-based strategies are exercised in contrast agent administration. As such, a diagnosis may be made not only between malignant and benign but also primary and metastatic lesions in oncologic applications to support the clinical decision in diagnosis, staging, therapeutic intervention and response assessment (Bae et al. 1998; Brink 2003a, 2003b; Bae 2003, 2010).

Aided by iodinated contrast agents, CT has led a paradigm shift in practice of contemporary medicine since the mid-1970s, which was further fortified by a series of technological leaps in CT instrumentation, such as the advancement from step-and-shoot to spiral/helical scan, single detector to multiple detectors, single source to dual source, the evolution in 3D spatial resolution from sub-centimeters to sub-millimeters, and the speeding of gantry rotation to approach 0.2 sec/rotation. We are at the verge of another technological leap in X-ray detection from energy integration to photon counting, which not only provides an unprecedented opportunity for iodinated contrast agents to find more applications in the clinic but also demands more innovations in the research and development of contrast agents to fulfill CT's potential in diagnostic imaging. To meet the challenges, it is essential for scientists and researchers in the field to sufficiently extend their exposure to the fundamentals of iodinated contrast agents, ranging from their physics and chemistry to physico-chemistry, pharmacokinetics, toxicity and pathophysiology, and their interplay with

CT physics. Additionally, it is important for the diagnostic medical physicist who is on the frontline of patient care to have a solid understanding of those factors and their interplay. Thus, comprehensive coverage on these facets of iodinated contrast agents for diagnostic imaging in CT is given in this chapter, followed by an outlook of the opportunities in the research and development (R&D) of novel contrast agents for diagnostic CT imaging in the future.

9.1 IODINATED CONTRAST AGENTS FOR MDCT: PHYSICAL, CHEMICAL AND PHYSIOCHEMICAL FUNDAMENTALS

Starting from its physics, we will cover the fundamentals related to iodinated contrast agents in this section, serving as a foundation for one to understand the materials presented in the following sections, particularly the interplay among those factors that are vital to optimizing CT performance in clinical practice.

9.1.1 IODINE AND ITS ATTENUATION BY X-RAY

In clinical CT, the vast majority of pathophysiologic lesion(s) are vascular or parenchymal anomalies in the head/neck, thorax, abdomen/pelvis and extremities. Via intravenous administration, the iodinated contrast agent that circulates in the capillary beds and diffuses into the extracellular space enhances the conspicuity of parenchymal lesions, while that in the systemic and pulmonary circulation boosts the contrast of vascular pathologies. As indicated earlier, the contrast in CT is generated at the atomic level and thus it is only the mass attenuation coefficient and density of the materials utilized in fabricating the agents that matter. Figure 9.1a is a representation of Figure 3.1 to show the profiles of mass attenuation coefficients corresponding to the soft tissues, bone, iodine and gold over the energy range 0–150 keV. In general, the X-ray photons interact with materials via photoelectric

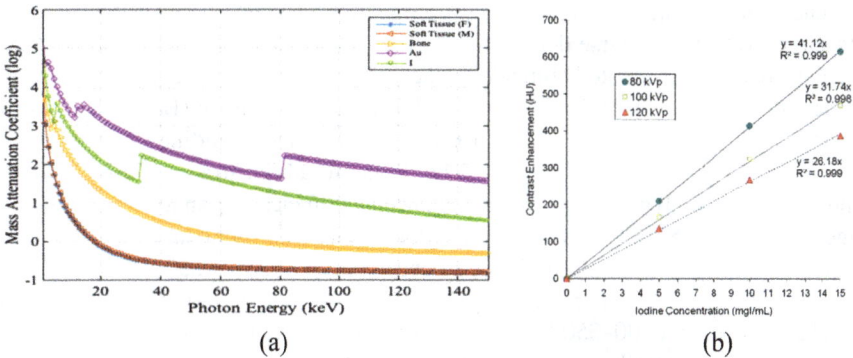

FIGURE 9.1   (a) Plotting of the mass attenuation coefficient corresponding to soft tissues, bone, iodine and gold in the energy range from 0 to 150 keV and (b) the attenuation of iodinated contrast agents. (Panel b is adopted from Bae 2010 with permission.)

absorption, Compton scattering and Raleigh scattering in the energy range for diagnostic imaging (20–150 keV). In fact, the coherent Raleigh scattering is negligibly small and thus can be neglected, while the attenuation of X-rays in soft tissue is mainly by Compton scattering, and that in bone, iodine and gold by photoelectric absorption. Notably, as the attenuation coefficient varies as a function of energy, there is an abrupt variation called the K-edge at 33.2 keV in iodine's attenuation profile, while two abruptions, which are called K-edge and L-edge, respectively, exist in gold's attenuation profile.

In a clinical CT, as indicated in Chapter 3, Section 3.3.1 (especially Figure 3.4b), the X-ray source spectrum is shaped via filtration by metal foils at adequate thickness to remove the X-ray photons that are doomed to have no chance to penetrate the human body, e.g., the X-ray photons at energy lower than 20 keV, from the beam. In practice, the effective energy of the X-ray source is roughly half the peak voltage (kVp) when the kVp is relatively low, e.g., 80 keV, and equal to one-third to half when the kVp is high, e.g., 120 or 140 keV. Figure 9.1a tells us that, to have optimal enhancement by the iodinated contrast agent, the peak voltage should go down toward 80 keV, as exemplified in CT perfusion of the brain parenchyma for imaging and functional assessment in acute ischemic stroke. However, if the anatomic site to be scanned is of large dimension, e.g., the thorax, abdomen or pelvis, the kVp should go up to 120–140 kVp, since the penetration of a sufficient number of X-ray photons in those settings is of highest relevance for scan (data acquisition) and image formation.

The iodinated contrast agent can be administered via four routes: intraarterial, intravenous, oral (including enteric) and direct injection (into targeted anatomic cavity). Under clinical settings, its administration in CT is dominantly intravenous, though oral administration is also common. In this chapter, we focus on the iodinated contrast agents in the form of small molecules and administered intravenously. The concentration of iodine in the commercially available contrast agent ranges from 150 to 400 mg/ml. Once injected, the agent propagates in the circulation system and undergoes continuous dilution and dispersion, with vascular and visceral parenchymal enhancements ramping up, going over the summit, and decaying to the baseline over a time course determined by the patient's cardiac output and hemodynamics. In a well-calibrated clinical CT, the iodine at 1 mg/ml concentration roughly generates 41, 31 or 26 HU at 80, 100 or 120 kVp, respectively (Bae 2010), and in general the contrast enhancement in CT is proportional to iodine's concentration (Figure 9.1b). Though it varies significantly due to administration timing and the individual's hemodynamics, a typical enhancement induced by an iodinated contrast agent can reach 250–350 HU in angiographic applications. For example, at adequate timing, enhancement by the iodinated contrast agent reaches 250–300 HU in the aorta, 300–350 HU in the pulmonary trunk, 250–350 HU in the vasculature of the head and neck, and 300–350 HU in the coronary, mesenteric and renal arteries, but goes down substantially in the peripheral vasculature (Bae 2010). In visceral CT, the enhancement in hepatic, pancreatic and renal parenchyma is at 50, 70–105 and 140–160 HU, respectively, in which the strategy of multi-phasic imaging strategy is usually exercised (Brink et al. 1995; Bae 2010).

9.1.2 CHEMICAL STRUCTURES OF IODINATED CONTRAST AGENTS FOR MDCT

Though they are under various generic and commercial names, all the commercially available iodinated contrast agents for CT are in the form of small molecules. They share the same basic unit of chemical structure – a tri-iodinated benzene ring in monomeric or dimeric structure, as illustrated in Figure 9.2a. A total of three iodine atoms are covalently bonded to every other vertex of the hexagonal ring, while the remaining vertexes are filled with organic functional groups that govern the molecule's physiochemical behavior, ranging from iconicity to osmolality, viscosity, clearance route and rate, hydrophilicity, lipophilicity, and ultimately to toxicity (Eloy et al. 1991; Shahid et al. 2020; Schöckel et al. 2020). For example, the R_1 group is mainly used for adjustment of hydrophilicity (water solubility) that is one of the primary determinants of toxicity, while the R_2 group decides the route of clearance for the contrast agent to be removed from the human body via renal excretion (glomerular filtration) or biliary excretion (macrophage collection) by the liver or spleen. A carboxylate (-COO-) functional group can be loaded at the site labeled as R_3 to decide the molecule's ionicity that in turn determines the molecule's osmolality. To increase the count of iodine atoms per molecule and accordingly the iodine concentration for stronger X-ray attenuation, two benzene rings can be covalently bonded together into a dimer with almost doubled molecular size in the manner exemplified in Figure 9.2b. Hence, depending on their ionicity and molecular structure, there are basically four types of iodinated contrast agents: (i) ionic monomer, (ii) nonionic monomer, (iii) ionic dimer and (iv) nonionic dimer, which lead to various physicochemical properties to be elucidated next (Eloy et al. 1991; Shahid et al. 2020; Schöckel et al. 2020).

9.1.3 PHYSICOCHEMICAL PROPERTIES OF IODINATED CONTRAST AGENTS

The molecules of iodinated contrast agents propagate in the plasma of the circulation system and thus it is mandate for them to be water soluble (i.e., hydrophilic). In addition, the following parameters are also essential in determining the physicochemical properties and accordingly the toxicity of iodinated contrast in clinical applications.

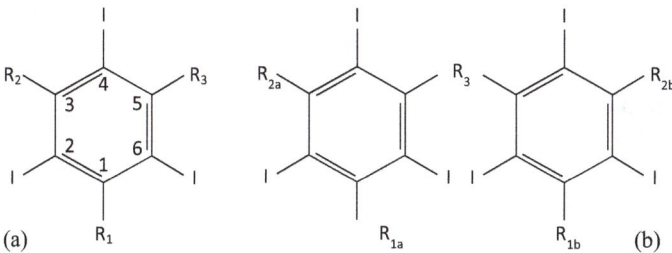

FIGURE 9.2 Schematic diagram showing the molecular structures of tri-iodinated benzene rings in (a) monomeric and (b) dimeric forms.

9.1.3.1 Ionicity

If it is soluble, the solute in a solution may exist in the form of a particle, e.g., atom, molecule or ion. In layman language, the ionicity can be perceived as the availability of ions in a solution, though it may refer to more specific measures that character-ize the ions' behavior in the sense of physical chemistry or chemical physics. Once administered into the circulation system, the ionic iodinated contrast exists in the plasma in the form of anions or cations, whereas nonionic ones in the form of mol-ecules that are neutral in polarity. Notably, given an identical molar concentration of solute, the number of particles in ionic contrast agent may double that of an nonionic agent.

9.1.3.2 Osmolality

In chemistry, the osmolality is defined as the osmole of solutes per kilogram of solvent; in layman language it refers to the number of particles (ions in the case of iodinated contrast agents) per unit weight of a solution. The osmolality of iodin-ated contrast agents is the primary determinant of its tolerance, biocompatibility and thus toxicity to the organ systems of the human body. The osmolality of ionic monomeric iodinated contrast agents is roughly twice that of nonionic monomeric agents. If you take the osmolality of blood (310 mOsm/kg) as the benchmark, ionic monomeric iodinated contrast is usually of high osmolality (1510–2000 mOsm/kg), while nonionic monomeric iodinated contrast is low in osmolality (860 mOsm/kg). Typically, the dimeric structure can further reduce the osmolality, as evidenced by the fact that the osmolality of nonionic dimeric iodinated contrast can be equal to or even lower than that of blood (290 mOsm/kg) (Shahid et al. 2020; Schöckel et al. 2020).

9.1.3.3 Viscosity

In principle, viscosity is defined as the intermolecular friction in liquid or fluid, i.e., a measure of the resistance to molecules' mobility or flow. In a non-linear man-ner, the viscosity of the iodinated contrast agent increases with its molecular size, concentration and interactions, but decreases with temperature. Additionally, the molecular shape is also an important determinant of viscosity, as evidenced by the fact that dimeric iodinated contrast agent is much more viscous than its monomeric counterpart at comparable iodine concentration (Eloy et al. 1991; Shahid et al. 2020; Schöckel et al. 2020).

9.1.3.4 Lipophilicity

In organic chemistry, opposite to hydrophilicity, lipophilicity characterizes the extent to which a substance interacts with lipids or proteins that are the essential biological components of cellular membrane and other tissues or organs. The lipo-philic constituents (mainly organic additives) of iodinated contrast agents may inter-act with the biological components of the cell membrane or affect diffusion through the brain–blood barrier (BBB), disturbing the metabolic pathways and thus inducing morbidity (Eloy et al. 1991; Shahid et al. 2020).

The relation between each of the physiochemical properties in iodinated contrast agents can be straightforward. For example, ionicity results in hydrophilicity proportionally, while viscosity is inversely proportional to osmolality. But the relation can also be complicated and the interplay between them may be critical to the contrast agent's pharmacokinetics and toxicity. For example, the interplay between hydrophilicity and lipophilicity has been taken advantage of for design and optimization of iodinated contrast agents, and readers are referred to publications in the literature (Shahid et al. 2020; Schöckel et al. 2020) for further information about physiochemical fundamentals of iodinated contrast agents.

In practice, the clinical utility of iodinated contrast agents is weighed on the trade-off over factors related to clinical indications, likelihood of adverse effects and cost. For example, due to its high osmolality, the earliest widely used ionic monomeric iodinated contrast agent – diatrizoate (Urografin) – is now employed only in gastrointestinal and cystourethral applications (Schöckel et al. 2020). All iodinated contrast agents that are routinely administered in the clinic are at low osmolality or iso-osmolality, using a protocol that is customized in injection duration, rate and volume, and iodine concentration, according to the specific clinical indication for vascular or parenchymal CT.

9.1.4 PHARMACOKINETICS OF IODINATED CONTRAST AGENTS

As iodinated contrast agent is in the form of small molecules, its distribution in the body is primarily "perfusion- (flow-) limited", rather than "diffuse-limited" (Bae 2010). In general, the contrast agent's distribution from the intravascular compartment to the interstitial compartment in well-perfused organs, e.g., the liver, pancreas or kidney, is fast (~2–5 minutes), whereas it is much slower in less perfused tissue or organs, e.g., bone and fat. Essentially, all iodinated contrast agents are unlikely to bind protein and thus the chance for its clinically relevant interference on metabolism is low. In patients with normal renal function, the half-life of iodinated contrast agents in the systemic circulation is in the range 90–120 minutes, prior to its clearance from the body via renal execration (mainly glomerular filtration). Nevertheless, in patients with preexisting renal conditions, e.g., renal insufficiency, the half-life can be as long as days or even weeks (Eloy et al. 1991; Shahid et al. 2020; Schöckel et al. 2020).

9.2 DISTURBANCE AND CHEMOTOXICITY OF IODINATED CONTRAST AGENTS THAT MAY INDUCE ADVERSE PHYSIOLOGICAL REACTIONS

Alongside its efficacy in increasing the vascular opacification and/or parenchymal enhancement in CT, iodinated contrast agents are associated with side effects that may disturb or impair a patient's physiologic status or trigger immediate and/or delayed hypersensitivity reactions (allergic-like or physiologic, or both). In practice, the intravenously administered iodinated contrast agents are usually nonionic at relatively low osmolality, but can still lead to, though rare, morbidity or even potentially life-threatening events in concert with or independent of existing clinical conditions, e.g., compromised hemodynamics and advanced chronic kidney or diabetic diseases. To have an in-depth understanding of the clinical consequences, one needs to know the iodinated contrast agent's toxicity at the plasmatic, cellular and molecular levels, regarding its disturbance on physiology, induction of hypersensitivity or impairment of renal functionality. The etiology of these adverse reactions has not been fully understood, though ionicity, osmolality and other chemotoxicities, e.g., molecular binding of iodinated contrast agent to certain activators (e.g., calcium), are assumed among the culprits (Eloy et al. 1991). The following sections provide concise coverage of the risks related to adverse physiologic reactions.

9.2.1 Disturbance on Hematology and Hemodynamics

As a connective tissue in liquid form, the blood circulates in the vasculature to transport oxygen, nutrients and metabolites; protect the human body from invading microorganisms (viruses, bacteria, etc.); and regulate the physiology. Blood volume, concentration and distribution of electrolytes and formed elements, and its osmolality and viscosity and their variation, are critical to the hematology and hemodynamics of systemic circulation.

9.2.1.1 Disturbance on Blood Volume and Erythrocyte Count

The average blood volume in a normal human circulation system is 4–6 liters (Saladin 2007a). The iodinated contrast agent injected at the antecubital site is usually about 60–120 ml, which is a relatively small increase (<3%) in blood volume (Eloy et al. 1991) and thus may only induce mild disturbance to the hemodynamics. However, though the osmolality of nonionic iodinated contrast currently administered in clinical practice is relatively low (600–800 mOsm/L), it is still significantly higher than that of blood (290 mOsm/L). Then, a large amount of water is drawn from cells and extracellular space into the blood plasma and increases the volume of blood by up to 10%–20%, which may significantly disturb the hemodynamics of systemic circulation. The initial enlargement in blood volume is proportional to iodinated contrast agent's osmolality, occurs about 2 minutes post injection and returns to the baseline in 20–60 minutes, owing to the renal excretion upregulated by the diuretic effect induced by the contrast agent's osmolality. In turn, the enlarged volume (and altered morphology and elasticity in the blood components, see later) may lead to a transient hematocrit – reduction in the counts of erythrocytes. Other clinical consequences include increased cardiac output, lifted intraventricular diastolic pressure, left atrial pressure, and even arterial and venous pulmonary pressure, which may further lead to escalated arterial and venous pulmonary pressure (Eloy et al. 1991; ACR 2021).

9.2.1.2 Disturbance on Intra-Plasma Electrolyte Distribution and pH

Via either direct or indirect complexing effects exerted by the molecules of the contrast agent itself, especially if it is ionic, or the additives in its clinical preparation, the contrast agent may decrease the concentration of electrolytes, K^+, Mg^{+2} and particularly Ca^{+2} (hypocalcemia), and accordingly reduce the plasmatic pH. As a result, the redistributed electrolytes may significantly decrease or even reverse the intra- and extra-cellular electrical potential cross the erythrocyte's plasmatic membrane that is essential to cellular metabolism and functionalities, such as cellular signaling and transportation via the ionic channels and/or pumps. Disturbance on the endothe- lial metabolic pathways and other functionalities may impair vascular contractility that is essential to maintenance of cardiovascular circulation (Eloy et al. 1991).

9.2.1.3 Disturbance on Peripheral Arterial Vasodilation

The intimate contact between molecules of the iodinated contrast agent and vascular wall may exert surgical (morphological) or pharmacological (e.g., atrophic, antihis- taminic or sympathicommimetic) interruption on or impairment of the functionality of vascular smooth muscles. The interrupted peripheral arterial vasodilation may clinically manifest as increased cardiac output, transient tachycardia or hypotension that occurs 1–2 minutes post contrast injection, in addition to the commonly reported sensation of warmth and/or pain during or post the injection. The extent to which the vasodilation is upregulated correlates with the contrast agent's osmolality, while other factors, e.g., chemotoxicity and viscosity, cannot be excluded. Notably, the pain associated with the administration of the iodinated contrast agent can be reduced by anesthetics, suggesting the nervous system's involvement, but the sensation of warmth, flushing or chilling cannot be altered by anesthetics, implying involvement of the body temperature controlling mechanism (Eloy et al. 1991; ACR 2021).

9.2.2 CHEMOTOXICITY TO BLOOD AT CELLULAR LEVEL

Blood mainly consists of plasma, electrolytes and formed elements (red and white blood cells) (Saladin 2007a). In addition to its direct disturbance on the blood vol- ume, electrolyte concentration and distribution, and vasoactivities, the iodinated contrast agent may interact with the blood components at the cellular level. Herein we talk about its interaction with erythrocytes and platelets, while that with leuko- cytes is deferred to the section focusing on the hypersensitivity reactions.

9.2.2.1 Chemotoxicity to Erythrocyte

Erythrocytes are the most abundant formed elements in blood (4.2–5.4 million/µl in females and 4.6–6.2 million/µl in males), claiming about 45% of the volume (Saladin 2007a). In systemic circulation, an erythrocyte is usually 7.5 µm in diameter (2 µm thick at its rim) and needs to pass through microvessels of 3–12 µm diameter or pores of 0.5–5 µm diameter on cell membrane. Thus the erythrocyte's deformability (or elasticity) is vital to the hematology and hemodynamics. Along with its disturbance on plasmatic viscosity, the contrast agent's relatively high osmolality may modu- late the erythrocyte's shape and other morphologic properties, leading to reduced deformability (or elasticity) and altered aggregability as the primary and secondary consequences, respectively. In a dose-dependent manner, these changes may further alter the blood flow (rheology) that is vital to systemic circulation (Eloy et al. 1991). Moreover, it has been reported that the iodinated contrast agent may increase the intracellular pH while it decreases the plasmatic pH. Fortunately, the disturbance or impairment is usually reversible and results in no clinically relevant consequences in the protocol (volume, concentration and injection rate) designed for intravenous administration in CT. However, it may be of concern in cases of pre-existing conditions, e.g., congenital cyanosis, sickle cell disease, hypoventilation or compromised peripheral or parenchymal vascularization, as the contrast agent may induce embolism or thrombosis in microcirculation, especially in the case of intra-arterial administration for angiography (Eloy et al. 1991).

9.2.2.2 Chemotoxicity to Platelets

Being the cell fragments of megakaryocytes, platelets are 2–4 μm in diameter and distribute in the blood at an average concentration 0.25 million/μl (Saladin 2007a). The platelet plays a variety of roles in physiology, including its engagement in defense via inflammation and phagocytosis, while its most prominent role is in hemostasis via adhesion, vasoconstriction, aggregation (plug formation) and coagulation (clotting) (Eloy et al. 1991). It has been observed that, in a manner related to injected dose, platelet aggregation may be inhibited as early as a couple of minutes post contrast agent injection, though the inhibition can be almost fully (up to 80%) recovered. Platelet adhesion may also be impaired due to the close contact with the iodinated contrast agent for a relatively long time (30–60 minutes) prior to recovery. Limited data has suggested that ionicity is the primary or direct culprit, though other indirect factors, such as hyperosmolality and pH, and in particular hypocalcemia due to interaction between the contrast agent and Ca^{+2}, may also play roles. Basically, they may disturb the platelet response by interfering with receptors on cell membrane, intracellular events and the transferring of cross-membrane signals that may activate platelet aggregation. The disturbance on or impairment of platelet functionality is usually of no clinical concern in intravenous contrast agent administration in CT, but may lead to clinically relevant complications in intra-artery administration in coronary angiography (Eloy et al. 1991).

9.2.3 Chemotoxicity to Vascular Endothelium

Being a tissue consisting of single-layer cells, the endothelium lines the vascular luminal surface. With a total area larger than 1000 m², the endothelium serves as not only a barrier but also a communication channel for interaction between blood and tissues (Saladin 2007a). Under well-controlled permeability, the endothelium in micro-circulation is more specific to ensuring intravascular transportation and cross-wall exchange of chemicals or molecules, along with its function as a barrier. In macro-circulation, the endothelium is more specific to maintaining resistance to thrombosis by regulating the tissue plasminogen activator to control the fibrinolytic system (Eloy et al. 1991). Moreover, the vascular endothelial cells may regulate the activation and/or inactivation of vasodilator, vasoconstrictor and other vasoactive chemicals, or even affect the function of the vascular smooth muscle. The blood's osmolality and ionicity may be increased by the iodinated contrast agent and thus disturb the endothelial permeability, leading to adverse reactions, such as the hypocalcemia mentioned earlier and local hyperemia induced by vasoactive chemicals, e.g., histamine, kinins and leukotrienes secreted by basophil cells in the blood and mast cells in the connective tissues. The local hyperemia may further cause extravasation, in which the iodinated contrast agent leaves the bloodstream via the so-called diapedesis process, though a correlative relationship between them has not be clinically established (ACR 2021). As reported in the literature, the iodinated contrast agent may also lead to cellular shrinkage, enlargement of extracellular space, expansion of intracellular cleft, disjoint of endothelial cells from sub-endothelial cells and inhibition of cellular proliferation. Fortunately, however, the cell's altered ultrastructure is reversible over a course of hours and days, as evidenced by the fact that the cells' viability is usually maintained without wide-spreading cell death (Eloy et al. 1991).

9.2.4 CHEMOTOXICITY TO BLOOD–BRAIN BARRIER

The BBB provides protection of the brain parenchyma from potentially harmful chemicals or molecules, e.g., antibodies and macrophages, in the systemic blood supply (Eloy et al. 1991). The endothelial cells forming the vascular endothelium and part of the basement membrane in the brain join so tightly that all the materials leaving the blood have to pass through the cells, while the intercellular passage almost fully closes. As such, the BBB is highly permeable to O_2, water, CO_2 and other lipophilic materials, but only slightly permeable to hydrophilic materials, e.g., sodium, potassium, chloride and other metabolic products. The protection is strictly enforced by impermeability, but may be compromised by the iodinated contrast agent's hyperosmolality or its disruption on blood flow due to its adverse influence on aggregation of blood cells. It has been reported that the iodinated contrast agent may be more than 1000 times more toxic to the central nerve system than to the circulation system. Moreover, the BBB is absent in areas surrounding the circumventricular organs that regulate body temperature, respiration, blood pressure and heartbeat rate, which may lead to clinically relevant consequences in physiology, such as nausea, vomiting, hypertension/hypotension, tachycardia or bradycardia, arrhythmia, or other vasovagal reactions (Eloy et al. 1991; ACR 2021).

9.2.5 CHEMOTOXICITY TO BLOOD AT MOLECULAR LEVEL

At the molecular level, the iodinated contrast agent and the additives in its clinical preparation may interact with plasmatic coagulation, the fibrinolytic system, the contact phase, the complement system and enzymes engaged in cellular metabolism and activities. In-depth coverage of them is beyond the scope of this chapter and interested readers are referred to the literature (e.g., Eloy et al. 1991).

9.2.6 IODINATED CONTRAST AGENTS AND RISK OF ADVERSE PHYSIOLOGICAL REACTION

A physiological adverse reaction can be systemic or organ specific, and commonly manifests as mild or moderate symptoms, such as tolerable pain at the injection site, limited extravasation, transient sensation of flushing, warmth or chills, headache and dizziness, and/or spontaneously resolvable vasovagal reactions. In clinical settings, they are usually self-limiting, and close clinical observation is sufficient. However, though extremely rare, severe adverse reactions that are potentially life threatening, e.g., angina, arrhythmia, cardiogenic pulmonary edema, compulsions and seizures, acute hypertension and treatment-resistant vasovagal reactions such as hypotension-induced unconsciousness, may unpredictably occur. With the severity depending on administered dose, the onset of adverse physiologic reaction can be acute (within 20 minutes) or delayed (ranging from 30–60 minutes to 1 week) (ACR 2021). A discussion on its incidence and clinical management is deferred to Section 9.3.4 in association with the discussion on hypersensitivity reactions.

Neither a pretest to predict or premedication to prevent the incidence of adverse physiological reaction to an iodinated contrast agent exists in the clinic. Hence, screening a patient for the risks of suffering from iodinated contrast agent-induced severe physiologic reaction based on the patient's medical history and current cardiac status is of clinical relevance. In general, the referral for contrast-enhanced CT should be weighed in on at least four aspects: (i) the administration of iodinated contrast agent appropriate to the patient and indication, (ii) the balance between the likelihood of adverse reaction and the benefit of the examination, (iii) promotion of efficient and accurate diagnosis and treatment, and (iv) preparedness for treatment of adverse reaction should one occur. In light of the risk of life-threatening events, though rare, a team of radiologists, technologists and emergency response personnel with familiarity to presentation and prompt treatment of the entire spectrum of adverse reactions must be in place. It is of paramount importance to differentiate the acute physiologic adverse reaction from acute hypersensitivity adverse reaction for clinical management (work flow). Importantly, the preparedness (personnel training, availability of equipment and medication) of the response team must be maintained via a quality assurance (QA) program and quality control practice with engagement of members of the emergency response (code) team (ACR 2021).

Correlated with the large volume and peripheral site of injection, the incidence of extravasation in the clinic induced by (either power or hand) injection of iodinated contrast in CT ranges between 0.1% and 1.2% (ACR 2021). The vast majority of extravasations is mild, only involving the surrounding tissues, typically the skin and subcutaneous tissues, with discomfort such as swelling or tightness and/or sting or burning pain. The extravasation usually recovers by itself without the need of clinical intervention, but it may cause acute severe local inflammatory injury and leading to skin ulceration and/or tissue necrosis that needs close clinical observation. Notably, the inflammatory injury may not fully manifest for hours or even days (24–48 hours), with the incidence of compartment syndrome as the most severe consequence that can lead to loss of limb function or even amputation if adequate surgical intervention is not promptly adopted. Notably, the likelihood of extravasation in patients with preexisting conditions, such as altered circulation due to atherosclerotic or diabetic vascular diseases and extensive surgery in the limb where the injection site is located at, is relatively higher, especially if the intravenous injection is administered at peripheral sites. In particular, severe extravasation is more likely to happen in patients with arterial insufficiency or compromised venous or lymphatic drainage in the affected limb. No premedication exists in the clinic for prophylaxis of iodinated contrast agent-induced extravasation. Once extravasation happens in the clinic, a physical evaluation, including the assessment of tenderness, swelling, erythema, active and passive finger motility and perfusion, should be performed. In the scenario of acute severe extravasation-induced compartment syndrome, prompt surgical consultation should be pursued (ACR 2021).

9.3 CHEMOTOXICITY OF IODINATED CONTRAST AGENTS THAT MAY INDUCE HYPERSENSITIVITY REACTIONS

Hypersensitivity reactions, which can be acute or delayed, may occur in clinical settings. Though the pathophysiology of hypersensitivity has not been fully understood, it has been presumed that the release of histamine by activation of the basophils in the circulation system and the mast cells in connective tissues in response to the contrast agent's hyperosmolality, hypertonicity and its complicated molecular structures, are among the etiologic factors (Eloy et al. 1991; Bush and Swanson 1991; Pasternak and Williamson 2012; ACR 2021).

9.3.1 LEUKOCYTE, LYMPHOCYTE AND IMMUNOLOGY

Ubiquitously existing in the environment, pathogens, e.g., bacteria, viruses, toxins and radiation, may invade the human body and cause pathophysiological lesions manifested as infection or disease. In addition to defense by the skin and mucous as a physical barrier, there are two other defense lines for humans to protect themselves from invading pathogens that may cause diseases (Saladin 2007b). The first line of defense is non-specific resistance, in which the leukocytes and macrophages play a dominant role against the invaded pathogens via the mechanisms of inflammation, immune clearance, phagocytosis and cytolysis. The second line of defense is specific immunity existing in two modes: cellular immunity and humoral immunity. In cellular immunity, the T lymphocytes (cytotoxic T_c, helper T_h and memory T_m cells) directly attack and kill the invading microorganisms, with the "3R" mechanism (recognition, react and remember) (Saladin 2007b). In the humoral immunity, still in the 3R manner, the B lymphocytes differentiate into plasma cells that produce a total of five classes of antibodies (immunoglobulin alpha (IgA), delta (IgD), epsilon (IgE), gamma (IgG) and mu (IgM)) to label the invading pathogenic agents for destruction by other processes or agents, e.g., complement fixation and phagocytosis, or rendering them into harmless forms by other measures. Given an antigen, the plasma cell produces IgM and establish the antigen–IgM complex in the first-time exposure, and produces IgG and forms the antigen–IgG complex while the next exposure occurs (Saladin 2007b).

9.3.2 HYPERSENSITIVITY: ANAPHYLAXIS (ALLERGIC) REACTIONS

Hypersensitivity is an excessive and thus detrimental immunological reaction to foreign pathogens, including the allergens that exist in the nature, such as dust, pollen, toxic agents in plants (pollen or poison ivy) and drugs (e.g., penicillin), and even in food (milk, eggs and shellfish). Depending on the respective mechanisms, four types of supersensitivity reactions have thus far been identified, with the first three types being associated with the humoral immunity and the rest with cellular hypersensitivity. Type I reaction is termed *anaphylaxis* and is the most common reaction that may occur immediately (in seconds to 30 minutes) following exposure to allergens. The allergen binds to IgE receptors on the surface of basophils and mast cells that activate the release of histamine and other vasoactive (either dilative or restrictive) agents (Saladin 2007b; Galli et al. 2005). Presumably, the onset of anaphylactic shock is not dose dependent once a certain but currently unknown threshold is exceeded. Type I hypersensitivity may lead to severe complications, such as bronchospasm, dyspnea, massive vasodilation, circulatory shock or even sudden death. In general, the clinical intervention with antihistamine drugs is not adequate to deal with the complications associated with type I reaction, but epinephrine can help relieve the symptoms by dilating the bronchioles, increasing cardiac output and restoring blood pressure. Types II and III hypersensitivities are sub-acute and usually occur 1–3 hours post exposure and lasts for about 10–15 hours. The IgG and IgM antibodies directly attack the antigens by activating the complement fixation in type II reaction, while the antigen–antibody (Ag-Ab) complex associated with IgG or IgM are formed in type III reaction to activate the complement fixation and intense inflammation for destruction of antigens. Associated with the cellular immunity and thus with the T lymphocyte's engagement, type IV supersensitivity is a delayed reaction that may occur 12 hours–3 days after exposure. Notably, the allergens that may induce type IV reaction include the haptens that may exist in cosmetics or the toxic agents in poison ivy (Saladin 2007b).

9.3.3 HYPERSENSITIVITY: ANAPHYLACTOID (ALLERGIC-LIKE) REACTIONS

An antigen can be any molecule that induces an immunologic response, and usually its molecular weight is larger than 10,000 amu. Though its weight is relatively small (<1000 amu), it is still likely for the molecule of an iodinated contrast agent, which is in relatively complex chemical structure, to trigger the activation, deactivation or inhabitation of a variety of vasoactive mediators (e.g., histamine – the inflammation mediator) or pathways (e.g., the complement or kinin system or contact phase) (Eloy et al. 1991). It has been reported in the literature that the iodinated contrast agent of low-osmolality nonionic monomers produces lower levels of histamine release from basophils compared with the iso-osmolality nonionic dimers. On average, hypersensitivity reaction occurs in a fraction of 1% of patients who are intravenously administered with an iodinated contrast agent for CT in clinical settings, with the symptoms being almost the same (e.g., urticaria) to that of the type I hypersensitivity mentioned earlier. The occurrence of urticarial and other cutaneous symptoms mean that histamine must have been released from basophils and mast cells in these hypersensitivity cases, but its pathogenicity can't been etiologically determined as an allergy, since, except in a very small fraction (4%), no antigen–IgE complex can be reliably identified in the vast majority of acute supersensitivity reaction cases, despite of the fact that the clinical manifestation is exactly the same as an allergy. Hence, the acute supersensitivity reaction induced by iodinated contrast agent has been termed "allergic-like", "anaphylactoid" or "idiosyncratic" in the literature. Most likely, the iodinated contrast agent-induced allergic-like reaction is not dependent on dose and concentration once an unknown threshold is exceeded (Bush and Swanson 1991; Pasternak and Williamson 2012; ACR 2021).

9.3.4 INCIDENCE OF HYPERSENSITIVITY REACTION AND CLINICAL MANAGEMENT

It has been reported that the aggregate (hypersensitivity + physiologic) incidence of acute adverse reaction induced by the low- or iso-osmolality iodinated contrast agent is low in clinical settings (<1% in adult and 0.5% in pediatric patients). The vast majority of the hypersensitivity reaction is mild, cutaneous and self-limiting, including local itching or hives, cutaneous edema, limited "itchy or scratchy" throat, nasal congestion or sneezing (ACR 2021). Hence, clinical attention via observation and/or supportive measures are usually sufficient. Unfortunately, however, though extremely rare, systemic and potentially life-threatening acute adverse reactions (morbidity: ~0.04%; mortality: <1:170,000), such as edema with dyspnea, erythema with hypotension, laryngeal edema with stridor and/or hypoxia, or bronchospasm (wheezing) with severe hypoxia, might occur and demand prompt clinical intervention by the emergency response team. If it happens, a potentially acute life-threatening reaction usually occurs within 20 minutes post intravenous injection. The onset of hypersensitivity reaction may be delayed in a fraction (0.5%–14%) of the patients for 3 hours to 2 days (ranging from 30–60 minutes to 1 week). The symptoms are usually cutaneous and self-limiting, but severe cutaneous reaction or fatalities, though rare, have been reported. It has also been reported that the incidence of delayed hypersensitivity reaction is modestly higher in iso-osmolality dimeric iodinated contrast agent than its low-osmolality counterpart, perhaps because of the dimeric agent's molecular complexity (ACR 2021).

As iodinated contrast agent-induced acute hypersensitivity is not IgE-mediated, the occurrence of a potentially fatal reaction is unpredictable in clinical practice. However, it has been reported that an iodinated contrast agent-induced anaphylactoid reaction is about five times more likely reoccur in the patient who has suffered a prior acute hypersensitivity event induced by the identical iodinated contrast agent (ACR 2021). Hence, premedication is recommended for prophylaxis of reoccurrence of acute hypersensitivity reaction in patients who have a history of hypersensitivity reaction under administration of exactly the same iodinated contrast agent, but not recommended for patients who have a history of mild delayed hypersensitivity reaction, due to the extreme rarity of severe delayed hypersensitivity reaction. In general, atopic individuals, especially those with multiple severe allergies, are at higher risk of hypersensitivity reaction to iodinated contrast agent, whereas patients who are allergic to shellfish are not at escalated risk. Moreover, certain preexisting conditions may increase the likelihood of a hypersensitivity reaction to an iodinated contrast agent, as evidenced by the fact that bronchospasm is a common adverse event in patients with asthma, while hemodynamic changes are more common in patients with severe cardiovascular diseases (ACR 2021).

9.4 NEPHROTOXICITY OF IODINATED CONTRAST AGENTS

In addition to the aforementioned adverse physiological reactions and hypersensitivity, acute kidney injury (AKI) is another major clinical consequence that may be induced by an iodinated contrast agent (Heinrichet al. 2005; Katzberg 2005; Seeliger et al. 2012; Bansal and Patel 2020). Rather than being a form of disease, AKI is actually an impairment of renal function (transit pathological status) with a sudden deterioration of renal function as the hallmark (Scholz et al. 2021; ACR 2021; Davenport 2020). Potentially, AKI may develop into chronic kidney disease (CKD) associated with fibrosis, vascular rarefaction, tubular loss, glomerular sclerosis or chronic inflammation, especially in patients with preexisting conditions, e.g., renal insufficiency or endothelial dysfunction in diabetes mellitus. Based on data published in the latest decade, the American College of Radiology (ACR) has been adapting its position on contrast-induced AKI (CI-AKI) and stated in its *Manual on Contrast Media* by its Committee on Drugs and Contrast Media that "the CI-AKI is a real, albeit rare, entity" (ACR 2021; Davenport et al. 2020).

9.4.1 DIAGNOSIS OF CONTRAST-INDUCED ACUTE KIDNEY INJURY

In the clinical sense, AKI should be diagnosed by quantitatively assessing the renal function gauged by the glomerular filtration rate (GFR). However, almost all solutes undergo reabsorption and/or secretion (transport activities) while they pass through the renal tubules, making a direct gauge of GFR difficult, if not infeasible, in clinical settings. Alternatively, the serum creatinine produced by skeletal muscle has been adopted as a surrogate of GFR for renal function assessment. With endorsement by the National Kidney Foundation in its *Kidney Disease Outcomes Quality Initiative*, the Kidney Disease Improving Global Outcomes (KDIGO) recommends the following criteria for diagnosis of AKI: (ACR 2021) (i) absolute increase in serum creatinine ≥ 0.3 mg/dl (>26.4 µmol/L); (ii) percentage increase in serum creatinine $\geq 50\%$ (1.5-fold above baseline); and (iii) urine output reduced to lower than 0.5 ml/kg/hour for at least 6 hours. This criterion has been adopted by the ACR Committee on Drugs and Contrast Media for diagnosis of CI-AKI within 48 hours of intravenous administration of iodinated contrast agent, if no other etiologies can be identified (ACR 2021). It should be noted that the level of serum creatinine is not an accurate indicator of AKI, as has been reported in the literature that it can remain unchanged until a nearly 50% reduction in the GFR (Scholz et al. 2021). One of the underlying reasons may be that the serum creatinine distributes over a large volume (the entire water compartment), which leaves the variation in serum creatinine behind that in GFR (see Figure 9.3). To date, the calculated estimation of GFR (eGFR) is a more accurate and thus gaining the clinical community's recognition as a potentially better indicator of AKI diagnosis.

As illustrated in Figure 9.3, a few biomarkers, such as cystatin C and NGAL (neutrophil gelatinase-associated lipocalin), can promptly follow the rapid drop in GFR

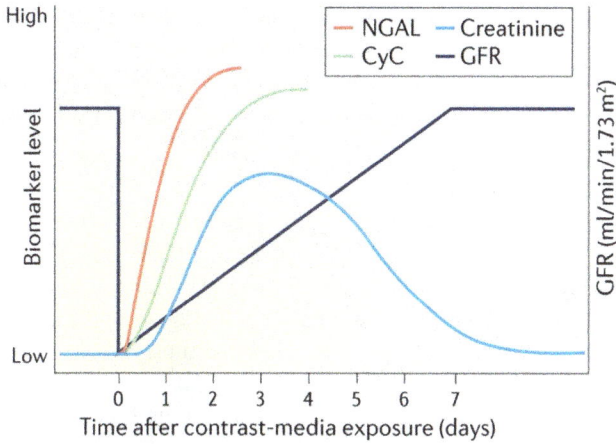

FIGURE 9.3 The variation of biomarkers in contrast-induced acute kidney injury. (Adopted from Fähling et al. 2017 with permission.)

due to renal impairment, and thus they should perform much better than the serum creatinine if they serve as the indicator of AKI in clinical settings (Scholz et al. 2021). The main reason behind the accuracy and promptness of cystatin C in following the variation in GFR is the fact that cystatin C only distributes in the extracellular space that is approximately one-third the entire water compartment in which serum creatinine distribute. The level of cystatin C gauged at the 24-hour temporal window can be a predictor of AKI severity. Moreover, NGAL is greatly upregulated in response to the impairment occurring in the distal nephron segment and thus the biomarker associated with the damage to the thick ascending limb of the Henle loop, distal tubule and the collecting duct (Saladin 2007c). Another biomarker, which is not included in the plotting presented in Figure 9.3, is called the phosphatidylserine receptor kidney injury molecule 1 (KIM-1) and may serve as an indicator of nephrotoxic injury to the proximal nephron segment. Once the tubular epithelium detects insult on the proximal nephron segment, it activates the phagocytosis in which the KIM-1 molecules play active roles. Nevertheless, although these biomarkers are very sensitive, all of them have not yet established themselves as point-of-care indicators in clinical settings, as more work is needed to improve their specificity regarding the loop in the pathophysiological chain that leads to AKI (Scholz et al. 2021).

9.4.2 RENAL ANATOMY AND PATHOPHYSIOLOGY

In a cascade of three stages (glomerular filtration, tubular reabsorption and secretion, and water conservation), the kidneys, as the most important and delicate organ in the urinary system, are responsible for two fundamental functions: (i) elimination of metabolic waste and (ii) homeostatic regulation of body fluid volume and composition (Saladin 2007c). The iodinated contrast agent is not a metabolic product but certainly a form of waste that is dominantly (if not exclusively) eliminated from the body via renal excretion, as its molecule is smaller than 3 nm (Eloy et al. 1991; Shahid et al. 2020; Schöckel et al. 2020). To have an in-depth understanding of the kidneys' susceptibility to iodinated contrast agent, we herein prepare ourselves with a brief review of the gross anatomy and general physiology of the kidneys.

9.4.2.1 Nephric Anatomy

There are roughly 1.2 million nephrons in a kidney and each nephron consists of two major components: renal corpuscle and renal tubule. Each renal corpuscle, located within the kidney cortex, is fed with an afferent arteriole coming from the inter-lobular artery that is supplied by the renal artery (Figure 9.4) (see Saladin 2007c for more details). Having passed through the glomerulus, the blood flow leaves the renal corpuscle via the efferent arteriole at the same side of the afferent arteriole and branches into the capillaries called vasa recta to surround the nephron loop on its way entering and turning back from the kidney medulla. Concurrently, on the oppo-site side of the corpuscle, the fluid and solutes filtrated by the glomerulus flow into the renal tubule that is roughly divided into four segments with distinct physiologic functions: (i) proximal convoluted tubule (PCT), (ii) nephron loop (loop of Henle), (iii) distal convoluted tubule (DCT) and (iv) collecting duct. In fact, the nephron can

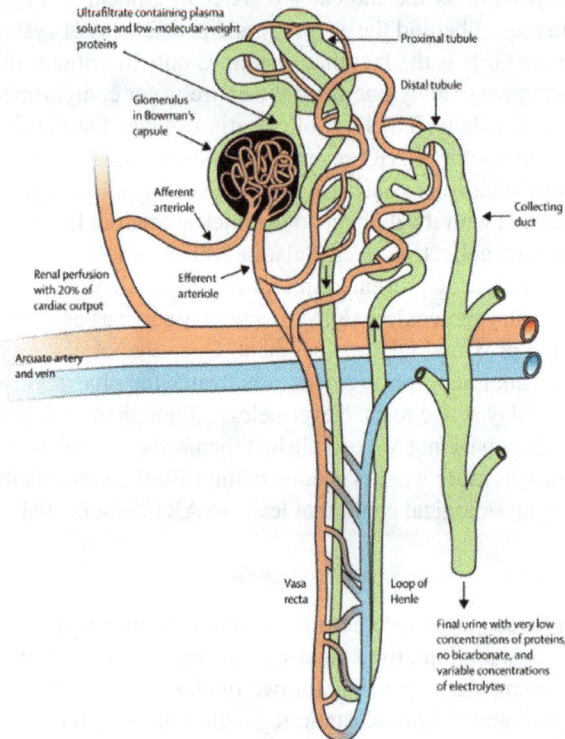

FIGURE 9.4 Schematic diagram showing the structure of a cortical (top half) and juxta-medullary (bottom half) nephron. (Adopted from Eckardt et al. 2013 with permission.)

be categorized as cortical or juxtamedullary (on the top and bottom of Figure 9.4, respectively), with the former located just beneath the renal capsule and the latter within the medulla. Notably, the cortical nephron loop is relatively short, while that of the juxtamedullary nephron is very long and extends to the apex of the renal pyramid, establishing and maintaining the salinity gradient that helps water conservation in the body. Readers who want to learn more about the kidney anatomy are referred to the related textbooks (e.g., Saladin 2007c).

9.4.2.2 Nephric Physiology

The kidneys carry out glomerular filtration, tubular reabsorption, secretion and water conservation through the following important renal components in a cascading manner (Saladin 2007c).

Glomerular filtration membrane: As blood passes through the glomerulus under hydrostatic pressure, the water and solutes that are smaller than 70–90 nm are filtered out the pores of the endothelial cells that line the glomerular capillary wall, whereas others, including formed elements and proteins, are retained in the plasma. As an interface between the glomerular capillary and capsule space, the filtration membrane further filtrates the fluid based on size and (negative) electrical repellent effect, ensuring that only the molecules that are smaller than 3 nm, such as water, electrolytes, glucose, fatty acids, amino acids, nitrogenous wastes and vitamins, can enter the capsule space. Notably, many chemicals at small molecular weight, such as Ga^{+2}, Na^+ and thyroid hormone, are retained in the blood circulation, as they are bound to plasma proteins that are too large to pass through the membrane. Under renal autoregulation, sympathetic control and hormone control, the glomerular filtration membrane maintains a stable GFR by adjusting the glomerular blood pressure.

Proximate convoluted tubule: In a normal male, the GFR is 125 ml/min (105 ml/min in female), which would be tantamount to 180 L/day urine (150 L/day in female), if the glomerular filtrate is unchecked and goes downstream for renal excretion. In fact, fortunately, 99% of glomerular filtrates, both water and solutes, are reabsorbed after they leave the glomerulus, leading to 1–2 L of urine per day in normal cases. Roughly two-thirds of the reabsorption is carried out in the PCT that comprises three segments (see S_1–S_3 in Figure 9.5). Via transcellular and paracellular routes, the glomerular filtrates enter the extracellular space in the base of tubular epithelial cells and are then taken up by the paratubular capillaries owing to gradient in the interstitial fluid pressure, blood hydrostatic pressure and colloid osmotic pressure. Notably, reabsorption in the PCT is carried out at a constant rate and thus is termed obligatory water reabsorption, while that in other parts of the tubular system is continually adjusted by hormones according to the body's hydration status. Moreover, the absorption in PCT is proportionate over the amount of water and solutes, and thus doesn't change the gross osmolality of the tubular fluid.

Among all the solutes reabsorbed in the PCT, of special note is the transport of sodium Na^+ via Na^+-K^+ pumping, in which energy (ATP) is consumed. It is the transport of Na^+ that establishes the osmotic and electrical gradient that is the foundation for other tubular transport activities. The reabsorption of glucose is also of note, in which all the glucose is supposed to be reabsorbed, unless the glucose concentration is so high to exceed the reabsorption threshold of 220 mg/dL, in situations such as diabetes mellitus. Moreover, the transport activity in the PCT is a two-way process, in which, in parallel to the reabsorption of water and solutes from the tubule to the paratubular capillaries, metabolic wastes, such as urea, uric acid, ammonia and creatinine, and chemicals (hydrogen and biocarbonate ions H^+ and HCO_3^-) and pollutants as well, are extracted from the blood stream in the capillaries and secreted into the PCT for the purpose of waste removal and maintenance of the acid–base balance.

Nephric loops: As illustrated in Figure 9.5, once it leaves the PCT, the tubular fluid goes through the nephron loop prior to its arrival at the DCT, the segment between the thick ascending limb and collecting duct, for further

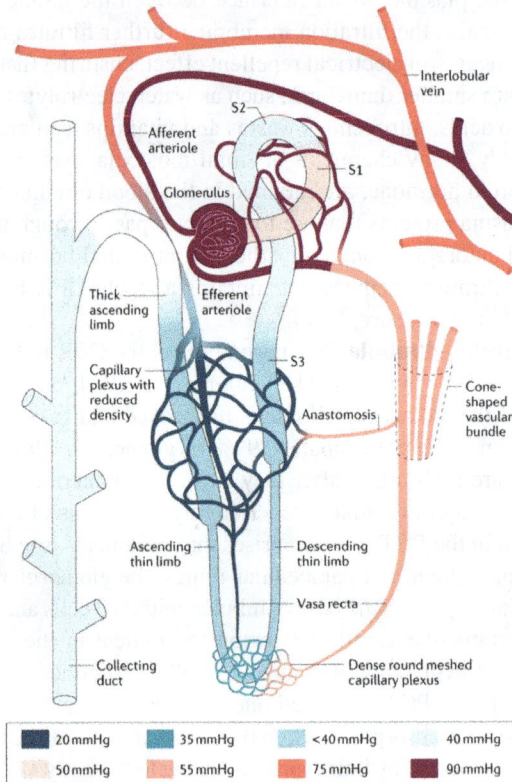

FIGURE 9.5 Schematic diagram showing the structure of juxtamedullary nephron loops and the distribution of partial pressure of oxygen. (Adopted from Scholz et al. 2021 with permission.)

resorption and secretion. The U-shaped nephron loop comprises three portions: (i) thick descending limb (TDL) articulated from PCT, (ii) thin limb around the bend of the U-shape and (iii) thick ascending limb (TAL) leading to the DCT. The vast majority (85%) of nephrons (cortical nephrons) have short or no nephron loop at all (see top half of Figure 9.4), while the rest (15%) (juxtamedullary nephrons) have relatively long loops (see bottom half of Figure 9.4). The nephron loop reabsorbs about 25% of the Na^+, K^+ and Cl^- ions, and 15% of the water from the glomerular filtrates, in addition to its major function of forming the salinity gradient for water conservation in the collecting duct. The salinity gradient is generated via the countercurrent multiplier mechanism implemented by the nephron loop itself, under the aid of the countercurrent exchange system implemented in the vasa recta that perfuse the nephron loop and other structures in the outer and inner strips of the medulla, as briefly delineated next.

- **Countercurrent multiplier**: Both the thick descending and ascending limbs are impermeable to water. In addition to the physical U-shape of the nephron loop, the key that enables the formation of the countercurrent multiplier is that the descending thin limb is very impermeable to water but not to salt (NaCl), and the ascending thin limb is very impermeable to NaCl and K^- via active transport pumps but not to water. Then, via osmosis, an increasing amount of water leaves the tubule and enters the extracellular space of tubular epithelial cells, along the way of tubular fluid from the cortex going downstream to the deep medulla. In contrast, along its way running from the deep medulla upstream to the cortex, Na^+, Cl^- and K^- ions are pumped into the extracellular space. Through such positive feedback, the salinity gradient is stably established in the kidneys: 300 mOsm/L at the end of the PCT, 1200 mOsm/L at the bend of the loop and 100 mOsm/L at the entrance of the DCT.

- **Countercurrent exchange system**: Physiologically, the supply of oxygen and other nutrients to and removal of metabolic wastes from the nephron loops are carried out in the paratubular capillaries called vasa recta. The vasa recta is also routed in the countercurrent fashion as such the salinity gradient formed by the nephron loops can spare the process of removing the metabolic wastes. Specifically, the blood flow in the vasa recta trades for more NaCl with water along its way from the cortex down to the deep medulla and vice versa, leaving the salinity gradient intact. Notably, in fact, the vasa recta carries away more water on its way out than it unloads on its way in, providing the passage for reclaiming water absorbed by the nephron loops from the tubular fluid and the collecting duct (see later) from the urine.

Distal convoluted tubule: After going through the PCT and nephron loops, the tubular fluid arrives at the entrance of the DCT at an amount that is still equal to ~20% of the water and 7% of the salt in the glomerular filtrates. Further reabsorption of water and solutes from the tubular fluid is needed, or the urine would be projected to be ~36 L/day. Notably, rather than reabsorption in the PCT that runs at a constant rate, the water absorption rate in DCT is variable and continuously under regulation of hormones, e.g., aldosterone, atrial natriuretic peptide and other antidiuretic and parathyroid ones, depending on the body's hydration status. Concurrently, the DCT extracts metabolic wastes, drugs, pollutants and other substances from the blood stream and secretes them into the nephric tubule for excretion.

Collecting duct: Within the renal cortex, the output of a number of nephrons drain into the collecting duct, in which, aided by the salinity established by the nephron loops as described earlier, the urine is concentrated by water reabsorption via osmosis, leading to the final amount of 1–2 L urine per day in a normal person. Notably, the reabsorption rate in the collecting duct is dependent on the body's hydration status. Under dehydrated conditions, the relatively high blood osmolality activates the release of antidiuretic hormone (ADH) that drives the nephron tubular cells to synthesize a water-channel protein called aquaporin to upregulate the transport of water across the epithelial plasma membrane. In extreme cases, the blood pressure of a dehydrated subject can be low enough to significantly reduce the GFR, leading to slower fluid in the tubules and thus a longer stay in the collecting duct for water reabsorption.

9.4.2.3 Nephropathy underlying AKI

As elucidated earlier, to fulfill its functions in the urinary system, the kidneys' anatomic structure is complex and delicate. They work at high load and receive up to 25% the entire cardiac output via the renal artery. Depending on the tubular transport activity, the kidneys consume a large amount of energy that is tantamount to ~7% the total energy generated by an adult under rest, especially in the PCT and DCT wherein reabsorption and secretion occur (Scholz et al. 2021). In accordance to the heterogeneity in the kidneys' structure and functions over nephron segments, there exists heterogeneity in their cellular metabolism sustained by oxygenation, energy production and consumption, and cellular protection. Specifically, as illustrated in Figure 9.6, the PCT can be divided into S_1, S_2 and S_3 segments, with the S_1 and S_2 segments being located in the cortex and the S_3 segment in the outer strip of the medulla. Also located in the outer medulla is the TAL of the DCT. Notably, the production of energy (ATP) in the PCT is carried out aerobically, whereas that in the DCT is mainly through anaerobic glycolysis (Scholz et al. 2021; Saladin 2007c). On the other hand, the blood stream enters the kidney via the interlobular artery and perfuses the cortex heterogeneously. From the efferent arteriole of the juxtamedullary nephron come the microvessels called vasa recta down to the medulla, forming a negative corticomedullary gradient of oxygen that is relatively low in pressure (~20 mmHg, as indicated in Figure 9.5), because of the vasa recta's countercurrent architecture. Additionally, the density of the vasa recta is relatively low, thus making the S_3 segment of the PCT and the TAL of the DCT distant from the peritubular capillaries, limiting its access to diffused oxygen in these two nephron areas that consume much energy.

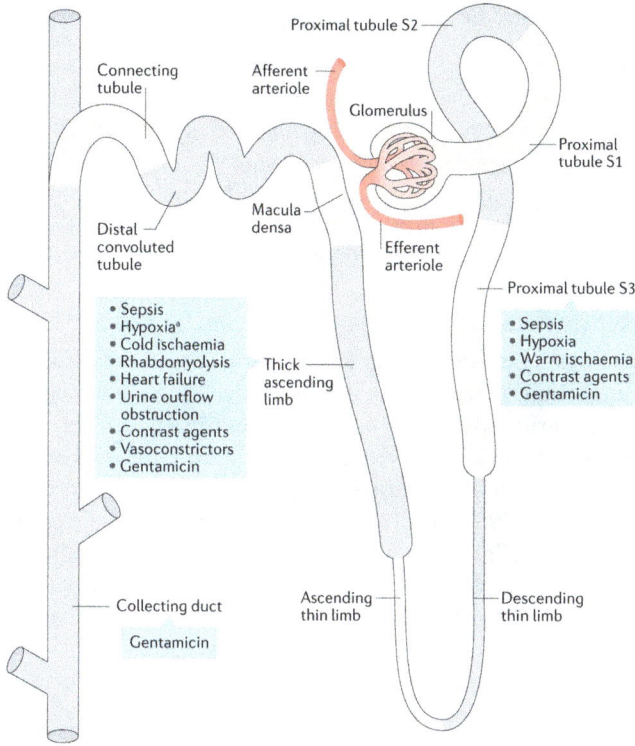

FIGURE 9.6 Schematic diagram showing the susceptibility of each nephric segments that may lead to various acute kidney injuries. (Adopted from Scholz et al. 2021 with permission.)

Under normal conditions, a balance between the supply and demand of oxygen and energy is maintained over the nephron components in the heterogeneous environment. However, such a balance may be disrupted by disturbance of the intrarenal hemodynamics, making the S_3 segment of the PCT and the TAL of the DCT, especially the former, vulnerable to hypoxia or compromised energy supply, triggering AKI that may further develop into CKD, in a manner that relies on the tubular transportation activity. The hemodynamic disturbance may be attributable to hypoperfusion induced by major surgery, heart failure, systemic vasodilation, systemic inflammation and/or inflammatory processes within the kidney, especially under pre-existing endothelial dysfunction in diabetes mellitus patients. External stimuli, e.g., exposure to vascular and/or tubular toxins, including medicine and iodinated contrast agent, are also factors that may disrupt the intrarenal hemodynamics and thus lead to AKI, especially during dehydration (volume depletion) (Scholz et al. 2021; Eloy et al. 1991; Saladin 2007c). Moreover, the difference in the mechanisms of cellular defense and repairing, such as anti-inflammatory or anti-oxidative response, may also be among the factors contributing to AKI. Notably, most of these etiologic factors are summarized in Figure 9.6.

9.4.3 Contrast Agent-Induced Nephrotoxicity

Once intravenously injected into the systemic circulation, the iodinated contrast agent starts to be removed from the body exclusively via renal excretion. Consequently, each nephron in the kidney is exposed to the toxicity associated with iodinated contrast agent. Having understood the renal anatomy, physiology and vulnerability attributable to its complexity in anatomy and heterogeneity in physiology, it is the time for to review the nephrotoxicity associated with iodinated contrast agent (Fähling et al. 2017; Davenport et al. 2020; ACR 2021).

9.4.3.1 Cytotoxicity to Vascular Endothelium and/or Tubular Epithelium

The direct cytotoxicity exerted by iodinated contrast agent on vascular endothelium and tubular epithelium is mainly the damage on cell membrane or impairment of cell membrane integrity, which includes nuclear protrusion, cell shrinkage, fenestration of the endothelial layer and formation of microvilli, ranging from cytoplasmic vacuolization, loss of membrane proteins, e.g., caveolin, and impairment to the Na^+/K^+-ATPase (Eloy et al. 1991; Scholz et al. 2021). For patients with pre-existing conditions, such as endothelial dysfunction in diabetes mellitus wherein the glycocalyx function is impaired, leaves the endothelial cells more vulnerable to the cytotoxicity associated with the iodinated contrast agent. It has been reported in animal models that, due to the cytotoxicity associated with iodinated contrast agent, viscous vesicles may be formed surrounding the vascular endothelial cells or tubular epithelial cells, leading to hypoperfusion and thus ischemia or hypoxia in the endothelium or epithelium, which further worsens the cytotoxic damage initially induced by the contrast media. Specifically, the tubular cells lying at the outer strip of the medulla bear the biggest vulnerability to hypoxia-induced cellular damage, due to heterogeneity in the oxygen supply, and consumption and exposure to the contrast media at high concentration and viscosity (Scholz et al. 2021). The iodinated contrast media may induce apoptosis via other pathways or an interplay of molecular pathways that need to be further investigated. On the other hand, the free iodine molecules have long been recognized as a septic (Sendeski 2011), but it is still under debate whether the trace amount of iodine molecules in the contrast media causes cellular damage (Eloy et al. 1991).

9.4.3.2 Disturbance on Intra-Renal Hemodynamics

The intravenously administered contrast agent may increase the blood viscosity and thus slow blood flow in the peritubular capillaries, especially the vasa recta, which triggers release of endothelin, angiotensin II and prostaglandin. Consequently, the decelerated flow may alter the delicate balance between oxygen supply and consumption, and lead to hypoperfusion and thus ischemia or hypoxia in endothelial cells. Meanwhile, in addition to the direct cytotoxicity mentioned earlier, the iodinated contrast media may disrupt the flow-mediated release of nitric oxide (NO), which is one of the reactive oxidative species (ROS) that acts as a vasodilator (Eloy et al. 1991; Sendeski 2011), leading to constriction of the peritubular capillaries (especially the vasa recta) that may aggravate the hypoperfusion and thus tip the balance between oxygen supply and energy consumption (Fähling et al. 2017; Scholz et al. 2021). Lowered NO production can be due to the loss of endothelial cell viability. Indeed, the constriction of vasa recta induced by iodinated contrast agent has been reported in the literature across all four types of iodinated contrast agent. Notably, the disturbance on intra-renal hemodynamics may also induce oxidative stress (Pizzino et al. 2017) that may be the cause or consequence of endothelial ischemia or hypoxia and further investigation is under way.

9.4.3.3 Disturbance on Intra-Renal Tubulodynamics

The iodinated contrast agent is left alone in the nephric tubules while water is being reabsorbed, which increases the tubular viscosity and leads to a longer stay of iodinated contrast agent in the tubules, i.e., the epithelial cells are exposed to more direct cytotoxicity, especially under the condition of dehydration-induced volume depletion. The elevated viscosity increases the tubular pressure that may lead to vasa recta compression and local vascular resistance to blood flow, aggravating the hypoperfusion, ischemia and/or hypoxia (Fähling et al. 2017; Scholz et al. 2021; Sendeski 2011). Moreover, the injured tubular epithelial cells may compromise the cross-talk between the medullary thick ascending limb (mTAL) and the descending vasa recta (DVR) that regulates the response to reduced blood flow in the DVR. The nephric tubulovascular cross-talk has been revealed in the literature as angiotensin II escalates the presence of intracellular Ca^{+2} in pericytes for vasoconstriction but diminishes its presence in endothelial cells for vasodilation; angiotensin II also elevates the intracellular presence of Ga^{+2} in tubular epithelial cells; catalyzed by nitric oxide synthase, the Ga^{+2} in tubular epithelial cells activates the production of NO; angiotensin II also activates the production of free radical superoxide O_2^- in tubular epithelial cells; with its bioavailability mediated by O_2^-, the NO diffuses from the tubular epithelial cells to the pericytes of DVR, buffering the pericytes' function as vasoconstrictors (Sendeski 2011; Fähling et al. 2017; Zhang and Edwards 2007; Zhao et al. 2014).

9.4.4 Incidence of Contrast-Induced Acute Kidney Injury and Clinical Management

The clinical consequence of CI-AKI has been drawing the community's attention from the very beginning, as evidenced by the papers and data published in the literature, in which the incidence of CI-AKI up to 22.1% was reported. However, it has not been realized that almost all the published data had been actually on the contrast-associated AKI (CA-AKI) until 2008 when Newhouse et al reported their finding that the incidence rate of AKI in patients who have not received intravenous administration of iodinated contrast agent for CT scan is actually comparable to those who did receive (Rao and Newhouse 2006; Newhouse et al. 2008; Newhouse and Roychoudhury 2013; McDonald 2013b). Since then, further studies with a control group and adjustment in the propensity score have been carries out, showing that the incidence of CI-AKI is substantially lower than what had been perceived in previous publications. For example, a study with a registry of 57,925 subjects reported that the incidence rate of clinically relevant CI-AKI is 0.8%–1.7%, confirming the epidemiologic relevance of separating CI-AKI from CA-AKI (ACR 2021).

A meta-analysis of the literature concerning the nephrotoxicity of iodinated contrast agent has shown that there is little difference in nephrotoxicity among the low-osmolality iodinated contrast agents that are currently utilized in clinical settings. By addressing the selection bias in their study design via propensity adjustment and matching, four large-scale studies (Davenport et al. 2013a, 2013b; McDonald et al. 2013a, 2014) published in 2013–2014 reported that intravenous administration of iodinated contrast agents in CT is not an independent risk factor of nephrotoxicity in patients with stable baseline eGFR $\geq$45 ml/min/1.73 m^2, while it is either not nephrotoxic or rarely so in patients with the baseline eGFR in the range 30–44 ml/min/1.73 m^2. In patients with baseline eGFR <30 ml/min/1.73 m^2 (stage IV and V chronic kidney disease), two of the studies found that the intravenous contrast agent is an independent risk factor of nephrotoxicity, while the other two did not (ACR 2021). In clinical practice, 30 ml/min/1.73 m^2 has been a plausible choice if a threshold in eGFR has to be set for stratifying the risk of CI-AKI, since it is consistent with the data published in the literature. Notably, however, eGFR <30 ml/min/1.73 m^2 is not an absolute contraindication for intravenous administration of iodinated contrast agent, and the decision is weighed on the benefits, risks and adequacy of alternative imaging modalities (ACR 2021).

In clinical practice, the screening of at-risk patients starts with checking the patient's medical history for chronic kidney disease, remote AKI, dialysis, kidney surgery, kidney ablation, diabetes mellitus or consumption of metformin or metformin-containing drugs, followed by stratification based on eGFR. In general, eGFR <30 ml/min/1.7 3m^2 is an indication for prophylaxis in the cases wherein the clinical benefits over the risks for intravenous administration of iodinated contrast agent is justified. Though prophylaxis is not indicated in the cases with eGFR $\geq$30 ml/min/1.7 3m^2, consideration should be given to the patients with borderline eGFR 30–44 ml/min/1.73 m^2 and multiple other risk factors. Periprocedural intravenous volume expansion with isotonic fluid such as 0.45% or 0.9% saline is the only evidence-supported prophylaxis regiment, which typically begin 1 hour prior to the CT examination and continues for 3–12 hours post the examination, though a longer regiment (12 hours before and after the examination) has been reported to be superior to the shorter regiment for risk mitigation (ACR 2021; Fähling et al. 2017).

Within the dose range of intravenous administration of iodinated contrast agent, there is no established relationship between the dose and nephrotoxicity, and thus any attempt to mitigate the risk of CI-AKI by reducing the contrast dose is not recommended. Typically, it takes about 20 hours for one administered dose of low osmolality iodinated contrast to be cleared from the circulation and thus a contrast-enhanced CT repeated in a short interval may increase the dose in the circulation and thus the risk of nephrotoxicity. Even though, if the benefits over the risks are clinically justified, a contrast-enhanced scan can be repeated according to clinical context, as long as greater caution is exercised, especially in high-risk patients, such as those with stage IV and V chronic kidney disease or acute kidney injury (ACR 2021; Davenport et al. 2020).

9.5 CONTRAST-ENHANCED MDCT UNDER CLINICAL SETTINGS

An iodinated contrast agent generates substantially better conspicuity in CT for detection and characterization of lesions, including both diseases and dysfunctions due to vascular anomalies and neoplasm, and thus has been utilized in the majority of CT scans in clinics. Given a patient's cardiovascular circulation and renal function, the ultimate goal of applying iodinated contrast agents in clinical CT is to achieve diagnostically adequate enhancement of contrast among the targeted tissues/organs, using the least amount of iodine injected at an acceptable rate, at a radiation dose that is as low as reasonably achievable (ALARA). To reach this goal, one needs to take into account numerous factors related to patient physiology (body weight, height, cardiovascular output and systemic circulation, gender/age, venous access site, hepatic pathophysiology and renal function) and contrast agent (injection duration, rate, concentration, bolus shaping and saline flush). In a contrast-enhanced CT scan, these factors jointly determine the time of contrast arrival and the time to peak contrast enhancement, which in turn demands an adequate design of the protocols for intravenous administration of iodinated contrast agent and CT scan (scan duration, direction and delay (either single phase or multi-phasic)) (Bae 2010).

In clinics, the iodinated contrast agent is usually injected at the antecubital vein, while the forearm or hand veins are options if the antecubital vein is not readily accessible. The route of contrast agent circulation is antecubital vein $\longrightarrow$ right heart $\longrightarrow$ pulmonary circulation $\longrightarrow$ left heart $\longrightarrow$ central arterial system. Under clinical settings, the behavior of contrast enhancement is usually assessed at the abdominal aorta and the liver for angiographic and parenchymal scans, respectively. It is important for us to keep the following points in mind prior to delving into more details:

- The molecules in an iodinated contrast agent are relatively small (~1–2 nm) and highly diffusible, and thus the contrast agent is basically "flow limited" or "perfusion limited", rather than "diffusion limited".
- The kidney, spleen and liver are well perfused organs and show high contrast enhancement in CT.
- As it propagates in the circulation system, the contrast agent dilutes and disperses in its arrival time and intensity because of hemodynamics.
- The contrast medium recirculates in the system via multiple routes and a normal recirculation time is in the range of 15–40 sec.
- For a very short injection (<15 sec), the recirculation contributes little to the peak aortic enhancement.
- In a typical clinical contrast agent injection last longer than 15 sec, the recirculation contributes about 10%–20% to the peak aortic enhancement.
- The propagation of a contrast agent in the body is governed by hemodynamic physiology, while the hemodynamic physiology is perturbed by the injected contrast agent, i.e., they interact with each other.

Through modeling the circulation system, a desired contrast enhancement profile can be achieved using a customized contrast agent injection protocol (Bae 2010).

In the following sections, concise and relatively deep coverage on the timing and interplay among the factors in physiology, contrast injection and CT scan are given.

9.5.1 OPTIMIZATION OF PROTOCOL PARAMETERS RELATED TO PHYSIOLOGY

In general, blood volume (BV) and cardiac output (CO) are the two most important patient-related factors to determine the magnitude and timing of contrast enhancement. Their relationship with body weight (W) and height (H) have been found to be (Bae 2010)

$$BV_{(ml,male)} = 23.6 \cdot H^{0.725} \cdot W^{0.425} - 1220 \tag{9.1}$$

$$BV_{(ml, female)} = 24.8 \cdot H^{0.725} \cdot W^{0.425} - 1954 \tag{9.2}$$

$$CO_{(ml,male \ \& \ female)} = 25.3 \cdot H^{0.725} \cdot W^{0.425} \tag{9.3}$$

Note that, there exists a significant difference in the blood volume between male and female, whereas their cardiac outputs are almost the same. Specifically, the following physiological parameters need to be considered in the design and optimization of protocols.

9.5.1.1 Body Weight

Body weight is the most important factor in determining the magnitude of contrast enhancement in CT. It is a common practice to adjust the amount of iodine mass according to the body weight in a 1:1 manner, i.e., doubled iodine mass should be administered to a patient with doubled body weight. However, such a linear proportion may lead to overestimation of contrast agent in obese patients, since body fat is usually less vascular and thus leads to modest dilution and dispersion of the contrast medium. Notably, as illustrated in Figure 9.7, body weight affects the magnitude of contrast enhancement significantly, while it does little to the timing of enhancement. Body height is also a factor that affects the enhancement magnitude, but to a weaker extent in comparison to the body weight. The so-called body mass index is commonly used in the clinic to adjust the total iodine mass needed in a CT scan, though it is a measure of body thinness, rather than body size. Hence, the body mass index alone should not be the basis for decision-making on iodine mass adjustment, and its coupling with other parameters, such as body weight and body surface area, should be taken into consideration. Actually, body surface area or lean body mass is the more reliable basis to make the decision on iodine mass adjustment, though they are not readily available in clinical practice (Bae 2010).

9.5.1.2 Cardiac Output and Cardiovascular Circulation

As illustrated in Figure 9.8, cardiac output is the most important factor affecting the timing of contrast enhancement. A reduction in the cardiac output slows

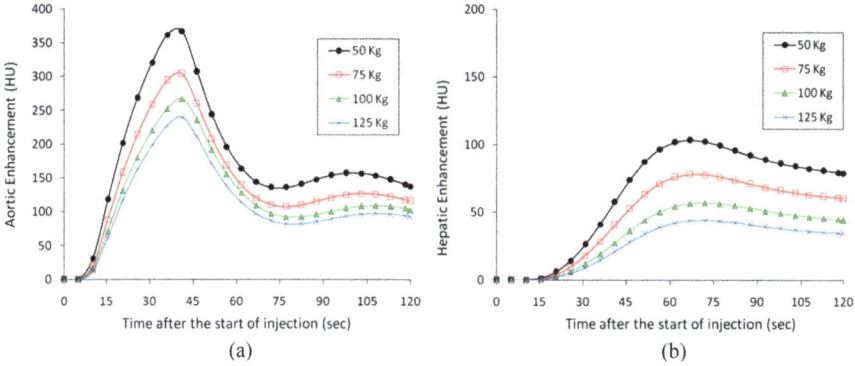

FIGURE 9.7 Typical contrast enhancement profiles as a function of time and their variation over body weight, simulated for a 70 kg, 30-year-old male with an injection volume of 125 mL contrast medium (iodine concentration: 350 mgI/ml) at injection rate 4 mL/sec: (a) aortic enhancement gauged at abdominal aorta, (b) hepatic enhancement gauged at liver. (Adopted from Bae 2010 with permission.)

cardiovascular circulation, leading to proportionally delayed bolus arrival and arterial/parenchymal enhancement, as the bolus washes in slowly and in turn washes out slowly, and the delayed clearance results in a stronger and longer enhancement. Notably, however, compared to a substantial increase in the peak arterial enhancement (Figure 9.8a), the increase in peak parenchymal enhancement due to cardiac output reduction is modest (Figure 9.8b). The typical transit time of contrast bolus from the injection site (antecubital vein) to the aorta is 14–32 sec (median 18 sec), while that from the aorta to the pedal arteries is 6–39 sec (median 15 sec). It also should be noted that vascular disorders, such as stenosis and aneurism, may severely affect the timing of contrast enhancement, especially in with peripheral and cerebral CT angiography or CT perfusion. A large variation in the downstream contrast bolus flow complicates the precise determination of enhancement timing, necessitating the customized scan delay for each patient, particularly in angiographic cases in which scan timing is of essence.

9.5.1.3 Gender and Age

In general, the blood volume of a female is 5%–10% smaller than that of a male, which is the reason behind the clinical observation that the contrast enhancement in the former is slightly stronger than that in the latter (Bae 2010). Furthermore, given the cardiac output that is virtually identical in both male and female, the contrast bolus arrives slightly earlier in a female patient compared to that in a male patient, due to the smaller blood volume. It is well known in physiology that cardiac output decreases with increasing age. Hence, it is not surprising to observe a delayed and stronger contrast enhancement in elderly patients in comparison to mid-age or young patients.

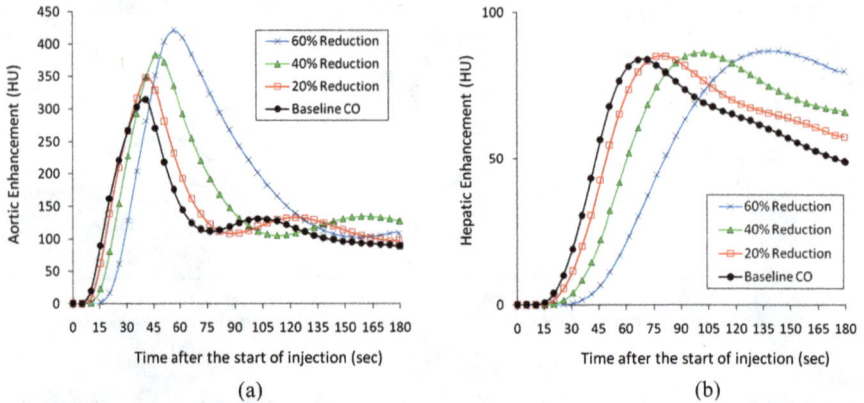

FIGURE 9.8 Typical contrast enhancement profiles as a function of time and their variation over cardiac output reduction, simulated for a 70 kg, 30-year-old male with an injection volume of 125 mL contrast medium (iodine concentration: 350 mgI/ml) at injection rate 4 mL/sec: (a) aortic enhancement gauged at abdominal aorta, (b) hepatic enhancement gauged at liver. (Adopted from Bae 2010 with permission.)

9.5.1.4 Other Factors

Other factors that may affect the magnitude and timing of contrast enhancement include hepatic diseases. For example, a reduction in the hepatic enhancement may be observed in patients with cirrhosis, due to parenchymal fibrosis and lowered portal venous perfusion (Bae 2010). An iodinated contrast agent could induce nephropathy in a clinical CT scan, especially in patients with renal dysfunction or deficiency. In general, the smaller the volume of contrast administered, the less the toxicity. However, it seems that no threshold exists in the volume of iodinated contrast agent, because it has been observed in the clinic that even a 30 ml contrast medium can cause contrast-induced nephropathy in high-risk patients. Hence, clinically speaking, the administration of less iodinated contrast agent in cases with preexisting renal dysfunction is desirable. In practice, as suggested by the Contrast-Induced Nephropathy Consensus Working Panel as a guideline (Bae 2010), preferably no more than a 100 ml contrast medium should be administered to a patient with a glomerular filtration rate below 60 ml/min/1.73 m^2.

9.5.2 OPTIMIZATION OF PROTOCOL PARAMETERS RELATED TO CONTRAST AGENT INJECTION

Having understood the physiology-related factors, we are ready for a brief review of the factors related to contrast agent injection (Bae 2010).

9.5.2.1 Injection Duration

In principle, the injection duration is the most crucial factor to impact both the magnitude and timing of contrast enhancement, and shown in Figure 9.9 are typical cases corresponding to arterial and parenchymal enhancement, respectively. In general, the injection duration should be determined by taking into account CT scanning conditions and clinical objectives, e.g., body size, targeted vessel or organ, and desired enhancement level, in a balanced manner. Listed next are the caveats that should be heeded while the injection duration for a clinical CT scan is being determined (Bae 2010).

- The injection duration directly alters the time to peak enhancement in a vessel or organ.
- It makes more sense to take the contrast injection ending point, rather than the starting point, as the temporal reference for design and optimization of protocols in the contrast injection and CT scan.
- It is advantageous to use a fixed injection duration, other than a fixed injection rate, as the basis for design and optimization of protocols in the contrast injection and CT scan.
- The determination of optimal injection duration in an arterial or angiographic CT scan is more challenging than that in a visceral parenchymal scan.
- Given the contrast agent volume, the injection duration may be shortened on purpose for injection at a high rate, which is particularly useful in arterial and angiographic scans, but is of little utility in venous and parenchymal scans, since the enhancement in the latter cases is mainly determined by the amount of administered iodine mass (see Figure 9.9).
- Because of contrast dispersion, reflux from the right atrium, the pressure performance of the power injector and the risk of stressing at high flow rate, the injection rate should not exceed 8–10 ml/sec, implying that an injection shorter than 15 sec is not recommended in the clinic (see more in next section).

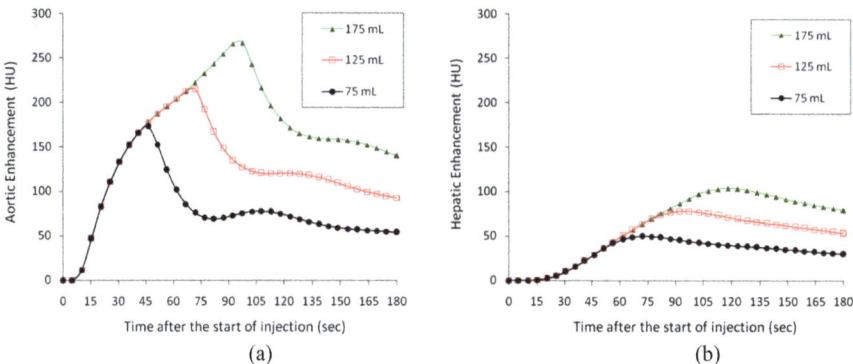

FIGURE 9.9 Typical contrast enhancement profiles as a function of time and their variation over injection duration, simulated for a 70 kg, 30-year-old male at injection rate 2 mL/sec (iodine concentration: 350 mgI/ml): (a) aortic enhancement gauged at abdominal aorta, (b) hepatic enhancement gauged at liver. (Adopted from Bae 2010 with permission.)

9.5.2.2 Injection Rate

Compared to that in single-detector CT, the injection rate used in multi-detector CT is significantly higher. An injection at a high flow rate is preferred in a multi-phasic scan of visceral organs, including the liver, pancreas and kidney, as it results in a larger temporal separation and thus improves the detection and characterization of lesions. However, a close inspection of Figure 9.10 tells us that the peak enhancement increases modestly when the injection rate exceeds 10 ml/sec and 3 ml/sec in arterial and parenchymal scans, respectively. It should be emphasized here that the injection rate in clinics should not exceed 8–10 ml/sec. Meanwhile, the following suggestions on the contrast injection rate in the clinic have been made in the literature (Bae 2010):

- Contrast bolus with the antecubital vein as the injection site at a rate of 2–5 ml/sec is common.
- Contrast bolus with central venous catheter access at a rate of 3–5 ml/sec is feasible and safe.
- Contrast bolus with central venous catheters, peripherally inserted central catheter or small-caliber catheter access at the forearm or hand vein at a 1.5–2.0 ml/sec injection rate is typical.
- A 5–10 ml/sec injection rate is usually administered in CT perfusion to generate a strong peak enhancement with a short peak time.

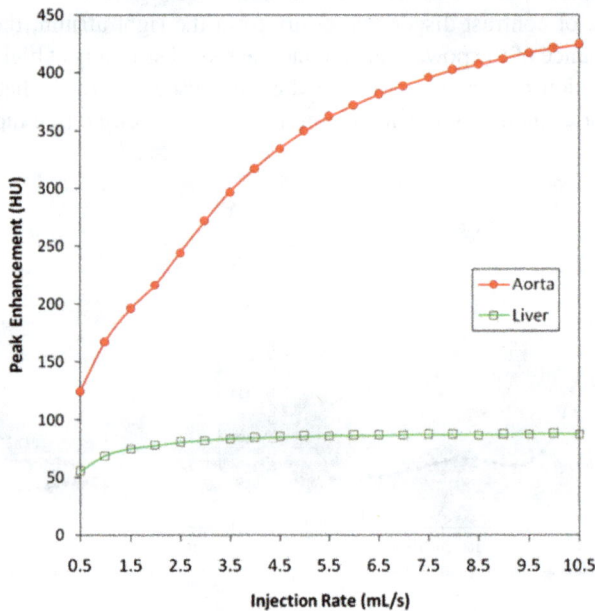

FIGURE 9.10   The profiles showing the distinct behavior between aortic and hepatic peak enhancement in response to injection rate, simulated for a 70 kg, 30-year-old male injected with a fixed amount of contrast volume of 125 ml (iodine concentration: 350 mgI/ml). (Adopted from Bae 2010 with permission)

9.5.2.3 Contrast Agent Concentration

With increasing scan speed, an MDCT demands the injected contrast agent concentration be 350 mgI/ml or higher (Bae 2010). Also, the following points are relevant in designing and optimizing the contrast injection protocol:

- An injection at high concentration is similar to that at high rate in terms of fast delivery of the contrast medium.
- If the volume, rate and duration of the contrast injection are fixed, the injection at high concentration results in stronger peak enhancement and a wider temporal window for CT scan.
- The time to peak enhancement is not altered by an injection of contrast agent at high concentration, if the injection duration and rate remain unchanged.
- Injection of the contrast agent at low concentration may be preferable in a number of clinical cases, especially in the scenario in which saline flush is not available.

It is a good practice to maximize the peak arterial enhancement via administering the iodinated contrast agent at low iodine concentration but high injection rate (i.e., a fast injection).

9.5.2.4 Saline Flush

With the availability of a double-barrel power injector and the increasing application of CT angiography, saline flush is now widely adopted in the clinic. By pushing the tail of injected contrast agent into the central blood volume and making use of the medium that would otherwise go unused in the injector tube and peripheral veins, a saline flush increases not only the efficiency of contrast agent usage but also the level of peak enhancement. Especially, the saline flush is beneficial in the cases wherein a small volume of contrast medium is administered. Notably, however, a saline flush at volume larger than 20–30 ml no longer helps improve the efficiency of contrast agent usage (Bae 2010).

9.5.2.5 Other Factors

The other main factors that should be taken into account in design and optimization of a contrast injection protocol include the shaping of the contrast bolus injection. Driven by clinical applications with recourse to the power injector, the shape of the contrast agent can be administered at a uni-phasic rate, bi-phasic rate and even tri-phasic rate. In clinical settings, to improve the detection and characterization of lesions, a desired contrast enhancement pattern can be achieved by adequately tailoring the bolus shape (Bae 2010).

9.5.3 OPTIMIZATION OF PROTOCOL PARAMETERS RELATED TO MDCT SCAN

Thus far, we have only discussed the factors that interactively determine the temporal variation, especially in magnitude and timing, of the administered contrast agent. It is not hard to understand that the ultimate goal of clinical CT can only be achieved if the scan starts and finishes at the right time, which means that a CT scan should follow the temporal variation of the administered contrast agent promptly and adequately.

9.5.3.1 Scan Duration

It is straightforward to understand that a longer CT scan requires a longer period of peak enhancement. It has been identified that scan duration is the most important factor in design and optimization of protocols for contrast injection. In MDCT, a typical contrast-enhanced scan can be conducted in approximately 10 sec, while the scans that demand much longer duration, such as peripheral run-off angiography, cardiac and coronary angiography, multi-phasic abdominal organ scan, and perfusion, do exist. In practice, the CT scan range is specified based on a scout image (also called a topogram) according to the order placed by the physician. The scan duration is calculated by taking into account the scan range and mode (axial or spiral/helical), X-ray beam aperture, gantry rotation speed and table speed (spiral/helical pitch).

9.5.3.2 Scan Direction

With respect to scan direction, a CT should scan along the direction that chases the contrast bolus flow, i.e., the scan starts at an upstream location with peak enhancement and moves downstream in pace with the bolus flow. However, exceptions exist in the clinic for special considerations. For example, to avoid the blurring caused by respiratory motion in the thoracic scan for detection and characterization of pulmonary emboli, the lower lobes, where the emboli occur most frequently, are usually scanned first (Bae 2010). Other exceptions are CT scans in which the beam-hardening artifacts caused by the massive contrast agent in the superior vena cava and carotid arteries need to be avoided.

9.5.3.3 Scan Phase

A multi-phasic scan is routinely carried out in the clinic to improve the detection and characterization of lesions in the liver, pancreas, kidney and associated vessels, which makes the determination of scan protocols more challenging. Due to space limitations, an in-depth introduction to the principles of the multi-phasic scan is omitted herein, and readers who are interested in the guidelines are referred to the literature (Bae 2010).

9.5.4 Contrast-Enhanced MDCT: A Concert of Physiology, Contrast Injection and CT Scan

With the scan duration determined, a sound strategy to acquire high-quality CT images is to match the mid-scan point with the instant at which the contrast enhancement reaches its pinnacle, i.e., the time from the beginning of contrast medium injection to the peak enhancement T_{peak}. Once T_{peak} is determined, the delay of scan relative to the beginning of contrast agent injection to match the mid-scan point and the peak enhancement is calculated as (Bae 2010)

$$T_{scan-delay} = T_{peak} - T_{scan-duration} / 2 \qquad (9.4)$$

In practice, the time to peak enhancement is defined as

$$T_{peak} = T_{ID} + T_{CTT}, \qquad\qquad (9.5)$$

where T_{ID} denotes the injection duration, and T_{CTT} is the time of contrast transit that is defined by taking the completion of contrast injection as the reference. It is not hard to understand that there is no guarantee of accurate estimation of either the T_{peak} or T_{CTT} because of the variety in patients' circulation systems and resultant variation in the contrast medium transit time, not to mention that pre-existing disorders in the circulation system, such as stenosis, aneurism, cirrhosis and renal dysfunction, may make the situation even worse. This means that, T_{peak} or T_{CTT} can only be reliably determined via an experimental process. In practice, it has been found that it is more feasible to gauge another time index called the contrast arrival time T_{arr}, which is a surrogate of T_{CTT}. Under clinical settings, the following two regiments are adopted to determine the T_{arr} (Bae 2010):

- **Test bolus**: In this approach, a small bolus (10–20 ml) of contrast agent is injected prior to the administration of a full bolus for diagnostic imaging. Once the injection of the test bolus is started, a series of images at low radiation dose are acquired at a temporal interval of roughly 2–3 sec, right at the starting end of the scan range specified in the topogram. A region of interest (ROI) of adequate size is placed in the targeted organ (usually aorta or cardiac chamber) to gauge the temporal variation in intensity. By analyzing the temporal profile, the time to peak enhancement of this small bolus is defined as the contrast arrival time T_{arr}.
- **Bolus tracking**: In this approach, a baseline image is acquired at the reference location specified in the topogram right before the injection of a full contrast bolus. At the beginning of an injection, a technologist stays in the scanner room to check the integrity of the injection site and makes sure there is no occurrence of extravasation. Once the technologist leaves the scanner room, a series of images at low radiation dose are acquired at an interval of roughly 2–3 scc at the starting end of scan range. Similar to what is done in the test-bolus approach, a temporal profile corresponding to an ROI placed in the targeted organ is recorded and displayed on the CT console. Immediately after the intensity reaches a preset threshold (50–150 HU), the bolus tracking process terminates and the elapsed time is recorded as T'_{arr}. After an additional delay, called diagnostic delay, the diagnostic CT scan starts.

The relationship among $T_{scan\text{-}delay}$, $T_{scan\text{-}duration}$, T_{peak}, T_{CT}, T_{arr} and T_{ID} can be understood using the schematic diagram presented in Figure 9.11. Furthermore, regarding the test-bolus and bolus-tracking methods, the following points are relevant (Bae 2010):

- The T'_{arr} gauged via the bolus-tracking approach with the threshold preset at 50 HU seems equivalent to the T_{arr} acquired using the test-bolus approach, i.e., $T'_{arr} \cong T_{arr}$.

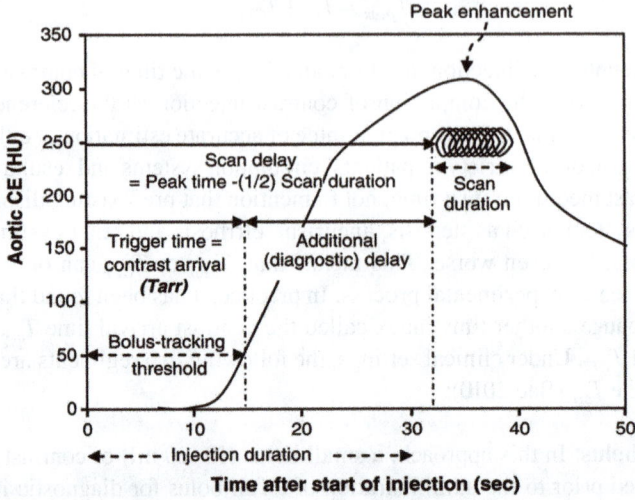

FIGURE 9.11 The schematic graph shows how the scan delay is determined in a clinical CT scan and the relationship among the temporal variables that plays an important role in the design and optimization of scan timing. (Adopted from Bae 2010 with permission.)

- The bolus-tracking approach is adopted in a vast majority of clinical CT scans, while the test-bolus method is preferable in cardiovascular imaging, especially CT coronary angiography, since the latter provides an opportunity to inspect the integrity of injection site, variation of heart rate over breath holding and whether beta-blocker should be administered.
- The test-bolus approach is preferable in the cases in which a very short (<10 sec) injection duration is needed.

Neither T_{arr} nor T'_{arr} is directly used as the scan delay. Rather, they should be used as the basis to customize the scan delay for individual patients by adding a post-trigger delay (diagnostic delay).

It has been empirically determined that there exists the following relationship between T_{CTT} and T_{arr} (Bae 2010):

$$T_{CTT} = k \cdot T_{arr} \pm \Delta T \tag{9.6}$$

Consequently, Equation 9.5 becomes

$$T_{peak} = T_{ID} + k \cdot T_{arr} \pm \Delta T \tag{9.7}$$

Note that both k and ΔT are dependent on the anatomic location to be scanned and the diagnostic purpose (angiographic or parenchymal). For example, the pulmonary angiography and abdominal aortic angiography share the following equation in calculating the time to peak enhancement:

$$T_{peak} = T_{ID} + T_{arr} - 5, \qquad (9.8)$$

where the corresponding T_{arr} is gauged at the main pulmonary artery and abdominal aorta, respectively. Notably, the determination of T_{peak} becomes more complicated in multi-phasic CT scans. For example, in a dual-phase hepatic CT scan with T_{arr} gauged at the abdominal aorta, the T_{peak} corresponding to the arterial phase is

$$T_{peak} = T_{ID} + T_{arr} - 5 \qquad (9.9)$$

while that corresponding to the hepatic phase accounting for the portal circulatory delay can be determined with either of the following two equations:

$$T_{peak} = T_{ID} + T_{arr} + 25 \qquad (9.10)$$

$$T_{peak} = T_{ID} + 2 \cdot T_{arr} + 5 \qquad (9.11)$$

With all the major points presented thus far, it should no longer be difficult for one to understand the scan timing of typical clinical CT scans, as presented in Figure 9.12 (Bae 2010).

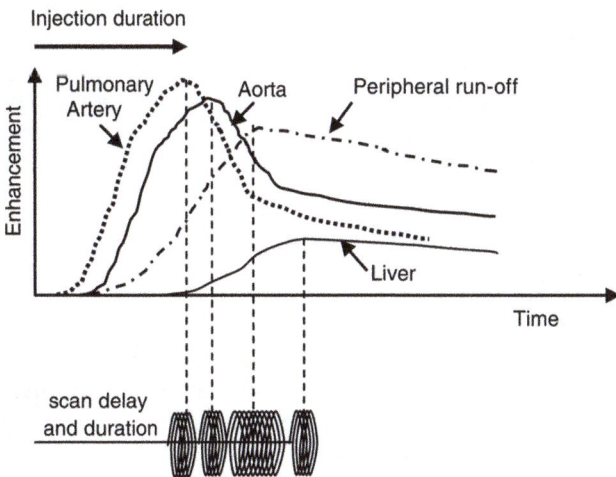

FIGURE 9.12 The schematic graph illustrates the scan timing in typical clinical CT scans that are routinely conducted in the clinic. (Adopted from Bae 2010 with permission.)

9.5.5 CLINICAL EXAMPLES

To appreciate the relevance and significance of timing and interplay among human physiology, contrast injection and CT scan in the protocols for contrast-enhanced CT in clinical settings, a few routine protocols corresponding to scanning of the head and neck, thorax, abdomen, peripheral run-off and angiography in 16-DCT and 64-DCT are presented in Tables 9.1–9.5, respectively, in which the image slice thickness plays an important role in the design and optimization (Bae 2010).

9.6 NOVEL CT CONTRAST AGENTS: PROGRESSION AND OUTLOOK

Using the effects of blood pool and body compartments, the iodinated contrast agent substantially increases the sensitivity and specificity (and thus clinical utility) of CT in detection and characterization of vascular and visceral parenchymal pathologies. Implemented in the form of small molecules, the iodinated contrast agent is indispensable to CT clinical applications, with its efficacy, safety and relatively low cost being greatly appreciated by the entire healthcare community. In the past three decades, research, e.g., the effort on iosimenol and GE-145 (Lusic and Grinstaff 2013), continues to make this relatively matured contrast agent even better for diagnostic CT, with the focus on improving the viscosity for a lowered likelihood of delayed adverse reaction in the non-ionic iso-osmolality iodinated contrast agent that is in the form of dimeric rings.

Among all the imaging modalities that are widely used in clinics, CT is certainly the one with its image qualities well balanced over contrast resolution (sensitivity), spatial resolution and temporal resolution, though its sensitivity (10^{-3} M) is considerably lower than MRI (10^{-5} M) and substantially lower than PET/SPECT (10^{-10} M) (Roessl et al. 2011; Kim et al. 2017). As elucidated next, in the past three decades, lifting CT's contrast resolution has been one of the most challenging tasks to be accomplished by the R&D community, through innovations in exploring more materials of higher X-ray attenuation, formulating contrast agent for longer half-life in the systemic circulation, boosting the local distribution via biomarker targeted delivery and uptake, and improving the profiles in bio-tolerability and toxicity.

9.6.1 MATERIALS ALTERNATIVE TO IODINE TO MAKE CONTRAST AGENTS FOR MDCT

Iodine has been the material for fabrication of the contrast agent used in X-ray–related modalities for a long time. However, it is still fair to state that the iodine is actually not optimal, particularly in CT, in terms of contrast generation, though it may be a good choice from other perspectives, such as biosafety, natural availability and cost. In clinical settings, to penetrate the body of an adult patient at average habitus, the peak voltage of CT for routine diagnostic imaging is set at 120 kVp, leading to an effective energy in the range between 40 and 60 keV (~1/3–1/2 kVp). This range misses iodine's K-edge (33.2 keV) at which the highest attenuation occurs, while

TABLE 9.1

Typical Protocols of Head and Neck CT for a 70 kg Patient

Exam	Contrast dose	IR	ID	SD	Fixed SD	Variable SD	Circulation-Adjusted SD	Saline
Brain parenchyma	80 ml of 300 mg I/ml (0.3–0.4 g I/kg)	1 ml/sec or hand injection	1–2 min	Variable	5 min	NA	NA	NE
Neck soft tissue	100 ml of 300 mg I/ml (0.4 g I/kg)	2 ml/sec	50 sec	Variable	50–90 sec	ID+10–SD/2	ID+T_{arr}–2–SD/2 (T_{arr} @ asce. aorta)	NE
Neck and brain angiography	100 ml of 350 mg I/ml (16-DCT) 75 ml of 350 mg I/ml (64-DCT)	4 ml/sec (16-DCT) 4.5 ml/sec (64-DCT)	25 sec (16-DCT) 17 sec (64-DCT)	10–15 sec (16-DCT) 5–10 sec (64-DCT)	15 sec (neck) 18–20 sec (brain)	ID+5–SD/2 (neck) ID+8–SD/2 (brain)	ID+T_{arr}–7–SD/2 (neck) ID+T_{arr}–4–SD/2 (brain) (T_{arr} @ asce. aorta)	E
Brain perfusion	50 ml of 300 mg I/ml	4–10 ml/sec	<10 sec	<60 sec	5 sec	5 sec	5 sec	E

Source: Bae 2010.

Note: SD, scan delay; ID, injection duration; IR, injection rate; min, minute; sec, second; E, essential; NE, non-essential.

TABLE 9.2

Typical Protocols of Thoracic CT Scans for a 70 kg Patient

Exam	Contrast Dose	IR	ID	SD	Fixed SD	Variable SD	Circulation-Adjusted SD	Saline
Routine chest	70 ml of 300–350 mg I/ml	2–3 ml/sec	30–40 sec	5–20 sec	40–60 sec	ID+5–SD/2	ID+T_{arr}−7–SD/2 (T_{arr} @asce. aorta)	NE
Pulmonary angiography	120 ml of 350 mg I/ml for venogram 100 ml of 350 mgI/ml	4–5 ml/sec	20–25 sec or 15 + SD	3–4 min for venogram 5–10 sec	15 sec (16-DCT) 20 sec (64-DCT)	ID+5–SD	ID+T_{arr}−5–SD (T_{arr} @main pulmonary aorta)	E
Aortic and coronary angiography	100 ml of 350 mg I/ml (16-DCT) 75 ml of 350 mg I/ml (64-DCT)	4 ml/sec (16-DCT) 4.5–5 ml/ sec (64-DCT)	25 sec (16-DCT) 15 sec (64-DCT) or 15+SD/2	10–15 sec (16-DCT) 5–10 sec (64-DCT) Longer for coronary	20 sec	ID+5–SD/2 (thora. aorta, coronary) ID+10–SD/2 (abdo. aorta)	ID+T_{arr}−7–SD/2 (thoracic aorta, coronary; T_{arr} @ asec. aorta) ID+T_{arr}−5–SD/2 (abdominal aorta, (T_{arr} @abdo. aorta)	E

Source: Bae 2010.

Notes: SD, scan delay; ID, injection duration; IR, injection rate; min, minute; sec, second; E, essential; NE, non-essential.

TABLE 9.3

Typical Protocols of Abdominal CT for a 70 kg Patient

Exam	Contrast Dose	IR	ID	SD	Fixed SD	Variable SD	Circulation-Adjusted SD	Saline
Liver and routine abdomen	100 ml of 350 mg I/ml (0.5 g/kg)	4 ml/sec (dual phase) 2–3 ml/sec (hepatic)	25–30 sec (dual phase) 35–50 sec (hepatic) 3–10 min (delayed)	10–15 sec (16-DCT) 5–10 sec (64-DCT)	30–35 sec (arterial) 65–70 sec (hepatic)	ID+10–SD/2 (arterial) ID+40–SD/2 (hepatic)	ID+T_{arr}–5–SD/2 (arterial, T_{arr} @ abdo. aorta) ID+T_{arr}+25–SD/2 or ID+2 T_{arr}+10–SD/2 (hepatic)	E (dual) NE (hepatic only)
Pancreas	100–120 ml of 50 mg I/ml (dual) 120–140 ml of 350 mg I/ml (single combined)	4–5 ml/sec (dual) 2.5–3 ml/sec (single)	25–30 sec (dual) 50 sec (single)	10–15 sec (16-DCT) 5–10 sec (64-DCT)	35–40 sec (pancreatic) 65–70 sec (hepatic) 60 sec (single)	ID+15–SD/2 (pancreatic) ID+40–SD/2 (hepatic)	ID+T_{arr}–SD/2 (pancreatic, T_{arr} @abdo. aorta) ID+T_{arr}+25–SD/2 or ID+2 T_{arr}+10–SD/2 (hepatic)	E (dual) NE (hepatic only)
Kidney	100–120 ml of 350 mg I/ml	4 ml/sec (CM phase) 2.5–3 ml/sec (no CM phase)	25–30 sec (CM phase) 30–50 sec (no CM phase)	10–15 sec (16-DCT) 5–10 sec (64-DCT)	35–45 sec (CM phase) 75–90 sec (NG phase) 10 min (UG phase)	ID+15-SD/2 (CM phase) ID+55–SD/2 (NG phase)	ID+T_{arr}–SD/2 (CM; T_{arr} @ abdo. aorta) ID+3 T_{arr}+10–SD/2 (NG phase)	E (CM)

Source: Bae 2010.

Notes: SD, scan delay; ID, injection duration; IR, injection rate; min, minute; sec, second; E, essential; NE, non-essential; CM: corticomedullary; NG: nephrographic; UG: urographic.

TABLE 9.4

Typical Protocols of Peripheral Run-Off CT for a 70 kg Patient

Exam	Contrast Dose	IR	ID	SD	Fixed SD	Variable SD	Circulation-Adjusted SD	Saline
Peripheral run-off angiography	125–140 ml of 350 mg I/ml	3.5–4 ml/sec or biphasic or exponentially decelerated	35 sec or 15 + SD/2	40 sec	NA	NA	$ID+T_{art}-5-SD/2$ (abdo. aorta); T_{art} @abdo. aorta)	Useful

Source: Bae 2010.

Notes: SD, scan delay; ID, injection duration; IR, injection rate; min, minute; sec, second; E, essential; NE, non-essential.

TABLE 9.5

Typical Protocols of CT Angiography for Patients in Various Groups of Body Weight

Scanner	Procedure	Body Weight (kg)	SD (sec)	ID/IR (sec)/(ml/sec)	Fixed SD (sec)	Adjusted SD (sec)
16-DCT	Pulmonary angiography	<60 60–90 >90	8–15	25/4 25/4.5 25/5	15–20	T_{arr} + 5 (bolus-tracking 100HU @ pulmonary artery; 1st scan @ 10 sec after injection starts)
	Aortic angiography	<60 60–90 >90	5–10	20/4 20/4.5 20/5	20	T_{arr} + 5 (bolus-tracking 50–100HU @ aorta)
	Peripheral run-off angiography (slow circulation)	<60 60–90 >90	40	35/3.5 35/4 35/4.5	NA	T_{arr} + 10 (bolus-tracking 50–100HU @ aorta)
64-DCT	Pulmonary angiography	<60 60–90 >90	5–7	20/4 20/4.5 20/5.5	20	T_{arr} + 10 (bolus-tracking 100HU @ pulmonary artery; 1st scan @ 10 sec after start of injection)
	Aortic angiography	<60 60–90 >90	3–5	15/4.5 15/5 15/5.5	20	T_{arr} + 5 (bolus-tracking 50–100 HU @ aorta)
	Peripheral run-off angiography (normal circulation)	< 60 60–90	20–30	25/4 25/5	NA	T_{arr} + 10 (bolus-tracking 50–100 HU @ aorta)

Source: Courtesy of KT Bae, MD, Radiology, 2010.

Notes: SD, scan delay; ID, injection duration; IR, injection rate.

the situation gets even worse in cases wherein 140 kVp (effective energy ~43–70 keV) has to be employed for scanning a patient at large habitus. Hence, it is rational to investigate the feasibility of other materials with K-edges within CT's effective energy range. Following is a summary of the candidate materials that have been studied in the literature.

- **Gadolinium**: Being an element of the lanthanide family, the K-edge of gadolinium ($Z = 64$) is at 50.2 keV, which is within CT's effective energy range and thus gadolinium is more appropriate than iodine to be the material for generation of contrast in a "per mole" manner (Gierada and Bae 1999). In its free ion form, Gd^{3+} is extremely toxic, as it competes with Ca^{2+} in biological systems and processes. However, if combined with polyaminocarbolxylic acid, the formed gadolinium chelating complex is quite stable thermomechanically and biologically. This is the reason underlying the fact that gadolinium-based contrast agents have been approved by the Food and Drug Administration for MRI in clinical applications. In theory, gadolinium would be a good choice as the material for fabricating CT contrast agent, whereas, in practice, the clinically tolerable concentration of gadolinium in MRI contrast agent is substantially lower than that of iodine in CT contrast agent, implying that, if used as a contrast agent in CT, the gadolinium-based contrast agent may not be as effective as the iodinated CT contrast agent. It has been found that to generate an attenuation in CT that is the same as that generated by iodinated CT contrast agent, the dose of gadolinium-based MRI contrast has to be at an extent that would be clinically unacceptable in terms of toxicity (Gierada and Bae 1999).
- **Gold**: With its K-edge at 81 keV, gold ($Z = 79$) is a much stronger attenuator of X-rays and thus generates much stronger contrast in CT in comparison to iodine (roughly 2.7-fold more attenuating per unit weight) (Lusic and Grinstaff 2013). Gold has long been identified as one of the most potential alternative materials to iodine to make a CT contrast agent (Chhour et al. 2017), as exemplified by the commercial availability of gold-based nanoparticulate (AuNP) for imaging vascular and visceral parenchymal lesions in animal models (see more details on nanoparticulate contrast agent in Section 9.6.2). Gold is biochemically stable in physiologic environments under various pH and temperature, and exhibits excellent in vitro and in vivo biocompatibility, though more in-depth studies of its toxicity are needed. Notably, the K-edge of gold is modestly too high for conventional CT, but may offer opportunities for spectral CT implemented via energy-integration or photon-counting detection of X-rays. Moreover, it should be mentioned that the price tag of gold in the marketplace may limit its chance to be the material for fabrication of CT contrast agent.
- **Bismuth**: Owing to its strong attenuation of X-rays, bismuth ($Z = 83$) has long been used as a material for shielding the reproductive organs from

X-rays in clinical settings. In light of gold's price tag, bismuth has been investigated as a substitute for gold in fabrication of CT contrast agents (Fu et al. 2020), especially in the form of nanoparticles (Lusic and Grinstaff 2013). In general, bismuth's profile of biochemical stability under physiological environments is not as good as that of gold, in addition to the difficulties in modifying the surface of bismuth-based nanoparticles. Furthermore, the K-edge of bismuth (91 keV) is even higher than that of gold, which is not optimal for diagnostic imaging with conventional CT, though, similar to the case of gold, it may offer the opportunity for spectral CT implemented via X-ray detection based on either energy integration or photon counting.

- **Tantalum**: Recently, tantalum ($Z = 73$) has been drawing attention as a material to make CT contrast agent for scanning of obese patients wherein a high peak voltage (140 kVp) has to be adopted for adequate penetration (Schöckel et al. 2020; Shahid et al. 2020). The K-edge of tantalum is at 67.4 keV, which falls well within the effective energy corresponding to 140 kVp (~43.3–70 keV). Using swine as the animal model, the tantalum-based contrast agent formatted as nanoparticles (carboxybetaine zwitterionic TaO oxide) at size 3.1±0.5 nm exhibits a strong range in vascular (aorta: 19%–49%) and parenchymal (hepatic: 26%–47%) contrast enhancement compared to nonionic monomeric iodinated contrast agent (iopromidine), if the injections are identical in terms of mass concentration. Notably, though the carboxybetaine zwitterionic tantalum is formatted as nanoparticles in the reported studies, its size is comparable to that of conventional iodinated contrast agent (nonionic monomer: ~1.9 nm; dimeric: ~2.2 nm) (FitzGerald et al. 2016). Thus, similarity in the pharmacological and pharmacokinetic profiles, such as half-time in systemic circulation, tissue retention and endothelial permeation, has been reported in the literature (Schöckel et al. 2020; Shahid et al. 2020).

- **Hafnium**: Hafnium ($Z = 72$) is tantalum's neighbor in the periodic table, with its K-edge at 65.3 keV, which is just slightly lower than that of tantalum (Schöckel et al. 2020; Shahid et al. 2020). It should be of no surprise that the performance of contrast enhancement by hafnium in CT is quite comparable to that of tantalum-based contrast agent, particularly in the cases in which the patient's habitus is large and the peak voltage has to be set high at 140 keV. In a way similar to the fabrication of gadolinium-based contrast agent, the hafnium-based contrast is formatted as a chelating complex, with its pharmacological and pharmacokinetic profiles being comparable to that of gadolinium (Schöckel et al. 2020).

It is interesting to note that other materials of high atomic number, e.g., ytterbium ($Z = 70$, K-edge: 61.3 keV) and tungsten ($Z = 74$, K-edge: 69.5 keV), have also been proposed as alternative materials to iodine, since they are more attenuating at their K-edges than iodine in the effective energy range of conventional CT. It also should be noted that the toxicity of those potential metal materials for fabrication of CT contrast agents should be further investigated in depth via animal models and eventually clinical trials, though lots of encouraging but incomplete data in this regard have been reported in the literature (Lusic and Grinstaff 2013; Schöckel et al. 2020; Shahid et al. 2020).

9.6.2 NANOPARTICULATED CONTRAST AGENTS FOR CT

Once an injection starts, the concentration of iodinated contrast agent is diluted in the blood pool due to dispersion in the intravascular space, extravasation to the extracellular space and renal excretion. To reach adequate enhancement of contrast in CT, the administration of iodinated contrast needs to be carried out using power injector at a sufficient injection duration and rate (Bae 2010). As shown in Figure 9.12, once the injection ends, the contrast enhancement in arteries drops immediately, as the extravasation to the extracellular space and renal excretion are still going on, which makes a match in timing between the contrast agent injection and CT scan critical to acquiring images of high quality in cardiovascular applications. In clinical workflow, slowing the declination of the iodinated contrast agent's concentration in the blood pool would be beneficiary. Moreover, an adequate longer stay (tens of minute, rather than tens of second) of iodinated contrast agents in the circulation may facilitate targeted delivery to and taking up by vascular and parenchymal pathologies. As introduced next, contrast agents in the form of nanoparticles may be one of the approaches toward this goal.

9.6.2.1 Variety in Nanoparticle Structures

Aimed at having a high payload as imaging probes or therapeutics, or both, and adequate half-time in systemic circulation, a variety of nanostructures have been proposed and investigated as the vehicle of delivering nanoparticulate agents in nanomedicine. They range from the simplest ones, such as nanosuspensions, nanoemulsions and liposomes, to more sophisticated forms, such as nanospheres, nanocapsules, nanorods, nanocages, micelles and dendrimers (Lusic and Grinstaff 2013; Kim 2017). There may or may not be solid cores in those structures, but, if there are, the cores are usually where the payloads are stored, though the payloads can in principle be attached to anywhere, including the surface, in the particle. In nanoparticulate CT contrast agents, there usually exists one (or multiple for multimodal imaging) core coated with lipid or polymer, in which the contrast-generating materials are loaded. In general, the structure of a nanoparticle can strongly influence its pharmacological properties, such as solubility, biodistribution, half-life of circulation and biocompatibility. Notably, it has been reported that certain nanostructures can induce hypersensitivity reactions that has been drawing the community's attention. Readers who are interested in more details regarding nanoparticle structures are referred to the literature (Lusic and Grinstaff 2013; Kim et al. 2017).

9.6.2.2 Manipulation of Nanoparticle Size

Nominally, the size of nanoparticles falls in the range of 1–1000 nm, which determines the route for them to get removed from the systemic circulation. Nanoparticles under 3 nm are rapidly excreted from the body via glomerular filtration in the kidneys, while those larger than 80 nm can be readily taken up by the liver and the spleen via the reticuloendothelial system (RES) in which macrophages and other phagocytic cells play the role of scavengers (Lusic and Grinstaff 2013). Hence, the RES response can be taken advantage of for detecting and characterizing hepatocellular carcinoma or malignance in the spleen if the nanoparticle size is large (80 nm). For those nanoparticles in between, their size can be manipulated to (i) maintain the enhancement of vascular contrast in the blood pool by adjusting the rates of renal excretion and/or endothelial permeation and (ii) facilitate the taking up by the targeted pathologies when the strategy of targeted delivery (see later) is adopted.

9.6.2.3 Coating of Nanoparticle Surface

The surface of the nanoparticulate contrast agent can be manipulated to alter its hydrophilicity, lipophilicity and other physiochemical properties. For example, with an aqueous core loaded with iodine, liposomes are in the form of nanospheres shelled by a lipid bilayer (Lusic and Grinstaff 2013). In the "stealth" liposomes, their surface are coated with polyethylene glycol (termed *PEGylation*) to shield the surface from aggregation, opsonization and phagocytosis, as such their half-life in the systemic circulation can be extended, while their immunogenicity can be mitigated. Recently, various polymers have been preferably utilized to form nanoparticles that are biodegradable for improving the profiles of biosafety in intended applications (see more details later) (Lusic and Grinstaff 2013).

9.6.3 FUNCTIONALIZATION FOR BIOMARKER-TARGETED DELIVERY

In addition to being coated for optimizing physiochemical properties, the surface of nanoparticles can be functionalized by molecular conjugation to guide their delivery toward atherosclerotic and/or neoplastic pathologies. A few paradigms based on the mechanism of antigen–antibody, enzyme–inhibitor or ligand–receptor interaction have been proposed thus far. For example, it has been reported in animal studies that the EGFR (epidermal growth factor receptor) conjugated AuNP can be taken up by squamous cell carcinoma, while that conjugated with the ligand bombesin (BBN) peptides can target prostate tumors wherein the receptor gastrin-releasing peptides are overexpressed (Lusic and Grinstaff 2013; Kim et al. 2017). Another example was via the enzyme–inhibitor interaction, in which the AuNP conjugated with lisinopril – a tripeptide ACE (angiotensin converting enzyme) inhibitor – can be taken up by pulmonary tissues wherein ACE is overexpressed in response to fibrosis. Of special note is the use of an escalated metabolic rate in

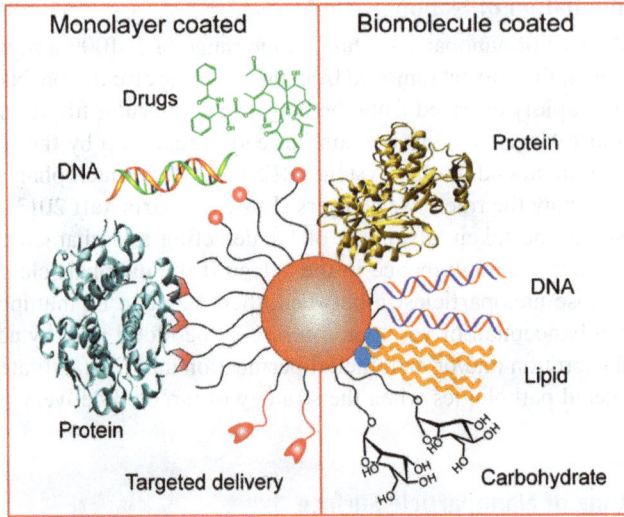

FIGURE 9.13 The schematic diagram showing the example of gold nanoparticles with a monolayer or biomolecule coating strategy for targeted delivery of contrast agents in CT. (Adopted from Rana 2012 with permission.)

cancerous cells, in which the AuNP conjugated with 2-deoxy-D-glucose (2-DG) can be selectively taken up. The biomarker-targeted delivery of the contrast agent may be a game changer in paradigm and many more studies are under way (Rana et al. 2012). As an example, Figure 9.13 shows the potential strategies that may be employed for biomarker-targeted delivery of AuNP as the CT contrast agent for diagnostic imaging.

9.6.4 BIODEGRADABLE NANOPARTICULATED CONTRAST AGENTS

In general, the nanoparticles that are relatively larger in size are taken up by RES, accumulated in the liver, and eventually may undergo hepatic metabolism and be removed from the body along with bile and feces. However, this may not be the case for nanoparticulate CT contrast agents when heavy metals, e.g., gold or bismuth, are used in the formulation. The concerns on the biosafety of metal-based nanoparticulate CT contrast can be mitigated if the nanoparticles, with or without biomarker-targeting capability, are biodegradable in controlled manners. Recently, the schemes of theranosis, wherein imaging probes and therapeutics are co-payloads and delivered to pathologies at the right timing and dose, are gaining attention from the community. Being biodegradable, nanoparticles can be naturally degraded under the physiological environment to release the payload at targeted sites while retaining its integrity at off-target sites. In making biodegradable nanoparticles, polymers have shown high biocompatibility and biosafety, and thus has been preferably adopted by either embedding or encapsulating the payloads within the polymeric matrix, or adsorbing them onto the surface. The degradation rate of polymeric nanoparticles are affected by many factors, including the particles' property, such as size, structure and molecular weight, and/or physiological conditions such as pH and temperature. Eventually, the degraded products become less toxic biologically and gradually excreted from the body via metabolism, making the biodegradable nanoparticulate CT contrast agent physiologically safe.

9.7 DISCUSSION

As the result of decades of R&D, iodinated contrast agents in the form of small molecules have been the state of the art for CT in clinical practice thus far and will continue to be state of the art in the foreseeable future. The success of non-ionic low-osmolality and iso-osmolality iodinated contrasts is grounded on their efficacy, biosafety, patient comfort, fit into the clinical workflow and low cost. To improve CT's patency, mainly the low contrast resolution for early detection and characterization of atherosclerotic and neoplastic diseases, advanced contrast agents with longer half-life in systemic circulation and stronger enhancement in local (lesion) contrast are needed. The biodegradable nanoparticulate contrast agents hold promise, since, potentially, they are physiochemically and biochemically stable to sustain longer half-life in systemic circulation, capable of controlling the rate of payload(s) release, and are non-toxic and non-immunogenic.

There exist two approaches for nanoparticulate contrast agents to increase contrast enhancement in CT. The first is to use high atomic number materials, e.g., gold or bismuth, as the payload(s), which is preferable in light of the limit in uptake by atherosclerotic or neoplastic lesions, while the second is to increase the density of payload(s) made of materials of moderate atomic number, such as calcium ($Z =$ 20), in consideration of biosafety. Notably, calcium in its ionic form may interfere with the physiologic process and thus is toxic, but it would be safe if it was packed as payload in a nanoparticulate format. If nanoparticulate contrast agents based on calcium (or other materials of moderate atomic number) are fabricated in a size that enables them to avoid renal excretion, sequentially, they may stay in the blood pool and extracellular space sufficiently long for lesion uptake, be degraded once they are done with their job as the imaging probes, go through the metabolic process, and eventually be excreted from the body. Apparently, a combination of the two approaches would be more efficient in increasing the contrast enhancement, but, certainly, this would pose more challenges.

Challenges to the success of biodegradable nanoparticulate contrast agents can never be overestimated, since multiple complex systems have lots of factors, many of which are conflicting, entangled and interacting. In particular, the spectral CT implemented in either energy integration or photon counting for X-ray detection adds an extra dimension to the complexity, since the optimal performance of spectral imaging in CT varies over the materials of various atomic numbers. Given different materials as the payload(s), the conditionings of basis materials and spectral channelization (see Chapter 8) in spectral CT should be tuned accordingly to reach the most achievable performance. It is believed that a synergy between spectral CT and biodegradable nanoparticulate contrast agents would be the ultimate solution to improve CT's sensitivity to detecting and characterizing atherosclerotic and neoplastic lesions at the earliest stage. Therefore, in addition to being an expert in CT technologies, scientists and researchers in the field of medical physics should expose themselves sufficiently to the fundamentals, state of the art and prospects of CT contrast agents, in the form of small molecules (iodinated contrast agents) and nanoparticles. This is the major reason behind the intent of providing this relatively long chapter in a book with scientists and researchers in medical physics being its primary audience.

10 Challenges and Opportunities in Photon-Counting Spectral MDCT

As presented in Chapter 8, Section 8.7, energy-integration spectral computed tomography (CT) has been increasingly accepted with its added value in increasing CT's clinical utility and reduction of radiation dose. Recognizing its advantages in suppression of electronic noise, separation of X-ray source spectra and inter-kVp spatial registration, future photon-counting spectral CT is anticipated to do a better job in accomplishing those clinical tasks. Objectively speaking, however, advancements made by spectral CT in the clinic so far can only be categorically delineated as incremental. To make more significant progress or even breakthroughs to fulfill the unmet needs in oncological, cardiovascular and neurovascular applications, continuous progress in the technologies enabling spectral CT, e.g., accurate modeling of spectral CT, optimal choice in basis materials in material decomposition and spectral channelization, task-specific image formation algorithms, extended spectral analysis endorsed by virtual monochromatic imaging, and their synergy, has to be made along the roads ahead. Following is a brief survey (or speculation) of the technologies that may make spectral CT more effective in the clinic, followed by a discussion on their pros and cons.

10.1 POTENTIAL TECHNOLOGICAL SOLUTIONS FOR IMAGE QUALITY IMPROVEMENT IN SPECTRAL MDCT

- **Accurate modeling of spectral CT**: To date, the decomposition of interaction proposed by Alvarez and Macovski has been the physical foundation of spectral CT, regardless of its implementation in energy integration or photon counting. As pointed out by them in their milestone paper (Alvarez and Macovski 1976), the decomposition of interaction into photoelectric absorption and Compton scattering is merely an approximation in which Rayleigh scattering is ignored. In practice, the imaging performance of spectral CT is short of what was initially anticipated. It is speculated that, in addition to other factors (e.g.. overlapping of X-ray source spectra), the ignorance of Rayleigh scattering in modeling the interaction decomposition may be the culprit in the first place. It is time for the community to conduct a deep investigation or at least revisit the modeling of interaction and material decompositions systematically.

DOI: 10.1201/9780429028465-10

- **Photon-counting X-ray detection with full spectral resolution**: In principle, the scheme of spectral weighting in spectral CT can be substantially facilitated if the energy of each X-ray photon is exactly known (full spectral resolution). However, such an attempt may be over-demanding in system design and thus costly in instrumentation. Moreover, as demonstrated in Section 8.6, the gain associated with full spectral resolution over that with energy binning is marginal, especially in light of the fact that the dimensionality of material space in spectral CT is at most four. More important, full spectral resolution is equivalent to infinitely narrow spectral channel (energy binning), which may lead to severe photon starvation in data acquisition. Hence, it is not necessary for spectral CT to have an X-ray photon-counting detector with full spectral resolution.
- **Enhancement of subject contrast and suppression of artifacts and noise**: In theory, there should not be any beam hardening artifacts in spectral CT images after material decomposition, but this has not been the case in practice (see Figure 8.1). The underlying reasons may include inaccuracies in modeling the interaction decomposition in the first place and the overlapping of X-ray source spectra. A fundamental solution has to start with addressing the inaccuracies, with the challenge that Rayleigh scattering is not straightforwardly separable as to what can be done in photoelectric absorption and Compton scattering (Williamson et al. 2006). In addition, noise is also a root cause and should be suppressed as much as possible, using various approaches available in the literature, especially the latest developments using convolutional neural network (CNN)-based machine (deep) learning.
- **Implementation of spectral CT with monochromatic X-rays**: If a monochromatic X-ray source is available, the spectral CT can be implemented by solving Equations 7.1.1–71.2, a system of linear equations, rather than a system of integral equations (Equations 7.2.1–7.2.2) or its polynomial approximation (Equations 7.14.1–7.14.2 or 7.16.1–7.16.2) (see Chapter 7). Moreover, with a monochromatic X-ray source, all the issues associated with spectral mis-registration in photon-counting spectral CT, including scattering and fluorescence, can be substantially reduced, if not totally eliminated. Hence, a monochromatic X-ray source with its output power viable for various clinical applications is the ultimate solution for spectral CT, especially in the implementation with photon-counting detection.

10.2 SYNERGY OF SPECTRAL MDCT WITH NOVEL CONTRAST AGENTS

The clinical utility of conventional CT has been substantially boosted by intravenous iodinated contrasts for not only subject contrast enhancement via the blood compartment effect but also hemodynamics, e.g., the arterial and portal phases, to detect and characterize the pathophysiology. It is the synergy of conventional CT with intravenous iodinated contrast agents that makes CT much more successful in the clinic than the use of conventional CT alone. Therefore, it is hoped that the clinical utility of spectral CT can be enhanced by contrast agents substantially too. Actually, due to its ability in material decomposition and virtual monochromatic imaging and analysis, the synergy of spectral CT with existing and new contrast agents may make their working together much more effective in fulfilling unmet needs in the clinic.

- **Potential materials for novel contrast agents in spectral CT**: Via the blood vasculature and body compartment mechanism, the iodinated contrast that is intravenously administered has had a strong record of safety in the clinic, though side effects may occur, especially in patients with pre-existing conditions. Other materials of higher atomic number, such as gadolinium, gold, platinum, xenon, bismuth, hafnium, tungsten and ytterbium, have been proposed to make contrast agents, and some of them may be less toxic to patients with compromised renal functionality, since their high atomic number leads to a smaller molar amount of agent needed to reach the desired contrast enhancement. Compared to conventional CT, the synergy of spectral CT with those non-iodinated contrast agents, especially their applications in K-edge imaging, can potentially be more successful than the iodinated contrast agents, if care is taken between spectral channelization in spectral CT and the materials' K-edge.
- **Multi-phasic spectral CT with novel multi-material contrast agents**: The current practice in multi-phasic CT is carried out by scanning in a temporally cascaded manner after a single administration of iodinated contrast agent, which leads to a doubled or higher radiation dose to patients. Moreover, there exists spatial mis-registration between the CT scans along the time course, which may compromise the characterization of lesions in clinical practice. With spectral CT, the contrast agents corresponding to different materials can be administered at different time points and one single CT scan is made at an adequate time. As such, the spatial mis-registration can be avoided while the radiation dose is being reduced.
- **Spectral CT with nanoparticulated contrast agents for molecular imaging**: The iodinated contrast agent in current clinical practice is in the form of small molecules, and its half-life in the circulation system is on the order of seconds. In recent years, nanoparticulated contrast agents using iodine, gold or other materials have been proposed to extend the half-life to, e.g., hours or even days, as the particles at nanometer scale can escape renal excretion. Moreover, the nanoparticulate contrast agents can be manipulated with the capability of targeting at biomarkers that may enable spectral CT for molecular imaging (Kim et al. 2017; Chhour et al. 2017).

The research and development in CT contrast agents with materials other than iodine in the form of macromolecules and nanoparticles are highly innovative. However, notably, all the investigations are in the early stage, with quite a few challenges, such as toxicity, and clinical trial and regulatory approval, to be addressed prior to establishing their clinical utility. In addition to the toxicity associated with the novel materials in macromolecular form, the nanoparticulated contrast agents bear extra toxicity, though strategies in optimizing particle size and making the nanoparticles biodegradable have been proposed. Hence, a strong push is anticipated for spectral CT's synergy with biomarker-targeting nanoparticulated contrast agents to play a role in molecular imaging.

10.3 CLOSING REMARKS

With the landscape of technological and clinical advancements in spectral CT sketched herein, it is fair to state that photon-counting spectral CT is gaining momentum in its research and development, while energy-integration spectral CT is ramping up for acceptance in the clinic. The technological advancements made in photon-counting spectral CT and the preliminary success made by energy-integration CT in the clinic are encouraging optimistic anticipation that, with the potential technological solutions to improve its imaging performance and its synergy with novel contrast agents, spectral CT, especially one that operates with photon counting, will be eventually able to advance CT's clinical utility in a manner that can be more significant than incremental, if not make breakthroughs. Via biomarker-targeted delivery, the subject contrast of pathological lesions, such as tumors and vulnerable plaques in atherosclerosis, may substantially increase. All these technological advancements encourage us to anticipate that axial MDCT/CBCT will play a more significant role in routine clinical practice in the future, and even a significant role in molecular imaging wherein the subject contrast is of essence.

References

Abbey CK and Bochud FO (2000), Chapter 11: Modeling visual detection tasks in correlated image noise with linear model observers, *The Handbook of Medical Image, Volume 1. Physics and Psychophysics* (Eds: Beutel J, Kundel HL and Van Metter RL), Bellingham: SPIE Press 629–654.

Abbey CK and Barrett HH (2001), Human- and model-observer performance in ramp-spectrum noise: Effects of regularization and object variability, *J. Opt. Soc. Am. A*, 18:473–488.

Abbey CK and Eckstein MP (2007), Classification images for simple detection and discrimination tasks in correlated noise, *J. Opt. Soc. Am. A*, 24(12):B110–B124.

Abbey CK and Eckstein MP (2019), Chapter 18: Observer models as a surrogate to perception experiments, *The Handbook of Medical Image Perception and Techniques* 2nd Edition (Eds: Samei E and Krupinski EA), Cambridge: Cambridge University Press 276–288.

ACR Committee on Drugs and Contrast Media (2021), ACR manual on contrast media, available at https://www.acr.org/-/media/acr/files/clinical-resources/contrast_media.pdf, accessed on 12/28/2022.

Agrawal MD, Pinho DF, Kulkarni NM, Hahn PF, Guimaraes AR and Sahani DV (2014), Oncologic applications of dual-energy CT in the abdomen, *RadioGraphics*, 34:589–612.

Alvarez RE (1976), *Extraction of energy-dependent information in radiography*, (Doctoral dissertation) Stanford University, Stanford, CA.

Alvarez RE (2019), Invertibility of the dual energy x-ray data transform, *Med. Phys.*, 46(1):93–103.

Alvarez RE and Macovski A (1976), Energy-selective reconstructions in x-ray computerized tomography, *Phys. Med. Biol.*, 21(5):733–744.

Alvarez RE and Seppi E (1979), A comparison of noise and dose in conventional and energy selective Computed Tomography, *IEEE Trans. Nuclear Sci.*, 26(2):2853–2856.

Alvarez RE, Seibert JA and Thompson SK (2004), Comparison of dual energy detector system performance, *Med. Phys.*, 31(3):556–565.

Alvarez RE (2010), Near optimal energy selective x-ray imaging system performance with simple detector, *Med. Phys.*, 37(2):822–841.

Alvarez RE (2011), Estimator for photon counting energy selective x-ray imaging with multi-bin pulse height analysis, *Med. Phys.*, 38(5):2324–2334.

Alvarez RE (2013), Dimensionality and noise in energy selective x-ray imaging, *Med. Phys.*, 40(11):111909, 13 pages.

Bae KT (2003), Peak contrast enhancement in CT and MR angiography: When does it occur and why? Pharmacokinetic study in a porcine model, *Radiology*, 227(3):809–816.

Bae K (2010), Intravenous contrast medium administration and scan timing at CT: Considerations and approaches, *Radiology*, 256(1):32–61.

Bae KT, Heiken JP and Brink JA (1998), Aortic and hepatic peak enhancement at CT: Effect of contrast medium injection rate-Pharmacokinetic analysis and experimental porcine model, *Radiology*, 206(2):455–464.

Baek J and Pelc NJ (2010), The noise power spectrum in CT with direct fan beam reconstruction, *Med. Phys.*, 37(5):2074–2081.

Baek J and Pelc NJ (2011), Local and global 3D noise power spectrum in cone-beam CT system with FDK reconstruction, *Med. Phys.*, 38(4):2122–2131.

Baek J, Pineda AP and Pelc NJ (2013), To bin or not to bin? The effect of CT system limiting resolution on noise and detectability, *Phys. Med. Biol.*, 58:1433–1446.

Bansal S and Patel RN (2020), Pathophysiology of contrast-induced acute kidney injury, *Interv. Cardiol. Clin.*, 9:293–298.

Barber RF, Sidky EY, Gilat-Schmidt T and Pan X (2016), An algorithm for constrained one-step inversion of spectral CT data, *Phys. Med. Biol.*, 61:3784–3818.

Barrett HH, Gordon SK and Hershel RS (1976), Statistical limitations in transaxial tomography, *Comput. Biol. Med.*, 6:307–323.

Barrett HH and Swindell W (1981), *Radiological Imaging: The Theory of Image Formation, Detection, and Process*, San Diego: Academic Press.

Barret HH, Yao J, Rolland JP and Myers KJ (1993), Model observer for assessment of image quality, *Proc. Natl. Acad. Sci. USA*, 90:9758–9765.

Barret HH and Myers KJ (2004), *Foundations of Image Science* 1st Edition, Hoboken: John Wiley & Sons.

Barrett HH (2009), NEQ: Its progenitors and progeny, *Proc. SPIE*, 7263, doi:10.1117/12.817795.

Behrendt FF, Schmidt B, Plumhans C, Keil S, Woodruff SG, Ackermann D, Mühlenbruch G, Flohr TG, Günther RW and Mahnken AH (2009), Image fusion in dual energy computed tomography effect on contrast enhancement, signal-to-noise ratio and image quality in computed tomography angiography, *Invest. Radiol.*, 44(1):1–6.

Benson JC, Rajendran K, Lane JI, Diehn, FE, Weber NM, Thorne JE, Larson NB, Fletcher JG, McCollough CH and Leng S (2022), A new frontier in temporal bone imaging: Photon-counting detector CT demonstrates superior visualization of critical anatomic structures at reduced radiation dose, *Am. J. Neuroradiol.*, 43:579–584.

Berger JO (1985), *Statistical Decision Theory and Bayesian Analysis*, 2nd Edition, New York: Springer-Verlag.

Besson G (1998), CT image reconstruction from fan-parallel data, *Med. Phys.*, 26:415–426.

Black MJ, Sapiro G, Marimont DH and Heeger D (1998), Robust anisotropic diffusion, *IEEE Trans. Imag. Proc.*, 7: 421–432.

Boedeker KL Cooper VN and McNitt-Gray MF (2007), Application of the noise power spectrum in modern diagnostic MDCT: Part I. Measurement of noise power spectra and noise equivalent quanta, *Phys. Med. Biol.*, 52:4027–4046.

Boedeker KL and McNitt-Gray MF (2007), Application of the noise power spectrum in modern diagnostic MDCT: Part II. Noise power spectrum and signal to noise, *Phys. Med. Biol.*, 52:4047–4061.

Bonnemain B and Guerbet M (1995), The history of Lipiodol (1901–1994) or How a medication may evolve with the times, *Rev. Hist. Pharm.*, 42(305):159–170.

Bornefalk H (2012), XCOM intrinsic dimensionality for low-Z elements at diagnostic energies, *Med. Phys.*, 39(2):654–657.

Bouman CA and Sauer KD (1993), A generalized Gaussian image model for edge-preserving MAP estimation. *IEEE Trans. Imag. Proc.*, 2: 296–310.

Bouman CA and Sauer KD (1996), A unified approach to statistical tomography using coordinate descent optimization. *IEEE Trans. Imag. Proc.*, 5:480–492.

Brenner DJ and Hall EJ (2007), Computed tomography–an increasing source of radiation exposure, *N. Engl. J. Med.*, 357(22):2277–2284.

Brink JA, Heiken JP, Forman HP, Sagel SS, Molina PL and Brown PC (1995), Hepatic spiral CT: Reduction of dose of intravenous contrast material, *Radiology*, 197(1):83–88.

Brink JA (2003a), Use of high concentration contrast media (HCCM): Principles and rationale - Body CT, *Euro. J. Radiol.*, 45(Suppl 1):S53–58.

Brink JA (2003b), Contrast optimization and scan timing for single and multidetector-row Computed Tomography, *J. Comp. Assi. Tomo.*, 27(Suppl 1):S3–8.

Brink JA (2003), Contrast optimization and scan timing for single and multidetector-row Computed Tomography, *Euro. J. Radiol.*, 45(Suppl 1):S53–58.

Brody WR, Butt G, Hall Anne and Macovski A (1981), A method for selective tissue and bone visualization using dual energy scanned projection radiography, *Med. Phys.*, 8(3):353–357.

Brooks B (1924), Intra-arterial injection of sodium iodine: Preliminary report, *JAMA*, 82(13):1016–1019.

Bruder H, Kachelrieβ M, Schaller S, Stierstorfer K and Kalender WA (2000), Single-slice rebinning reconstruction in spiral cone-beam computed tomography, *IEEE Trans. Med. Imag.*, 19:873–87.

Burgess AE (1994), Statistically defined background: Performance of a modified nonprewhitening observer model, *J. Opt. Soc. Am. A*, 11:1237–1242.

Burgess AE (1999), The Rose model, revisited, *J. Opt. Soc. Am. A*, 16(3):633–646.

Bush WH and Swanson DP (1991), Acute reactions to intravascular contrast media: Types, risk factors, recognition, and specific treatment, *American Journal of Roentgenology*, 157(12):1153–1161.

Bushberg JT, Seibert JA, Leidholdt EM and Boone JM (2012), *The Essential Physics of Medical Imaging* 3rd Edition, Philadelphia: Lippincott Williams & Wilkins.

Buzug TM (2008), *The Computed Tomography from Photon Statistics to Modern Cone-Beam CT* 1st Edition, Verlag Berlin Heidelberg: Springer.

Cahn RN, Cederström, DM, Hall A and Lundqvist (1999), Detective quantum efficiency dependence on X-ray energy weighting in mammography, *Med. Phys.*, 26(12):2680–2683.

Cai C, Rodet T, Legoupil S and Mohammad-Djafari A (2013), A full-spectral Bayesian reconstruction approach based on the material decomposition model applied in dual-energy computed tomography, *Med. Phys.*, 40(11):111916, 16 pages.

Chandra N and Langan DA (2011), Gemstone detector: Dual energy imaging via fast kVp switching, *Dual Energy CT in Clinical Practice* (Eds: Johnson T, Fink C, Schönberg SO and Reiser MF), Berlin, Heidelberg: Springer Berlin Heidelberg 35–41.

Charkraborty DP (2013), A brief history of free-response receiver operating characteristic paradigm data analysis, *Acad. Radiol.*, 20:915–919.

Chen B, Zhang Z, Xia D, Sidky EY, Zhang Z and Pan X (2018), Non-convex Chambolle-Pock algorithm for multispectral CT, Proceedings 5th International Conference on Image Formation in X-ray Computed Tomography, 377–381.

Chen J (1992), A theoretical framework of regional cone-beam tomography, *IEEE Trans. Med. Imag.*, 11:342–350.

Chhour P, Kim J, Benardo B, Tovar Λ, Mian S, Litt HI, Ferrari VΛ and Cormode DP (2017), Effect of gold nanoparticle size and coating on labeling monocytes for CT tracking, *Bioconjugate Chem.*, 28(1):260–269.

Choi S and Baek J (2015), Comparison of cone beam artifacts reduction: Two pass algorithms vs TV-based CS algorithm, *SPIE Proc.*, 9412:94124O, 6 pages, doi:10.1117/12.2081363.

Chuang K-S and Huang HK (1988), Comparison of four dual energy image decomposition methods, *Phys. Med. Biol.*, 33(4):455–466.

Clack R and Defrise M (1994), Overview of reconstruction algorithms for exact cone-beam tomography, *Proc. SPIE*, 2299:230–241.

Cody DD, Stevens DM. and Ginsberg LE (2005), Multi-detector row CT artifacts that mimic diseases, *Radiology*, 236:756–61.

Cowan G (1998), *Statistical Data Analysis*, Oxford: Oxford University Press.

Cullen DE, Hubbell JH and Kissel L (1997), EPDL97: The evaluated photon data library, *Lawrence Livermore National Laboratory Report UCRL-50400*, vol 6, rev 5.

Crawford CR and King KF (1990), Computed tomography scanning with simultaneous patient translation, *Med. Phys.*, 17:967–982.

Cunningham IA and Shaw R (1999), Signal-to-noise optimization of medical imaging system, *J. Opt. Soc. Am. A*, 16(3):621–632.

Cunningham IA (2000), Chapter 2: Applied linear-systems theory, *The Handbook of Medical Image, Volume 1. Physics and Psychophysics* (Eds: Beutel J, Kundel HL and Van Metter RL), Bellingham: SPIE Press 79–159.

Danad I, Fayad ZA, Willemink MJ and Min JK (2015), New applications of cardiac computed tomography: Dual-energy, spectral, and molecular CT imaging, *JACC: Cardiovasc. Imag.*, 8(6):710–723.

Danielsson PE, Edholm P, Eriksson J and Magnusson-Seger M (1997), Towards exact 3D-reconstruction for helical cone-beam scanning of long objects: A new arrangement and a new completeness condition, *International Meeting on Fully Three-dimensional Image Reconstruction in Radiology and Nuclear Medicine*, (Pittsburgh) ED Townsend and Kinahan 25–28.

Danielsson M, Persson M and Sjlin M (2021), Photon-counting x-ray detectors for CT, *Phys. Medi. Biol.*, 66:03TR01, 35 pages.

Davenport MS, Khalatari S, Dillman JR, Cohan RH, Caoili EM and Ellis JH (2013a), Contrast medium-induced nephrotoxicity and intravenous low-osmolality iodinated contrast material, *Radiology*, 267(1):94–105.

Davenport MS, Khalatari S, Cohan RH, Dillman JR, Myles JD and Ellis JH (2013b), Contrast material-induced nephrotoxicity and intravenous low-osmolality iodinated contrast material: Risk stratification by using extimated glomerular filtration rate, *Radiology*, 268(3):719–728.

Davenport MS, Perazella MA, Yee J, Dillman JR, Fine D, McDonald RJ, Rodby RA, Wang CL and Weinreb JC (2020), Use of intravenous iodinated contrast media in patients with kidney disease: Consensus statements from the American College of Radiology and the National Kidney Foundation, *Radiology*, 294(3):660–668.

Defrise M and Clack R (1994), A cone-beam reconstruction algorithm using shift-variant filtering and cone-beam backprojection, *IEEE Trans. Med. Imag.*, 13:186–195.

Di Chiro G, Brooks RA, Kessler RM, Johnston GS, Jones AE, Herdt JR and Sheridan WT (1979), Tissue signatures with dual-energy computed tomography, *Radiology*, 131(2):521–523.

Duan X, Arbique G, Guild J, Xi Y and Anderson J (2018), Technical note: Quantitative accuracy evaluation for spectral images from a detector-based spectral CT scanner using an iodine phantom, *Med. Phys.*, 45(5):2048–2053.

Durrett R (2019), *Probability: Theory and Examples*, 4th ed., Cambridge: Cambridge University Press.

Eckardt K-U, Coresh J, Devuyst O, Johnson RJ, Köttgen A, Levey AS and Levin A (2013), Evolving importance of kidney disease: from subspecialty to global health burden, *The Lancet*, 382(9887):158–169.

Eckstein MP, Abbey CK and Bochud FO (2000), Chapter 10: A practical guide to model observers for visual detection in synthetic and natural noisy images, *The Handbook of Medical Image, Volume 1. Physics and Psychophysics* (Eds: Beutel J, Kundel HL and Van Metter RL), Bellingham: SPIE Press 593–628.

Eckstein MP, Bartroff JL, Abbey CK, Whiting JS and Bochud FO (2003), Automated computer evaluation and optimization of image compression of x-ray coronary angiograms for signal known exactly detection tasks, *Opt. Express*, 11:460–475.

Ehn SSL (2017), Photon-counting hybrid-pixel detectors for spectral X-ray imaging applications (Doctoral dissertation). Retrieved from https://mediatum.ub.tum.de/doc/1363593/1363593.pdf.

Eloy R, Corot C and Belleville J (1991), Contrast media for angiography: Physicochemical properties, pharmacokinetics and biocompatability, *Clin. Mater.*, 7:89–197.

Fähling M, Seeliger E, Patzak A and Persson PN (2017), Understanding and preventing contrast-induced acute kidney injury, *Nat. Rev. Nephrol.*, 13(3):169–180.

Fan M, Zhou Z, Bruesewitz M, McCollough C and Yu L (2023), Evaluation of low-contrast detectability of photon-counting-detector CT using channelized Hotelling observer and an ACR accreditation phantom, *Proc. SPIE* 12463:1246348, pages; 10.1117/12.2655619

Faulkner K and Moores BM (1984), Analysis of x-ray computed tomography images using the noise power spectrum and autocorrelation function, *Phys. Med. Biol.*, 29:1343–1352.

Feldkamp LA, Davis LC and Kress JW (1984), Practical cone-beam algorithm, *J. Opt. Soc. Am. A*, 1(6):612–619.

Fessler JA and Booth SD (1999), Conjugate-gradient preconditioning methods for shift-variant reconstruction. *IEEE Trans. Med. Imag.*, 8:688–699.

Fessler JA (2009), Statistical image reconstruction methods for transmission tomography, *Handbook of Medical Imaging* (Eds: Sonka M and Fitzpatrick JM), Bellingham: SPIE Press 1–70.

Figueiredo M, Nowak R and Wright S (2007), Gradient projection for sparse reconstruction: Applications to compressed sensing and other inverse problems, *IEEE J. Sel. Top. Signal Processing*, 1:586–597.

FitzGerald PF, Butts MD, Roberts JC, Colborn RE, Torres AS, Lee BD, Yeh BM, and Bonitatibus PJ (2016), A proposed CT contrast agent using carboxybetaine zwitterionic tantalum oxide nanoparticles: Imaging, biological, and physicochemical performance, *Invest. Radiol.*, 51(12):786–796.

Flohr TG and Ohnesorge B (2000), Heart rate adaptive optimization of spatial and temporal resolution for electrocardiogram-gated multislice spiral CT of the heart, *J. CAT*, 27:907–923.

Flohr TG and Ohnesorge BM (2008), Imaging of the heart with computed tomography, *Basic Res. Cardiol.*, 103:161–173.

Flohr TG, Bruder H, Stierstorfer K, Petersilka M, Schmidt B and McCollough CH (2008), Image reconstruction and image quality evaluation for a dual source CT scanner, *Med. Phys.*, 35:5882–5897.

Flohr TG, Petersilka M, Henning A, Ulzheimer S, Ferda J and Schmidt B (2020), Photon-counting CT review, *Physica Medica*, 79:126–136.

Flohr TG, Stierstorfer K, Bruder H, Simon J., Polacin A and Schaller S (2003), Image reconstruction and image quality evaluation for a 16-slice CT scanner, *Med. Phys.*, 30:2650–2662.

Flohr TG, Stierstorfer K, Suss C, Schmidt B, Primak AN and McCollough CH (2007), Novel ultrahigh resolution data acquisition and image reconstruction for multi-detector row CT, *Med. Phys.*, 34:1712–1723.

Flohr TG, Stierstorfer K, Ulzheimer S, Bruder H, Primak AN and McCollough CH (2005), Image reconstruction and image quality evaluation for a 64-slice CT scanner with z-flying focal spot, *Med. Phys.*, 32:2536–2547.

Forghani R, De Man B and Gupta R (2017a), Dual-energy computed tomography physical principles, approaches to scanning, usage, and implementation: Part 1, *Neuroimag. Clin. North Am.*, 27:371–384.

Forghani R, De Man B and Gupta R (2017b), Dual-energy computed tomography physical principles, approaches to scanning, usage, and implementation: Part 2, *Neuroimag. Clin. North Am.*, 27:385–400.

Forghani R, Srinivasan A and Forghani B (2017c), Advanced tissue characterization and texture analysis using dual-energy computed tomography: Horizons and emerging applications, *Neuroimag. Clin. North Am.*, 27:533–546.

Forthmann P, Grass M and Proksa R (2009), Adaptive two-pass cone-beam artifact correction using a FOV-preserving two-source geometry: A simulation study, *Med. Phys.*, 36:4440–4450.

Fu J, Guo J, Qin A, Yu X, Zhang Q, Lei X, Huang Y, Chen M, Li J, Zhang Y, Liu J, Dang Y, Wu D, Zhao X, Lin Z, Lin Y, Li S and Zhang L (2020), Bismuth chelate as a contrast agent for X-ray computed tomography, *J Nanobiotechnol*, 18:110.

Galli SJ, Nakae S and Tsai M (2005), Mast cells in the development of adaptive immune response, *Nat. Immunol.*, 6(2):135–142.

Gerig G, Kübler O, Kikinis R and Jolesz FA (1992), Nonlinear anisotropic filtering of MRI Data, *IEEE Trans. Med. Imag.*, 11: 221–232.

Gierada DS and Bae KT (1999), Gadolinium as a CT contrast agent: Assessment in a porcine model, *Radiology*, 210(3):829–834.

Giersch J, Niederlöhner D and Anton G (2004), The influence of energy weighting on X-ray imaging quality, *Nucl. Instrum. Methods Phys. Res. A*, 531:68–74.

Grangeat P (1991), Mathematical framework of cone beam 3D reconstruction via the first derivative of the radon transform, *Mathematical Methods in Tomography, Lecture Notes in Mathematics 1497* (Eds: Herman GT, Luis AK, Natterer F), New York: Springer Verlag, 66–97.

Hainfeld, JF, Slatkin, DN, Focella, TM and Smilowitz, HM (2006), Gold nanoparticles: A new x-ray contrast agent, *Br. J. Radiol.*, 79:248–253.

Han X, Bian J, Eaker DR, Kline TL, Sidky EY, Ritman EL, Pan X (2011), Algorithm-enabled low-dose micro-CT imaging, *IEEE Trans. Med. Imag.*, 30:606–620.

Han D, Siebers JV and Williamson JF (2016), A linear, separable two-parameter model for dual energy CT imaging of proton stopping power computation, *Med. Phys.*, 43(1):600–612.

Han D, Porras-Chaverri MA, O'Sullivan JA, Politte DG and Williamson JF (2017), Technical note: On the accuracy of parametric two-parameter photon cross-section models in dual energy-CT applications. *Med. Phys.*, 44(6):2338–2346.

Han M and Baek J (2020), A convolutional neural network-based anthropomorphic model observer for signal-known-statistically and back-ground-known-statistically detection tasks, *Phys. Med. Biol.*, 65:225025, 16 pages.

Hanson KM (1979), Detectability in computed tomography images, *Med. Phys.*, 6:441–451.

Hanson KM (1980), Spectral analysis of non-stationary CT noise, International Symposium and Course on Computed Tomography, Las Vegas, April 7–11, available at https://kmh-lanl.hansonhub.com /talks/ct80vgr.pdf, accessed on 12/28/2022.

Hanson KM (1981), Chapter 113: Noise and contrast discrimination in computed tomography images, *Radiology of the Skull and Brain, Vol. 5: Technical Aspects of Computed Tomography* (Eds: Newton TH and Potts DG), St. Louis: C. V. Mosby.

Heinrich MC, Kuhlmann MK, Grgic A, Heckmann M, Kramann B and Uder M (2005), Cytotoxic effects of ionic high-osmolar, nonionic monomeric, and nonionic iso-osmolar dimeric iodinated contrast media on renal tubular cells in vitro, *Radiology*, 235(3):843–849.

Heismann BJ, Lepert J and Stiertorfer (2003), Density and atomic number measurements with spectral x-ray attenuation method, *J. Appl. Phys.*, 94(8):2073–2079.

Heron M (2021), Deaths: Leading causes for 2019, *Natl. Vital. Stat. Rep.*, 70(9):1–113.

Heuscher D (2002), Cone beam scanner using oblique surface reconstructions. US Patent Pub., 2002/0122529 A1.

Heuscher D, Brown K and Noo F (2004), Redundant data and exact helical cone-beam reconstruction, *Phys. Med. Biol.*, 49:2219–2238.

Holmes DR, Fletcher JG, Apel A., Huprich JE, Siddiki H, Hough DM, Schmidt B, Flohr TG, Robb R, McCollough CH, Wittmer M and Eusemann C (2008), Evaluation of non-linear blending in dual-energy computed tomography, *Eur. J. Radiol.*, 68:409–413.

Hounsfield GN (1973), Computerized transverse axial scanning (tomography): Part I. Description of system, *Br. J. Radiol.*, 46:1016–1022.

Hsieh J, Mollthen RC, Dawson CA and Johnson RH (2000a), An iterative approach to the beam hardening correction in cone beam CT, *Med. Phys.*, 27:23–29.

Hsieh J (2000b), A two-pass algorithm for cone beam reconstruction, *SPIE Proc.*, 3979:533–540.

Hsieh M (2009), *Computed Tomography Principles, Design, Artifacts, and Recent Advances*, 2nd Edition, Heboken: John Wiley & Sons.

Hsieh SS and Pelc NJ (2013), The feasibility of a piecewise-linear dynamic bowtie filter, *Med. Phys.*, 40(3):031910, 12 pages.

Hsieh J, Chao E, Grekowicz B, Horst A, McOlash SM and Myers TJ (2004), Novel approach to extend the scanner coverage beyond detector field-of-view, *Proc. SPIE*, 5368, 7 pages, doi:10.1117/12.534421.

Hsieh J, Londt J, Vess M, Li J, Tang X and Okerlund D (2006), Step-and-shoot data acquisition and reconstruction for cardiac x-ray computed tomography, *Med. Phys.*, 33:4236–4248.

Hu H (1995), A new cone beam reconstruction algorithm for the circle-and-line orbit, Proceeding of International Meeting on Fully 3D Image Reconstruction in Radiology and Nuclear Medicine, 303–310.

Hu H (1996), An improved cone-beam reconstruction algorithm for the circular orbit, *Scanning*, 18:572–582.

Hu H (1997), Exact regional reconstruction of longitudinally-unbounded objects using the circle-and-line cone beam tomographic system, *Proc. SPIE*, 3032:441–444.

Hu H (1998), Multi-slice helical CT: Scan and Reconstruction, *Med. Phys.*, 26:5–18.

Hubbell JH and Seltzer SM (2004), X-Ray mass attenuation coefficients, *NIST Standard Reference Database* 126. https://dx.doi.org/10.18434/T4D01F.

Huda W and Abrahams (2016), *Review of Radiologic Physics*, 4th Edition, Philadelphia: Wolters Kluwer.

ICRU (International Commission on Radiological Unit and Measurement) (April 1996), *Report 54: Medical Imaging: The Assessment of Image Quality*, ISBN 0-913394-53-X., Maryland.

Jin Y (2011), Implementation and optimization of dual energy computed tomography (Doctoral dissertation). Retrieved from https://d-nb.info/1011260859/34.

Johns HE and Cunningham JR (1983), *The Physics of Radiology*, 4th Edition, Springfield: Charles C Thomas.

Joseph PM and Spital RD (1978), A method for correcting bone induced artifacts in computed tomography scanners, *J. Comput. Assist. Tomogr.*, 2:100–108.

Joseph PM and Ruth C (1997), A method for simultaneous correction of spectrum hardening artifacts in CT images containing both bone and iodine, *Med. Phys.*, 24:1629–1634.

Kachelrieβ M, Schaller S and Kalender WA (2000), Advanced single-slice rebinning in cone-beam spiral CT, *Med. Phy.*, 27: 754–72.

Kalayoglu MV (2011), 64-slice CT and the new Age for cardiac diagnostics, http://www.med-compare.com/spotlight.asp?spotlightid=147, accessed September 28, 2011.

Kalender WA, Klotz E and Kostaridou L (1988), Algorithm for noise suppression in dual energy CT material density images, *IEEE Trans. Med. Imag.*, 7(3):218–224.

Kalender WA, Seissler W and Vock P (1989), Single-breathhold spiral volumetric CT by continuous patient translation and scanner rotation, *Radiology*, 173:414.

Kalender WA, Seissler W, Klotz E and Vock P (1990), Spiral volumetric CT with single-breathhold technique, continuous transport, and continuous scanner rotation, *Radiology*, 176:181–83.

Kak AC and Slaney M (1988), *Principals of Computerized Tomographic Imaging*, New York: IEEE Press 177–201.

Kalender WA, Perman WH, Vetter JR and Klotz (1986), Evaluation of a prototype dual-energy computed tomographic apparatus I: Phantom studies, *Med. Phys.*, 13(3):334–339.

Katsevich A (2002a), Analysis of an exact inversion algorithm for spiral cone-beam CT, *Phys. Med. Biol.*, 47:2583–2598.

Katsevich A (2002b), Theoretically exact filtered backprojection-type inversion algorithm for spiral CT, *SIAM J. Appl. Math.*, 62:2012–2026.

Katzberg RW (2005), Contrast medium-induced nephrotoxicity, *Radiology*, 235(3):752–755.

Kelcz F, Joseph PM and Hilal SK (1979), Noise consideration in dual energy CT scanning, *Med. Phys.*, 6(5):418–425.

Kijewski MF and Judy PF (1987), The noise power spectrum of CT images, *Phys. Med. Biol.*, 32(5):565–575.

Kim J, Chhour P, Hsu J, Litt HI, Ferrari VA, Popovtzer R and Cormode DP (2017), Use of nanoparticle contrast agents for cell tracking with computed tomography, *Bioconjugate Chem.*, 28(6):1581–1597.

Kim SK, Lee JM, Kim SH, Kim KW, Kim SJ, Cho SH, Han JK and Choi BI (2010), Image fusion in dual energy computed tomography for detection of hypervascular liver hepatocellular carcinoma, *Investig. Radiol.*, 45(3):149–157.

Köhler T and Roessl E (2011), Noise properties of grating-based x-ray phase contrast computed tomography, *Med. Phys.*, 38:S106–116.

Krillov AA (1961), A problem of I. M. Gel'fand, *Dokl. Akad. Nauk SSSR*, 137(2):276–277.

Kudo H and Saito T (1991), Helical-scan computed tomography using cone-beam projections, IEEE Conference Record of the 1991 Nuclear Science Symposium and Medical Imaging Conference, New York, 1958–1962.

Kudo H and Saito T (1994a), An extended completeness condition for exact cone-beam reconstruction and its application, IEEE Conference Record of the 1994 Nuclear Science and Medical Imaging Symposium, Norfolk, VA, 1710–1714.

Kudo H and Saito T (1994b), Derivation and implementation of a cone-beam reconstruction algorithm for non-planar orbit, *IEEE Trans. Med. Imag.*, 13:196–211.

Kupinski M (2019), Chapter 19: Implementation of observer models, *The Handbook of Medical Image Perception and Techniques* 2nd Edition (Eds: Samei E and Krupinski EA), Cambridge: Cambridge University Press 289–299.

Kyriakou Y, Meyer E, Prell D and Kachelriess M (2010), Empirical beam hardening correction (EBHC) for CT, *Med. Phys.*, 37:5179–5187.

La Rivière PJ, Bian J and Vargas PA (2006), Penalized likelihood sinogram restoration for computed tomography, *IEEE Trans Med Imaging*, 25:1022–1036.

Lange K and Carson R (1984), EM reconstruction algorithms for emission and transmission tomography. *J. Comp. Assisted Tomo.*, 8:306–316.

Lange K and Fessler JA (1995), Globally convergent algorithms for maximum a posteriori transmission tomography. *IEEE Trans. Imag. Proc.*, 4:1430–1450.

Larson GL, Ruth CC and Crawford CR (1998), Nutating slice CT image reconstruction, US Patent, 5,802,134.

Latchaw RE, Payne JT and Gold LH (1978), Effective atomic number and electron density as measured with a computed tomography scanner: Computation and correlation with brain tumor histology, *J. Comput. Assist. Tomogr.*, 2:199–208.

Lauzier PT, Tang J and Chen G-H (2012), Prior image constrained compressed sensing: Implementation and performance evaluation, *Med. Phys.*, 39:66–80.

Lehmann LA and Alvarez RE (1986), *Energy-Selective Radiography: A Review.* New York: Plenum Press 145–187.

Lehmann LA, Alvarez RE, Macovski A, Brody WR, Pelc NJ, Riederer SJ and Hall AL (1981), Generalized image combinations in dual kVp digital radiography, *Med. Phys.*, 8(5):659–667.

Leng S, Yu L, Wang J, Fletcher JG, Mistretta CA and McCollough CH (2011), Noise reduction in spectral CT: Reducing dose and breaking the trade-off between image noise and energy bin selection, *Med. Phys.*, 38(9):4946–49579.

Leng S, Yu L, Chen L, Zhang Y, Carter R, Toledano AY and McCollough CH (2013), Correlation between model observer and human observer performance in CT imaging when lesion location is uncertain, *Med. Phys.*, 40(8):081908, 9 pages.

Leng S, Yu L, Fletcher JG and McCollough CH (2015), Maximizing iodine contrast-to-noie ratios in abdominal CT imaging through use of energy domain noise reduction and virtual monoenergetic dual-energy CT, *Radiology*, 276(2):562–570.

Leng S, Brucewitz M, Tao S, Rajendra K, Halaweish AE, Fletcher JG and McCollough CH (2019), Photon-counting detector CT: System design and clinical applications of an emerging technology, *RadioGraphics*, 39:729–743.

Leon SJ (2006), *Linear Algebra with Applications*, 7th Edition, Pearson: Prentice Hall.

Liang Y and Kruger RA (1996), Dual-slice spiral versus single-slice spiral scanning: Comparison of the physical performance of two computed tomography scanners, *Med. Phys.*, 23:205–220.

Liu X, Primak AN, Yu L, McCollough CH and Morin RL (2008), Quantitative imaging of chemical composition using dual-energy, dual-source CT, *Proc. SPIE*, 6913:6913Z, 7 pages.

Liu X, Primak AN, Yu L, McCollough CH and Morin RL (2009), Quantitative imaging of element composition and mass fraction using dual-energy CT: Three-material decomposition, *Med. Phys.*, 36(5):1602–1609.

Long Y and Fessler JA (2014), Multi-material decomposition using statistical image reconstruction for spectral CT, *IEEE Trans. Med. Imag.*, 33(8):1614–1626.

Lusic H and Grinstaff MW (2013), X-ray computed tomography contrast agents, *Chem. Rev.*, 113:1641–1656.

Maass C., Baer M. and Kachelriess M. (2009), Image-based dual energy CT using optimized precorrection functions: A practical new approach of material decomposition in image domain, *Med. Phys.*, 36(8):3818–3829.

Macovski A (1983), *Medical Imaging Systems*, Hoboken: Prentice Hall.

Malusek A, Karlsson M, Magnusson M and Carlsson GA (2013), The potential of dual-energy computed tomography for quantitative decomposition of soft tissues to water, protein and lipid in brachytherapy, *Phys. Med. Biol.*, 58:771–785.

Marshall WH, Alvarez RE and Macovski A (1981), Initial results with prereconstruction dual-energy computed tomography (PREDECT), *Radiology*, 140:421–430.

Mattrey RF and Aguirre DA (2003), Advances in contrast media research, *Acad. Radiol.*, 10:1450–1460.

McCollough CH, Yu L, Kofler JM, Leng S, Zhang Y, Li Z and Carter RE (2015a), Degradation of CT low-contrast spatial resolution due to the use of iterative reconstruction and reduced dose levels, *Radiology*, 276(2):499–506.

McCollough CH, Leng S, Yu L and Fletcher JG (2015b), Dual- and multi-energy CT: Principles, technical approaches, and clinical applications, *Radiology* 276(3):637–653.

McDonald RJ, McDonald JS, Bida JP, Carter RE, Fleming CJ, Misra S, Williamson EE and Kallmes DF (2013), Intravenous contrast material-induced nephropathy: Causal or coincident phenomenon? *Radiology*, 267(1):106–118.

McDonald JS, McDonald RJ, Comin J, Williamson EE, Katzberg RW, Murad MH and Kallmes DF (2013b), Frequency of acute kidney injury following intravenous contrast medium administration: A systematic review and beta-analysis, *Radiology*, 267(1):119–128.

McDonald JS, McDonald RJ, Carter RE, Katzberg RW, Kallmes DF and Williamson EE (2014), Risk of intravenous contrast material-mediated acute kidney injury: A propensity score-matched study stratified by baseline glomerular filtration rate, *Radiology*, 271(1):65–73.

Metz CE, Wagner RF, Doi K, Brown DA, Nishikawa RM and Myers KJ (1995), Toward consensus on quantitative assessment of medical imaging systems, *Med. Phys.*, 22:1057–1061.

Metz CE (2000), Chapter 15: Fundamental ROC analysis, *The Handbook of Medical Image, Volume 1. Physics and Psychophysics* (Eds: Beutel J, Kundel HL and Van Metter RL), Bellingham: SPIE Press 751–796.

Molen AJ and Geleijns J (2006), Overranging in multisection CT: Quantification and relative contribution to dose – Comparison of four 16-section CT scanners, *Radiology*, 242:208–216.

Mory C, Sixou B, Si-Mohamed S, Boussel L and Rit S (2018), Comparison of five one-step reconstruction algorithms for spectral CT, *Phys. Med. Biol.*, 63:235001.

Myers KJ (2000), Chapter 9: Ideal observer models of visual detection, *The Handbook of Medical Image, Volume 1. Physics and Psychophysics* (Eds: Beutel J, Kundel HL and Van Metter RL), Bellingham: SPIE Press 559–592.

Myers KJ and Barret HH (1987), Addition of a channel machenism to the ideal-observer model, *J. Opt. Soc. Am. A*, 4:2447–2457.

Nakada K, Taguchi K, Fung GSK and Amaya K (2015), Joint estimation of tissue types and linear attenuation coefficients for proton counting CT, *Med. Phys.*, 42(9):5329–5341.

Natterer F (1986), *The Mathematics of Computerized Tomography*, New York: John Wiley & Sons.

Nett BE, Zhuang T, Leng S, Chen G-H (2007), Arc-based cone-beam reconstruction algorithm using an equal weighting scheme, *J. X-ray Sci. Tech.*, 15:19–48.

Newhouse JH, Kho D, Rao QA, Starren J (2008), Frequency of serum creatinine changes in the absence of iodinated contrast material: Implications for studies of contrast nephrotoxicity, *Am. J. Roent.*, 191(2):376–382.

Newhouse JH and Roychoudhury A (2013), Quantitating contrast medium-induced nephropathy: Controlling the control, *Radiology*, 267(1):4–8.

Niederlöhner D, Karg J, Giersch J. and Anton G (2005), The energy weighting technique: Measurement and simulations, *Nucl. Instrum. Methods Phys. Res. A*, 546:37–41.

Nielson M (2018), Neural networks and deep learning, https://static.latexstudio.net/article/2018/0912/neuralnetworksanddeeplearning.pdf

Nik SJ, Meyer J and Watts R (2011), Optimal material discrimination using spectral X-ray imaging, *Phys. Med. Biol.*, 56:5969–5983.

Ning R, Tang X, Conover D and Yu R (2003), Flat panel detector-based cone beam computed tomography with a circle-plus-two-arcs data acquisition orbit: Preliminary phantom study, *Med. Phys.*, 30, 1694–1705.

Noguchi K, Itoh T, Naruto N, Takashima S, Tanaka K and Kuroda S (2017), A novel imaging techniques (X-Map) to identify acute ischemic lesions using noncontrast dual-energy computed tomography, *J. Stroke Cerebrovasc. Dis.*, 26(1):34–41.

Noo F, Clack R, White TA and Roney TJ (1998), The dual-ellipse cross vertex path for exact reconstruction of long objects in cone-beam tomography, *Phys. Med. Biol.*, 43:797–810.

North DO (1943), Analysis of the factors which determine signal-to-noise discrimination in pulsed carrier systems, *Med. RCA Tech. Rep. PTR6C, Phys.*, reprinted in *Proc. IRE.*, 51:1016–1028 (1963).

Ohnesorge B, Flohr TG, Becker C, Kopp AF, Schoepf UJ, Baum U, Knez A, Klingenbeck-Regn K and Reiser MF (2000b), Cardiac imaging by means of eletrocardiaographically gated multisection spiral CT: Initial experience, *Radiology*, 217:564–571.

Orlov SS (1975), Theory of three dimensional reconstruction. I. Condition for a complete set of projections, *Sov. Phys. Crystallogr.*, 20:312.

Osborne ED, Sortherland CG, Scholl AJ and Rowntree LG (1923), Roentgenography of urinary tract during excretion of sodium iodine, *JAMA*, 80(6):368–373.

Pan X, Sidky EY and Vannier M (2009), Why do commercial CT scanner still employ traditional, filtered back-projection for image reconstruction? *Inverse Probl.*, 25:123009 (36pp).

Pan X, Chen B, Sidky EY, Zhang Z and Xia D (2018), Non-convex optimization-based reconstruction in multispectral CT, Proceedings of the 5th International Conference on Image Formation in X-ray Computed Tomography, 373–376.

Parker D (1982), Optimal short scan convolution reconstruction for fan beam CT, *Med. Phys.*, 9:254–257.

Pasternak JJ and Williamson EE (2012), Clinical pharmacology, uses, and adverse reactions of iodinated contrast agents: A primer for the non-radiologist, *Mayo Clin. Proc.*, 87(4):390–402.

Patino M, Prochowski A, Agrawal M, Simeone FJ, Gupta R, Hahn PF and Sahani DV (2016), Photon-counting detector CT: System design and clinical applications of an emerging technology, *RadioGraphics*, 36:1087–1105.

Perona P and Malik J (1990), Scale-space and edge detection using anisotropic diffusion, *IEEE Trans. Pattern Anal. Mach. Intell.*, 12: 629–639.

Persson M and Pelc NJ (2018), A framework for performance characterization of energy-resolving photon-counting detectors, *Med. Phys.*, 45(11):4897–4915.

Petersilka M, Bruder H, Krauss B, Stierstorfer K and Flohr TG (2008), Technical principles of dual source CT, *J. Eur. Radiol.*, 68:362–368.

Phantom Lab (2023), *Catphan® 500 and 600 Manual.* viewed June 19, 2023. https://static1 .squarespace.com/static/5367b059e4b05a1adcd295c2/t/622a29a2e82e60660bbb9afb /1646930339465/CTP500600ProductGuide20220308.pdf.

Pizzino G, Irrera N, Cucinotta M, Pallio G, Mannino F, Arcoraci V, Squadrito F, Altavilla D and Bitto A (2017), Oxidative stress: Harms and benefits for human health, *Oxid. Med. Cell. Longev.*, 2017:8416763, 13 pages.

Popescu LM (2011), Nonparametric signal detectability evaluation using an exponential transformation of the FROC curve, *Med. Phys.*, 38(10):5690–5702.

Popescu LM and Myers KJ (2013), CT image assessment by low contrast signal detectability evaluation with unknown signal location, *Med. Phys.*, 40(11):111908, 10 pages.

Primak AN, Ramirez JC, Liu X., Yu L. and McCollough CH (2009), Improved dual-energy material discrimination for dual-source CT by means of additional spectral filtration, *Med. Phys.*, 36(4):1359–1369.

Rana S, Bajaj A, Mout R and Rotello VM (2012), Monolayer coated gold nanoparticles for delivery applications, *Adv. Drug Deliv. Rev.*, 64:200–216.

Rao QA and Newhouse JH (2006), Risk of nephropathy after intravenous administration of contrast material: A critical literature analysis, *Radiology*, 239(2):392–397.

Raupach R and Flohr TG (2011), Analytic evaluation of the signal and noise propagation in x-ray differential phase-contrast computed tomography, *Phys. Med. Biol.*, 56:2219–2244.

Ren L, Allmendinge T, Halaweish A, Schmidt B, Flohr T, McCollough CH and Yu L (2021), Energy-integrating-detector multi-energy CT: Implementation and phantom study, *Med. Phys.*, 48(9):4857–4871.

Ren Y, Xie H, Long W, Yang X and Tang X (2020), Optimization of basis material selection and energy binning in three material decomposition for spectral imaging without contrast agents in photon-counting CT," *SPIE Proc.*, 11312: 113124X, 8 pages, doi: 10.1117/12.2549678.

Ren Y, Xie H, Long W, Yang X and Tang X (2021), On the conditinaing of spectral channelization (energy binning) and its impact on multi-material decomposition based spectral imaging in photon-counting CT, *IEEE Trans. Biomed. Engi.*, 68(9):2678–2688.

Richard S, Husarik DB, Yadava G, Murphy SN and Samei E (2012), Towards task-based assessment of CT performance: System and object MTF across different reconstruction algorithms, *Med. Phys.*, 39(7):4115–4122.

Riederer SJ and Mistretta CA (1977), Selective iodine imaging using K-edge energies in computerized x-ray tomography, *Med. Phys.*, 4(6):474–481.

Riederer SJ, Norbert NJ and Chesler DA (1978), The noise power spectrum in computed X-ray tomography, *Phys. Med. Biol.*, 23:446–454.

Rizo P, Grangeat P, Sire P., Lemasson P and Melennec P (1991), Comparison of two three-dimensional x-ray cone-beam-reconstruction algorithms with circular source trajectories, *J. Opt. Soc. Am. A*, 8:1639–1648.

Roessl E, Ziegler A and Proksa R (2007), On the influence of noise correlations in measurement data on basis image noise in dual-energy like x-ray imaging, *Med. Phys.*, 34(3):959–966.

Roessl E and Proksa R (2007), K-edge imaging in x-ray computed tomography using multi-bin photon counting detectors, *Phys. Med. Biol.*, 52:4679–4695.

Roessl E, Brendel B, Engel K-J, Schlomka J-P, Thran A and Proksa R (2011), Sensitivity of photon-counting based K-edge imaging in x-ray computed tomography, *IEEE Trans. Med. Imag.*, 30(9):1678–1690.

Roessl E and Herrmann C (2009), Cramér-Rao lower bound of basis image noise in multiple-energy x-ray imaging, *Phys. Med. Biol.* 54: 1307–1318.

Roessl E, Kraft E and Proksa R (2011), A comparative study of a dual-energy-like imaging technique based on counting-integrating readout, *Med. Phys.* 38(12):6416–6428.

Rose A (1946), A unified approach to the performance of photographic film, television pickup tubes and the human eye, *J. Soci. Motion Pict. Engi.*, 47:273–294.

Rose A (1948a), The sensitivity performance of the human eye on an absolute scale, *J. Opt. Soci. Am.*, 38:196–208.

Rose A (1948b), Television pickup tubes and the problem of vision, *Advances in Electronics and Electron Physics* (Eds: Marton L), Academic, New York, 1:131–166.

Rose A (1953), Quantum and noise limitations of the visual process, *J. Opt. Soci. Am.*, 43:715–716.

Roth E. (1984), *Multiple-Energy Selective Contrast Material Imaging* (Doctoral dissertation) Stanford University, Stanford, CA.

Rybicki RF, Otero HJ, Steigner ML, Vorobiof G, Nallamshetty L, Mitsouras D, Ersoy H, Mather RT, Judy PF, Cai T, Coyner K, Schultz K, Whitmore AG and Di Carli MF (2008), Initial evaluation of coronary images from 320-detetor row computed tomography, *Int. J. Cardiovasc. Imag.*, 24:535–46.

Rydberg J, Buckwalter KA, Caldemeyer KS, Phillips MD, Conces DJ, Aisen AM, Persohn SA and Kopecky KK (2000), Multisection CT: Scanning techniques and clinical applications, *RadioGraphics*, 20:1787–1806.

Saladin KS (2007a), Chapter 18 the circulatory system: Blood, *Anatomy and Physiology: The Unity of Form and Function*, 4th Edition, New York: McGraw-Hill.

Saladin KS (2007b), Chapter 21 the lymphatic and immune system, *Anatomy and Physiology: The Unity of Form and Function*, 4th Edition, New York: McGraw-Hill.

Saladin KS (2007c), Chapter 23 the urinary system, *Anatomy and Physiology: The Unity of Form and Function*, 4th Edition, New York: McGraw-Hill.

Sandrik JM and Wagner RF (1982), Absolute measures of physical image quality: Measurement and application to radiographic magnification, *Med. Phys.*, 9:540–549.

Saquib SS, Bouman CA and Sauer KD (1996), ML parameter estimation for Markov random fields with applications to Bayesian tomography, *IEEE Tans. Imag. Proc.*, 7: 480–492.

Schardt P, Deuringer J, Freudenberger J, Hell E, Knüpfer W, Mattern D and Schild M (2004), New x-ray tube performance in computed tomography by introducing the rotating envelope tube technology, *Med. Phys.*, 31(9):2699–2706.

Schlomka JP, Roessl E, Dorscheid R, Dill S., Martens G, Istel T, Bauümer C, Herrmann C, Streadmann R, Zeitler G, Livne A and Proksa R (2008), Experimental feasibility of multi-energy photon-counting K-edge imaging in preclinical computed tomography. *Phys. Med. Biol.*, 53:4031–4047.

Schmidt TG (2009), Optimal "image-based" weighting for energy-resolved CT, *Med. Phys.*, 36(7):3018–3027.

Schöckel L, Jost G, Seidensticker P, Lengsfeld P, Palkowitsch and Pietsch (2020), Developments in X-ray contrast media and the potential impact on computed tomography, *Invest. Radiol.*, 55(9):592–597.

Scholz H, Boivin FJ, Schmidt-Ott KM, Bachmann S, Eckardt K-U, Scholl UI and Persson PB (2021), Kidney physiology and susceptibility to acute kidney injury: Implications for renoprotection, *Nat. Rev. Nephrol.*, 17(5):335–349.

Seeliger E, Sendeski M, Rihal CS and Persson PB (2012), Contrast-induced kidney injury: Mechanism, risk factors, and prevention, *Eur. Heart J.*, 33:2007–2015.

Sendeski MM (2011), Pathophysiology of renal tissue damage by iodinated contrast media, *Clin. Exp. Pharm. Physiol.*, 38:292–299.

Shahid I, Lancelot E and Desché P (2020), Future of diagnostic computed tomography: An update on physicochemical properties, safety and development of X-ray contrast media, *Investig. Radiol.*, 55(9):598–600.

Shaw R (1963), The equivalent quantum efficiency of the photographic process, *J. Photographic. Sci.*, 11:199–204.

Shepp L and Vardi Y (1982), Maximum likelihood reconstruction for emission tomography. *IEEE Trans. Med. Imag.*, 1:113–122.

Shikhaliev PM (2005), Beam hardening artifacts in computed tomography with photon counting, charge integrating and energy weighting detectors: A simulation study, *Phys. Med. Biol.*, 50:5813–5827.

Shikhaliev P (2006), Tilted angle CZT detector for photon counting/energy weighting x-ray CT imaging, *Phys. Med. Biol.*, 51:4267–4287.

Shikhaliev P (2012), Photon-counting spectral CT: Improved material decomposition with K-edge-filtered x-rays, *Phys. Med. Biol.*, 57:1595–1615.

Shutterstock, https://www.shutterstock.com/image-illustration/human-body-anatomy -242876218.

Sidky EY and Pan X (2006b), Image reconstruction in circular cone-beam computed tomography by constrained, total-variation minimization, *J. X-ray Sci. Tech.*, 14:119–139.

Sidky E and Pan X (2008), Image reconstruction in circular cone-beam computed tomography by constrained, total-variation minimization, *Phys. Med. Biol.*, 53: 4777–4807.

Sidky EY, Pan X, Reiser IS and Nishikawa RM (2009), Enhanced imaging of microcalcifications in digital breast tomosynthesis through improved image-reconstruction algorithms, *Med. Phys.*, 36:4920–4932.

Sidky EY, Duchin Y, Pan X and Ullberg C (2011), A constrained, total-variation minimization algorithm for low-intensity x-ray CT, *Med. Phys.*, 38(Supplement 1):s117–s125.

Siewerdsen JH, Cunningham IA and Jeffray DA (2002), A framework fornoise-power spectrum analysis of multidimensional images, *Med. Phys.*, 29:2655–2671.

Silver MD (2000), A method for including redundant data in computed tomography, *Med. Phys.*, 27:773–774.

Smith BD (1985), Image reconstruction from cone-beam projections: Necessary and sufficient conditions and reconstruction methods, *IEEE Trans. Med. Imag.*, 4:14–25.

Smith BD (1990), Cone-beam tomography: Recent advances and a tutorial review, *Opt. Eng.*, 29:524–534.

Sodickson AD, Keraliya A, Czakowski B, Primak A, Wortman J and Uyeda JW (2021), Dual energy CT in clinical routine: How it works and how it adds value, *Emerg. Radiol.*, 28:103–117.

Sones RA and Barnes GT (1989), Noise correlations in images acquired simultaneously with a dual-energy sandwich detector, *Med. Phys.* 16(6):858–861.

Srinivasan A, Parker RA, Manjunathan A, Ibrahim M, Shah GV and Mukherji SK (2013), Differentiation of benign and malignant neck pathologies: Preliminary experience using spectral computed tomography, *J. Comput. Assist. Tomogr.*, 37(5):666–672.

Stierstorfer K, Rauscher A, Boese J, Bruder H, Schaller S and Flohr TG (2004), Weighted FBP: A simple approximate 3D FBP algorithm for multislice spiral CT with good dose usage for arbitrary pitch, *Phys. Med. Biol.*, 49:2209–2218.

Strang G (2006), *Linear Algebra and its Applications*, 4th Edition, Houghton Mifflin Harcourt. ISBN: 9780030105678.

Sturm RE and Morgan RH (1948), Screen intensification systems and their limitations, *Am. J. Roentgenol.*, 62:617–634.

Sukovle P and Clinthorne NH (1999), Basis material decomposition using triple-energy x-ray computed tomography, Proceedings of the 16th IEEE Instrumentation and Measurement Technology Conference, 1615–1618.

Swank RK (1973), Absorption and noise in x-ray phosphors, *J. Applied Phys.*, 44(9):4199–4203.

Szczykutowicz TP and Mistretta CA (2013a), Design of a digital beam attenuation system for computed tomography: Part I. System design and simulation framework, *Med. Phys.*, 40(2):021905, 12 pages.

Szczykutowicz TP and Mistretta CA (2013b), Design of a digital beam attenuation system for computed tomography: Part II. Performance study and initial results, *Med. Phys.*, 40(2):021906, 9 pages.

Taguchi K (2020), Multi-energy inter-pixel coincidence counters for charge sharing correction and compensation in photon counting detectors, *Med. Phys.*, 47(5):2085–2098.

Taguchi K and Aradate H (1998), Algorithm for image reconstruction in multi-slice CT system, *Med. Phys.*, 25:550–565.

Taguchi K. and Iwanczyk JS (2013), Vision 20/20: Single photon counting x-ray detectors in medical imaging, *Med. Phys.*, 40(10):100901, 19 pages.

Taguchi K, Chiang B and Hein I (2006), Direct cone-beam cardiac reconstruction algorithm with cardiac banding artifact correction, *Med. Phys.*, 33:521–539.

Taguchi K, Chiang B and Silver M (2004), New weighting scheme for cone-beam helical CT to reduce the image noise, *Phys. Med. Biol.*, 49:2351–2364.

Taguchi K, Frey EC, Wang X, Iwanczyk JS and Barber WC (2010), An analytical model of the effects of pulse pileup on the energy spectrum recorded by energy resolved photon counting x-ray detectors. *Med. Phys.*, 37(8):3957–3969.

Taguchi K, Polster C, Segars WP, Aygun N and Stierstorfer K (2022), Model-based pulse pileup and charge sharing compensation for photon counting detectors: A simulation study, *Med. Phys.* 49(8):5038–5051.

Tam KC (1995), *Three-dimensional computerized tomography scanning methods and system for large objects with smaller area detectors*, US Patent, 5,390,112.

Tang X (2001), *Flat panel imager based cone beam volumetric CT*, Ph.D. thesis, University of Rochester, USA.

Tang X (2003), Matched view weighting in tilted-plane-based reconstruction algorithms to suppress helical artifacts and optimize noise characteristics, *Med. Phys.*, 30:2912–2918.

Tang X (2014), Chapter 11: Multi-detector row CT, *Cone Beam Computed Tomography* 1st Edition, CRC Press, Taylor & Francis Group, Boca Raton, FL.

Tang X and Hsieh J (2007), Handling data redundancy in helical cone beam reconstruction using a cone-angle-based window function and its asymptotic approximation, *Med. Phys.*, 34:1989–1998.

Tang X and Ning R (2001), A cone beam filtered backprojection (CB-FBP) reconstruction algorithm for a circle-plus-two-arc orbit, *Med. Phys.*, 28:1042–1055.

Tang X and Pan T (2004), CT cardiac imaging: Evolution from 2D to 3D backprojection, *Proc. SPIE*, 5369:44–50.

Tang X and Ren Y (2021), On the conditioning of basis materials (functions) and its impact on multi-material decomposition based spectral imaging in photon-counting CT, *Med. Phys.*, 48(3):1100–1116.

Tang S and Tang X (2012), Statistical CT noise reduction with multiscale decomposition and penalized weighted least squares in the projection domain, *Med. Phys.*, 39:5498–44.

Tang S and Tang X (2016), Axial cone beam reconstruction by weighted BPF/DBPF and orthogonal butterfly filtering, *IEEE Trans Biomedical Engineering*, 63:1895–1903.

Tang X and Xie H (2018), Chapter 32: X-ray computed tomography for diagnostic imaging—From single-slice to multi-slice, *Handbook of X-ray Imaging Physics and Technology*, 1st Edition (Ed: Russo P), Roca Baton: CRC Press, Taylor & Francis Group 637–667.

Tang X and Yang Y (2014), Internal noise in channelized Hoteling observer (CHO) study of detectability index – Differential phase contrast CT vs. conventional CT, *SPIE Proc.*, 9033:903326, 11 pages, doi: 10.1117/12.2043251.

Tang X, Hsieh J, Dong F, Fan J and Toth TL (2008b), Minimization of over-ranging in helical CT scan via hybrid cone beam image reconstruction: Benefits in dose efficiency, *Med. Phys.*, 35:3232–3238.

Tang X, Hsieh J, Nilsen RA, Dutta S, Samsonov D and Hagiwara A (2006), A three-dimensional weighted cone beam filtered backprojection (CB-FBP) algorithm for image reconstruction in volumetric CT: Helical scanning, *Phys. Med. Biol.*, 51:855–874.

Tang X, Hsieh J, Nilsen RA, Hagiwara A, Thibault J-B and Drapkin E (2005), A three-dimensional weighted cone beam filtered backprojection (CB-FBP) algorithm for image reconstruction in volumetric CT under a circular source trajectory, *Phys. Med. Biol.*, 50:3889–3905.

Tang X, Hsieh J, Seamans J, Dong F and Okerlund D (2008a), Cardiac imaging in diagnostic volumetric CT using multi-sector data acquisition and image reconstruction: Step-and-shoot scan vs. helical scan, *Proc. SPIE*, 6913:69131H–1, 11 pages, doi:10.1117/12.769908.

Tang X, Krupinski EA, Xie H and Stillman AE (2018), On the data acquisition, image reconstruction, cone beam artifacts, and their suppression in axial MDCT and CBCT – A review, *Med. Phys.*, 45(9): e761–e782.

Tang X, Narayana S, Hsieh J, Pack JD, Mcolash SM, Sainath P, Nilsen RA and Taha B (2010), Enhancement of in-plane spatial resolution in volumetric CT with focal spot wobbling: Overcoming the constraint on number of projection view per gantry rotation, *J. X-ray Sci. Tech.*, 18:251–265.

Tang X, Ren Y and Xie H (2023), Noise correlation and its impact on performance of multi-material decomposition-based spectral imaging in photon-counting CT, *J. Appl. Clini. Med. Phys.*, 24:e13830. https://doi.org/10.1002/acm2.13830.

Tang X, Ren Y, Xie H and Long W (2020), Three material decomposition for spectral imaging without contrast agent in photon-counting CT–Modeling and feasibility study, *SPIE Proc.* 11312:113124W, 9 pages, doi: 10.1117/12.2549660.

Tang X, Yang Y and Tang S (2011), Characterization of imaging performance in differential phase contrast CT compared with the conventional CT–Noise power spectrum NPS(k), *Med. Phys.*, 38(7):4386–4395.

Tang X, Yang Y and Tang S (2012), Characterization of imaging performance in differential phase contrast CT compared with the conventional CT–Spectrum f noise equivalent quanta NEQ(k), *Med. Phys.*, 39(7):4467–4482.

Tanguay J, Kim HK and Cunningham IA (2010), The role of x-ray Swank factor in energy-resovling photon-counting imaging, *Med. Phys.*, 37(12):6205–6211.

Tanguay J, Yun S, Kim HK and Cunningham IA (2013), The detective quantum efficiency of photon-counting x-ray detectors using cascaded-systems analyses, *Med. Phys.*, 40(4):041913, 15 pages.

Tanguay J, Yun S, Kim HK and Cunningham IA (2015), Detective quantum efficiency of photon-counting x-ray detectors, *Med. Phys.*, 42(1):491–509.

Tapiovaara MJ and Wagner RF (1985), SNR and DQE analysis of broad spectrum x-ray imaging, *Phys. Med. Biol.*, 30(6):519–529.

Thibault J, Sauer KD, Bouman CA, Hsieh J (2007), A three-dimensional statistical approach to improved image quality for multislice helical CT, *Med. Phys.*, 34:4526–4544.

Thilander-Klang A, Ledenius K, Hansson J, Sund P and Båth M (2010), Evaluation of subjective assessment of the low-contrast visibility in constancy control of computed tomography. *Radiat. Prot. Dosim.*, 139:449–454.

Tlustos L (2010), Spectroscopic X-ray imaging with photon counting pixel detector, *Nuclear Instrumentation and Methods in Physics Research A*, 623:823–828.

Tong YL (1990), Chapter 2: The bivariate normal distribution, *The Multivariate Normal Distribution* (Ed: Tong YL), New York: Springer-Verlag, 6–22.

Toth TL, Ge Z and Daly P (2007), The influence of patient centering on dose and image noise, *Med. Phys.*, 34: 3093–101.

Tourassi G (2019), Chapter 15: Receive operating characteristic analysis: Basic concepts and practical applications, *The Handbook of Medical Image Perception and Techniques* 2nd Edition (Eds: Samei E and Krupinski EA), Cambridge: Cambridge University Press 227–244.

Tuy HK (1983), An inverse formula for cone-beam reconstruction, *Siam J. Appl. Math.*, 43:546–552.

Tward DL and Siewerdsen JH (2009), Noise aliasing and the 3D NEQ of flat-panel cone-beam CT: Effect of 2D/3D apertures and sampling, *Med. Phys.*, 36(8):3830–3843.

Tzedakis A, Damilakis J, Perisinakis K and Stratakis J (2005), The effect of z overscanning on patient effective dose from multidetector helical computed tomography examinations, *Med. Phys.*, 32:1621–1629.

Vaishnav JY, Jung WC, Popescu LM, Zeng R and Myers KJ (2014), Objective assessment of image quality and dose reduction in CT iterative reconstruction, *Med. Phys.*, 41(7):071904, 12 pages.

Vembar M, Garcia MJ, Heuscher DJ, Haberl R, Matthews D, Böhme GE and Greenberg NL (2003), A dynamic approach to identifying desired physiological phase for cardiac imaging using multislice spiral CT, *Med. Phys.*, 30:1683–1693.

Vetter JR, Perman WH, Kalender WA, Mazess RB and Holden JE (1986), Evaluation of a prototype dual-energy computed tomographic apparatus II: Determination of vertebral bone mineral content, *Med. Phys.*, 13(3):340–343.

Vlassenbroek A (2011), Dual Layer CT, *Dual Energy CT in Clinical Practice* (Eds: Johnson T, Fink C, Schönberg SO and Reiser MF), Berlin, Heidelberg: Springer Berlin Heidelberg 21–34.

Wagner RF (1977), Toward a unified view of radiological imaging system. Part II: Noisy images, *Med. Phys.*, 4(4):279–296.

Wagner RF, Brown DG and Pastel MS (1979), Application of information theory to the assessment of computed tomography, *Med. Phys.*, 6:83–94.

Wagner RF and Brown DG (1985), Unified SNR analysis of medical imaging systems, *Phys. Med. Biol.*, 30:489–518.

Wald A (1942), Chapter II: The Neyman-Pearson theory of testing a statistical hypothesis, *The Notre Dame Math. Lectures*, 1:10–20.

Wang A and Pelc NJ (2011), Sufficient statistics as a generalization of binning in spectral X-ray imaging, *IEEE Trans. Med. Imag.*, 30(1):84–93.

Wang X and Ning R (1999), A cone-beam reconstruction algorithm for circle-plus-arc data acquisition geometry, *IEEE Trans. Med. Imag.*, 18:815–824.

Weaver JB and Huddleston AL (1985), Attenuation coefficient of body tissues using principal-components analysis, *Med. Phys.*, 12(1):40–45.

Wiggins WF, Potter CA and Sodickson AD (2019), Dual-energy CT to differentiate small foci of intracranial hemorrhage from calcium, *Radiology*, 294(1):293–312.

Willemink MJ, Person M, Pourmorteza A and Pelc NJ (2018), Photon-counting CT: Technical principle and clinical prospects, *Radiology*, 289:293–312.

Williamson JF, Li S, Devici S, Whiting BR and Lerma FA, (2006), On two-parameter models of photon cross sections: Application to dual-energy CT imaging, *Med. Phys.*, 33(11):4115–4129.

Wilson JM, Christianson OL, Richard S and Samei E (2013), A methodology for image quality evaluation of advanced CT systems, *Med. Phys.*, 40(3):031908, 9 pages.

Woodard HQ and White DR (1986), The composition of body tissues, *Br. J. Radiol.*, 59(12):1209–1219.

Wunderlich A and Noo F (2008), Image covariance and lesion detectability in direct fan-beam x-ray computed tomography, *Phys. Med. Biol.*, 53:2471–2493.

Wunderlich A and Noo F (2011), Confidence intervals for performance assessment of linear observers, *Med. Phys.*, 38(7) Supplement 1:S57–S68.

Wunderlich A and Abbey CK (2013), Utility as a rationale for choosing observer performance assessment paradigms for detection tasks in medical imaging, *Med. Phys.*, 40(11):111903, 11 pages.

Xie H and Tang X (2017), Optimization of data acquisition in axial CT under the framework of sampling on lattice for suppression of aliasing artifacts with algorithmic detector interlacing, *Med. Phys.*, 44(12):6239–6250.

Xie H, Ren Y, Long W, Yang X and Tang X (2021), Principal component analysis in projection and image domains–Another form of spectral imaging in photon-counting CT, *IEEE Trans. Biomed. Eng.*, 68(3):1074–1083.

Xu J, Mahesh M and Tsui BMW (2009), Is iterative reconstruction ready for MDCT? *J. Amer. Coll. Radiol.*, 6: 274–276.

Xu Q, Yu H, Mou X, Zhang L, Hsieh J and Wang G (2012), Low-dose X-ray CT reconstruction via dictionary learning, *IEEE Trans Med. Imag.*, 31:1682–1697.

Yan X and Leahy RM (1992), Cone beam tomography with circular, elliptical and spiral orbits, *Phys. Med. Biol.*, 37:493–506.

Yang H, Li M, Koizumi K and Kudo H (2005), A FBP-type cone-beam reconstruction algorithm with Radon space interpolation ability for axially truncated data from a circular orbit, Proceedings of the Eighth International Meeting on Fully Three-dimensional Image Reconstruction in Radiology and Nuclear Medicine, 401–404.

Yang H, Lu K, Lyu X and Hu F (2019), Two-way partial AUC and its properties, *Stat. Methods Med. Res.*, 28(1):184–195.

Yu L, Primak AN, Liu X. and McCollough CH (2009), Image quality optimization and evaluation of linearly mixed images in dual-source, dual detector CT, *Med. Phys.*, 36(3):1019–1024.

Yu L, Leng S, Chen L, Kofler JM, Carter RE and McCollough CH (2013), Prediction of human observer performance in a 2-alternative forced choice low-contrast detection task using channelized Hotelling observer: Impact of radiation dose and reconstruction algorithms, *Med. Phys.*, 40(4):041908, 9 pages.

Yu L, Chen B, Koefler JM, Favaza CP, Leng S, Kupinski MA and McCollough CH (2017), Correlation between 1 2D channelized Hotelling observer and human observers in a low-contrast detection task with multislice reading in CT, *Med. Phys.*, 44(8):3990–3999.

Zeng GL and Gullberg GT (1992), A cone-beam tomography algorithm for orthogonal circle-and-line orbit, *Phys. Med. Biol.*, 37:563–577.

Zhang R, Thibault JB, Bouman CA, Sauer KD and Hsieh J (2014), Model-based iterative reconstruction for dual-energy x-ray CT using a joint quadratic likelihood model, *IEEE Trans. Med. Imag.*, 33(1):117–134.

Zhang S, Han D, Politte DG, Williamson JF and O'Sullivan JA (2018), Impact of joint statistical dual-energy CT reconstruction of proton stopping power images: Comparison
to Image- and sinogram-domain material decomposition approaches, *Med. Phys.*,
45(5):2129–2142.

Zhang Y, Pham BT and Eckstein MP (2007), Evaluation of internal noise methods for
Hotelling observer models, *Med. Phys.*, 34:3312–3322.

Zhang W and Edwards A (2007), A model of nitric oxide tubulovascular cross talk in a renal
outer medullary cross section, *Am. J. Physiol. Renal. Physiol.*, 292:F711–F722.

Zhao W, Vernekohl D, Han F, Han B, Peng H, Yang Y, Xing L and Min JK (2018), A unified
material decomposition framework for quantitative dual- and triple-energy CT imaging, *Med. Phys.*, 45(7):2964–2977.

Zhao Y, Zhao X and Zhang P (2015), An extended algebraic reconstruction technique
(E-ART) for dual spectral CT, *IEEE Trans. Med. Imag.*, 34(3):761–768.

Zhao Z, Schmerbach K, Lu Y, Perlewitz Andrea, NT, Cantow K, Seeliger E, Persson PB,
Patzak A, Liu R and Sendeski MM (2014), Iodinated contrast media cause direct tubular cell damage, leading to oxidative stress, low nitric oxide, and impairment of tubulo-
glomerular feedback, *Am. J. Physiol. Renal. Physiol.*, 306:F814–F872.

Zhuang T, Zambelli J, Nett BE, Leng S and Chen G-H (2008), Exact and approximate cone-
beam reconstruction algorithms for C-arm based cone-beam CT using a two-concen-
tric-arc source trajectory, *Proc. SPIE*, 6913:691321, 12 pages, doi:10.1117/12.772390.

Zou Y and Pan X (2004a), Exact image reconstruction on PI-lines from minimum data in
helical cone-beam CT, *Phys. Med. Biol.*, 49(6):941–959.

Zou Y and Pan X (2004b), Image reconstruction on PI-lines by use of filtered backprojection
in helical cone-beam CT, *Phys. Med. Biol.*, 49: 2717–2731.

Index

For Product Safety Concerns and Information please contact our EU
representative GPSR@taylorandfrancis.com
Taylor & Francis Verlag GmbH, Kaufingerstraße 24, 80331 München, Germany